ARBA In-depth:
Health and Medicine

ARBA In-depth Series:

Children's and Young Adult Titles
Economics and Business
Health and Medicine
Philosophy and Religion

ARBA In-depth:
Health and Medicine

Dr. Martin Dillon, EDITOR IN CHIEF

Shannon Graff Hysell, ASSOCIATE EDITOR

LIBRARIES
UNLIMITED
A Member of the Greenwood Publishing Group

Westport, Connecticut • London

British Library Cataloguing in Publication Data is available.

ISBN: 1–59158–122-2

First published in 2004

Libraries Unlimited, 88 Post Road West, Westport, CT 06881
A Member of the Greenwood Publishing Group, Inc.
www.lu.com

Printed in the United States of America

The paper used in this book complies with the
Permanent Paper Standard issued by the National
Information Standards Organization (Z39.48–1984).

10   9   8   7   6   5   4   3   2   1

Contents

Introduction

The staff of *American Reference Books Annual* is pleased to announce the first edition of *ARBA In-depth: Health and Medicine*. The second in this series of companion volumes to ARBA, this work is designed to assist academic, public, and corporate health libraries in the systematic selection of suitable reference materials for their collections. As with all publications in this series, its purpose is to aid in the evaluation process by presenting critical and evaluative reviews in all areas of health and medicine. The increase in the publication of reference resources in the United States and Canada, in combination with the decrease in library budgets, makes this guide an invaluable tool.

ARBA In-depth: Health and Medicine consists of reviews chosen from the past seven volumes of *American Reference Books Annual* (ARBA)—years 1997-2003. This work provides reviews of reference books, CD-ROMs, and Websites published in the United States and Canada, along with English-language titles from other countries. ARBA has reviewed more than 55,000 titles since its inception in 1970. Because it provides comprehensive coverage of reference resources in all subject areas, not just selected or recommended titles, many titles in ARBA are of interest only to large academic and public libraries. Thus, *ARBA In-depth: Health and Medicine* has been developed as an abridged version of ARBA with selected reviews of resources that are candidates for academic and public health collections as well as corporate health libraries. Titles reviewed in *ARBA In-depth: Health and Medicine* include dictionaries, encyclopedias, directories, bibliographies, guides, and other types of ready-reference tools.

This volume provides 473 unabridged reviews selected from ARBA 1997 through ARBA 2003. Some 100 subject specialists throughout the United States and Canada have contributed these reviews. Reviewers are asked to examine the resources and provide well-documented critical comments, both positive and negative. Coverage usually includes the usefulness of a given work; organization, execution, and pertinence of contents; prose style; format; availability of supplementary materials (e.g., indexes, appendixes); and similarity to other works and previous editions. All reviews provide complete ordering and bibliographic information, including title, publisher, price, and ISBN. References to all reviews published in periodicals during the year of coverage are appended to the reviews (see page xiii for journals cited). All reviews are signed and the title and affiliation of all reviewers at the time the review was published can be found on page ix. Comprehensive author/title and subject indexes can be found at the end of the volume.

The present volume contains 9 chapters that follow the organization of ARBA. Chapter 1, "General Works," is subdivided by form: bibliography, biography, dictionaries and encyclopedias, handbooks and yearbooks, and so on. The remaining chapters are arranged alphabetically by subject (e.g., medicine, nursing, nutrition, pharmacy and pharmaceutical sciences) and then by reference type (e.g., dictionaries and encyclopedias, handbooks and yearbooks).

The ARBA staff is continually striving to improve both the accessibility and timeliness of this resource, while at the same time retaining the quality reviews that librarians have come to expect. ARBA and its companion volume *Recommended Reference Books for Small and Medium-sized Libraries and Media Centers* have been favorably reviewed in such journals as *Library Journal*, *Booklist*, and *Journal of Academic Librarianship*. In 2002, Libraries Unlimited launched ARBAonline (www.arbaonline.com), a searchable database that provides more than 11,000 reviews of both print and electronic resources from the past seven years. The editors continue to strive to make the companion volumes in this series valuable acquisition tools for academic, public, and special libraries as well.

On behalf of our readers and Libraries Unlimited, I would like to express my gratitude to the contributors whose reviews appear in this volume. ARBA and its companion volumes would not be possible without their dedication and continued involvement. I would also like to thank the staff members of Libraries Unlimited who have been instrumental in the preparation of this work, and particularly Associate Editor Shannon Hysell, for her contribution to this volume.

Martin Dillon, Editor in Chief

Contributors

Alan Asher, Art/Music Librarian, Univ. of Northern Iowa, Cedar Falls.

Mark T. Bay, Electronic Resources, Serials, and Government Documents Librarian, Hagan Memorial Library, Cumberland College, Williamsburg, Ky.

Leslie M. Behm, Reference Librarian, Michigan State Univ., Libraries, East Lansing.

George H. Bell, Assoc. Librarian, Daniel E. Noble Science and Engineering Library, Arizona State Univ., Tempe.

Laura J. Bender, Science Librarian, Univ. of Arizona, Tucson.

Teresa U. Berry, Reference Coordinator, Univ. of Tennessee, Knoxville.

Barbara M. Bibel, Reference Librarian, Science/Business/Sociology Dept., Main Library, Oakland Public Library, Calif.

Adrienne Antink Bien, Medical Group Management Association, Lakewood, Colo.

Mary Pat Boian, Assoc. Editor, *Foster's Botanical & Herb Review*, Beaver, Ark.

Georgia Briscoe, Assoc. Director and Head of Technical Services, Law Library, Univ. of Colorado, Boulder.

Natalie Brower-Kirton, (formerly) Staff, Libraries Unlimited.

Sheila Bryant, Reference Librarian, Michigan State Univ., East Lansing.

Luiz Alberto Cardoso, D.D.S., Governors Park Dental Group, Denver, Colo.

Harriette M. Cluxton, (formerly) Director of Medical Library Services, Illinois Masonic Medical Center, Chicago.

Marianne B. Eimer, Interlibrary Loan/Reference Librarian, SUNY College at Fredonia, N.Y.

Jonathon Erlen, Curator, History of Medicine, Univ. of Pittsburgh, Pa.

Lorraine Evans, Instruction and Reference Librarian, Auraria Library, Denver, Colo.

Elaine Ezell, Library Media Specialist, Bowling Green Jr. High School, Ohio.

Eleanor Ferrall, Librarian Emerita, Hayden Library, Arizona State Univ., Tempe.

Lynne M. Fox, Information Services and Outreach Librarian, Denison Library, Univ. of Colorado Health Sciences Center, Denver.

Thomas K. Fry, Assoc. Director, Public Services, Penrose Library, Univ. of Denver, Colo.

Denise A. Garofalo, Director for Telecommunications, Mid-Hudson Library System, Poughkeepsie, N.Y.

Anthony Gottlieb, Asst. Clinical Professor, Univ. of Colorado School of Medicine, Denver.

Rachael Green, Reference Librarian, Noel Memorial Library, Louisiana State Univ., Shreveport.

Laurel Grotzinger, Professor, Univ. Libraries, Western Michigan Univ., Kalamazoo.

Stephen Haenel, (formerly) Staff, Libraries Unlimited.

Susan B. Hagloch, Director, Tuscarawas County Public Library, New Philadelphia, Ohio.

Patrick Hall, Assoc. Librarian for Public Affairs, Penn State Univ., Middletown, Pa.

Mary Hemmings, Technical Services Librarian, Law Library, Univ. of Calgary, Alberta.

Carol D. Henry, Librarian, Lyons Township High School, LaGrange, Ill.

Janet Hilbun, Student, Texas Woman's Univ., Denton.

Marilynn Green Hopman, Librarian, NASA Johnson Space Center, Scientific and Technical Information Center, Houston, Tex.

Shannon Graff Hysell, Staff, Libraries Unlimited.

Barbara Ittner, Staff, Libraries Unlimited.

Elaine F. Jurries, Coordinator of Serials Services, Auraria Library, Denver, Colo.

Vicki J. Killion, Asst. Professor of Library Science and Pharmacy, Nursing and Health Sciences Librarian, Purdue Univ., West Lafayette, Ind.

Diane Kovacs, Internet Consultant/Library School Faculty, Kent State Univ., Ohio.

Betsy J. Kraus, Librarian, Lovelace Respiratory Research Institute, National Environmental Respiratory Center, Albuquerque, N.Mex.

Marlene M. Kuhl, Library Manager, Baltimore County Public Library, Reisterstown Branch, Md.

Natalie Kupferberg, Biological Sciences/Pharmacy Library, Ohio State Univ., Columbus.

Michael R. Leach, Director, Physics Research Library, Harvard Univ., Cambridge, Mass.

Brenda Leeds, (formerly) Staff, Libraries Unlimited.

Polin P. Lei, Silver Springs, Md.

Eric v. d. Luft, Curator of Historical Collections, SUNY Upstate Medical Univ., Syracuse, N.Y.

Theresa Maggio, Head of Public Services, Southwest Georgia Regional Library, Bainbridge.

Glenn Masuchika, Senior Information Specialist, Rockwell Collins Information, Iowa City, Iowa.

Judy Gay Matthews, (formerly) Staff, Libraries Unlimited.

Dana McDougald, Lead Media Specialist, Learning Resources Center, Cedar Shoals High School, Athens, Ga.

Lynn M. McMain, Instructor/Reference Librarian, Newton Gresham Library, Sam Houston State Univ., Huntsville, Tex.

Sue Lyon Mertl, President, Lyon Consulting Group, Inc., Marietta, Ga.

Lillian R. Mesner, Mesner Information Connections, Lexington, Ky.

Gerald D. Moran, Director, McCartney Library, Geneva College, Beaver Falls, Pa.

Betty J. Morris, Assoc. Professor, State Univ. of West Georgia.

Paul M. Murphy III, Director of Marketing, PMX Medical, Denver, Colo.

Madeleine Nash, Reference Librarian, Spring Valley, N.Y.

Deborah D. Nelson, Serials Librarian, Univ. of Denver, Colo.

Rita Neri, Health Sciences Librarian, Long Island Univ., Brooklyn Campus, N.Y.

Carol L. Noll, Volunteer Librarian, Schimelpfenig Middle School, Plano, Tex.

Lambrini Papangelis, Health Sciences Librarian, Western Kentucky Univ., Bowling Green.

Elizabeth Patterson, Head, Reference and Computer Reference Services, Robert W. Woodruff Library, Emory Univ., Atlanta, Ga.

Gari-Anne Patzwald, Freelance Editor and Indexer, Lexington, Ky.

Pete Prunkl, Freelance Writer, Hickory, N.C.

Nancy P. Reed, Information Services Manager, Paducah Public Library, Ky.

Constance Rinaldo, Ernst Magr Library, Museum of Comparative Zoology, Harvard Univ., Hanover, N.H.

Cari Ringelheim, (formerly) Staff, Libraries Unlimited.

Melissa Rae Root, (formerly) Staff, Libraries Unlimited.

Bertram H. Rothschild, Asst. Chief of Psychology, V.A. Medical Center, Denver, Colo.

Edmund F. SantaVicca, Librarian, Phoenix College, Ariz.

Margretta Reed Seashore, Professor of Genetics and Pediatrics, Yale Univ. School of Medicine, New Haven, Conn.

Susan K. Setterlund, Science/Health Science Librarian, Florida Atlantic Univ., Boca Raton.

Mary Ellen Snodgrass, Freelance Writer, Charlotte, N.C.

Sandhya D. Srivastava, Asst. Professor, Serials Librarian, Hofstra Univ., Hempstead, N.Y.

Bronwyn Stewart, Reference Librarian, Sam Houston State Univ., Huntsville, Tex.

Martha E. Stone, Coordinator for Reference Services, Treadwell Library, Massachusetts General Hospital, Boston.

Susan D. Strickland, (formerly) Staff, Libraries Unlimited.

Bruce Stuart, Professor and Parke-Davis Chair, Univ. of Maryland, Baltimore.

Mila C. Su, Senior Asst. Librarian, Pennsylvania State Univ., Altoona.

Marit S. Taylor, Reference Librarian, Auraria Libraries, Univ. of Colorado, Denver.

Mary Ann Thompson, Asst. Professor of Nursing, Saint Joseph College, West Hartford, Conn.

Linda D. Tietjen, Senior Instructor, Instruction and Reference Services, Auraria Library, Denver, Colo.

Leanne M. VandeCreek, Social Sciences Reference Librarian, Northern Illinois Univ., DeKalb.

Ed Volz, Director, Estes Park Public Library, Estes Park, Colo.

Graham R. Walden, Assoc. Professor, Information Services Dept., Ohio State Univ., Columbus.

Michael Weinberg, Reference Librarian, Ronald Williams Library, Northeastern Illinois Library, Chicago.

Arlene McFarlin Weismantel, Reference Librarian, Michigan State Univ., East Lansing.

Lucille Whalen, Dean of Graduate Programs, Immaculate Heart College Center, Los Angeles, Calif.

Eveline L. Yang, Manager, Information Delivery Programs, Auraria Library, Univ. of Colorado, Denver.

Hope Yelich, Reference Librarian, Earl Gregg Swem Library, College of William and Mary, Williamsburg, Va.

Anita Zutis, Adjunct Librarian, Queensborough Community College, Bayside, N.Y.

Journals Cited

FORM OF CITATION	JOURNAL TITLE
AG	*Against the Grain*
ARBA	*American Reference Books Annual*
BL	*Booklist*
BR	*Book Report*
C&RL	*College and Research Libraries*
C&RL News	*College and Research Libraries News*
Choice	*Choice*
EL	*Emergency Librarian*
JAL	*Journal of Academic Librarianship*
LJ	*Library Journal*
RUSQ	*Reference & User Services Quarterly*
RBB	*Reference Books Bulletin*
SLJ	*School Library Journal*
SLMQ	*School Library Media Quarterly*
TL	*Teacher Librarian*
VOYA	*Voice of Youth Advocates*

1 General Works

ATLASES

1. **Atlas of Anatomy.** English ed. Hauppauge, N.Y., Barron's Educational Series, 1997. 104p. illus. index. $19.95. ISBN 0-7641-5000-6.

Every medical and university library, as well as many public and high school libraries, contains one or more atlases of basic human anatomy. Although the creators of this small, inexpensive volume recognize that there are a number of high-quality, very detailed atlases on this topic currently available, they intend their reference text for an intermediate-level audience, such as high school students or members of the general public who may find advanced atlases too technical.

The body of this volume, which is an English translation of a 1995 Spanish publication, is composed of 84 pages of attractive color plates illustrating normal human anatomy. The plates are organized by body systems (e.g., skeletal, muscular, circulatory, nervous, reproductive). Each plate is clearly labeled, although limited if any explanatory materials are included. There are no illustrations depicting changes caused by pathological conditions.

This volume is well indexed, thus making it easy to use. Public and high school libraries will find this new human anatomy atlas a worthwhile acquisition for their patrons.—**Jonathon Erlen**

2. **The Dartmouth Atlas of Health Care 1998.** Chicago, American Hospital Association, 1996. 305p. maps. $350.00. ISBN 1-55648-217-5.

The chief author of this reference work, Dartmouth Medical School professor John E. Wennberg, has published previously in *Science*, *Scientific American*, the *Journal of the American Medical Association*, the *New England Journal of Medicine*, and the *Lancet*. The information in his book is authoritative; there is no question about that. The question is, will readers use it?

Librarians should note that the reference questions they would use this book to answer would tend to be highly specialized. Take, for example, the section on the U.S. physician workforce. It could not be used to answer any hypothetical reference questions about who U.S. physicians are (e.g., "What percentage of U.S. physicians are women, African American, or over the age of 65?") or the specialties they practice (e.g., "What medical specialty pays the most?") . Rather it goes into detail about the physician workforce in different areas of the United States, specifically the various hospital referral regions into which the nation is divided. Over and over again in this book, a map of the United States showing the division into its 306 hospital referral regions is shown, and information for those regions is given that varies according to the title of the map. At the end of each chapter there is a multipage table that gives statistics, again for the 306 U.S. hospital referral regions. This kind of detail is the strength of the book. If reference questions dealing with U.S. health care statistics at the substate level are rare, the library may want to consider another work, such as the *Statistical Record of Health & Medicine* (see entry 124), whose statistics are primarily at the national level. However, if the library supports degree programs in health care administration, is a hospital library, or is a special library in a managed care corporation, there may be plenty of reasons to purchase *The Dartmouth Atlas of Health Care.*—**Lambrini Papangelis**

3.   **The Johns Hopkins Atlas of Human Functional Anatomy.** 4th ed. George D. Zuidema, ed. Baltimore, Md., Johns Hopkins University Press, 1997. 166p. illus. index. $39.95; $22.95pa. ISBN 0-8018-5651-5; 0-8018-5652-3pa.

The study of human anatomy is basic to medical and premedical education as well as the fields of dentistry, nursing, and many of the allied health sciences. This reasonably priced, attractively presented volume serves as a worthwhile introduction to this subject.

This reference work combines the clear illustrations drawn by the noted medical illustrator Leon Schlossberg, with the anatomical knowledge provided by a number of the Johns Hopkins University School of Medicine faculty. The text is comprised of 29 chapters, each covering a specific part of the body. There are 79 plates, mostly in color, which present sharp, detailed images of human anatomy and are the main strength of this volume. This 4th edition of the reference tool includes 16 new plates with accompanying text that, like the rest of the textual material in this book, is concisely and clearly written.

Although there are a number of excellent, lengthy texts available on human anatomy, including several outstanding atlases, this new edition of the Johns Hopkins University human anatomy atlas is a useful addition as an introductory work on this subject for health care, science, and public libraries.—**Jonathon Erlen**

4.   **The Ultimate Human Body Version 2.0.** [CD-ROM]. New York, DK Multimedia, 1996. Minimum system requirements: IBM or compatible 486DX/33MHz. Double-speed CD-ROM drive. Windows 3.1x. 8MB RAM (12MB recommended for Windows 95). 22MB hard disk space. 640 x 480 pixels, 256-color monitor (16 bit colors preferred). Mouse. 8 bit sound card. Loudspeakers or headphones. $39.95. ISBN 0-7894-1204-7.

The first version of this CD-ROM, published in 1994, won critical acclaim. This revised version uses a three-dimensional scanner to provide in-depth views of the body and its various systems. Animated sequences show how various organs look from any angle, including a cross-section. "Pop-up" models of each organ can also be dissected. Each view is accompanied by brief descriptions, and sound provides the correct pronunciation. As the user scrolls through the body, the names of various bones and organs are shown on a window in the frame. The program also contains a link to the Body Online Website, the publisher's subscription online "Health Club." The Body Quiz provides an interactive vehicle for exploration of human anatomy.

Aimed at users aged 10 and up, the information is easy to understand, yet comprehensive enough for school reports through high school age. Younger children will also be able to use it if their verbal skills are at 4th-grade level or above, although they will get more out of the disc if it is used with a parent's guidance. The price makes this an appropriate choice for school and public libraries, as well as for home use.—**Susan B. Hagloch**

5.   **The Virtual Body.** [CD-ROM]. Minneapolis, Minn., IVI Publishing, 1995. Minimum system requirements: IBM or compatible 486/33MHz. Double speed CD-ROM drive. Windows 3.1. 8MB RAM. Hard disk. 256-color VGA monitor (640 x 480 mode). Mouse. Sound Blaster 16 or compatible sound card. Speakers or headphones. $59.95. ISBN 1-884899-11-0.

This animated view of the human body and its workings is well worth the price for libraries, schools, and families seeking quality software to enthrall and educate young thinkers. The basic menu offers eight choices—seven on the body's systems and an eighth as a multiuse browser. Self-explanatory instructions guide the user to full-color cutaway reproductions of human systems (e.g., the male and female reproductive organs). Choices of activities include straightforward presentation; for example, an animated view of a leg and a hip in action to demonstrate how muscles and joints move the limbs and trunk. The narrator describes the coordination of contracted muscles and hinged joints to produce basic motion. Other detailed data call up interactive screens and vernacular speech to explain the origin of goose bumps, how a sphygmomanometer measures both diastolic and systolic blood pressure, and why the stomach does not digest itself.

The editors of *The Virtual Body* tap into the kinds of information the beginning student of anatomy needs to know and the questions that are likely to evolve from intense study of body parts, digestion, nerves and brain, respiration, and reproduction. Narration avoids the cutesiness found in less serious programs. Instructions and use of multipurpose screens invite manipulation and study according to personal need, interest, and preference. One weakness is the pictorial browser, which displays unidentified close-ups of cells, bones, and tissue and halts the flow of access while the user decodes the small cells. Overall, *The Virtual Body* is a must for student health reference.
—**Mary Ellen Snodgrass**

BIBLIOGRAPHY

6. **Bibliography of Bioethics. Volume 26.** LeRoy Walters and Tamar Joy Dahn, eds. Washington, D.C., Kennedy Institute of Ethics/Georgetown University Press, 2000. 740p. $70.00. ISBN 1-883913-06-3. ISSN 0363-0161.

There have been scattered sources on the various topics in bioethics. This epic work singularly provides the most complete and best indexing in the field. The scope of this bibliography covers the systematic study of 77 major topics in health care delivery and in biomedicine, of which 23 are further divided by subheadings. It also includes specific bioethical issues that have received worldwide attention, such as euthanasia, cloning, human and animal experimentation, genetic engineering, abortion, organ donation and transplantation, AIDS, managed health care, fraud, and reproductive technologies. The *Bibliography* made a successful attempt to cite most of the English-language materials that discuss ethical aspects of these topics. The materials include a variety of media and literary forms, such as journals, newspaper articles, monographs, book chapters, court decisions, bills, laws, audiovisual materials, and unpublished manuscripts. The scope is comprehensive; however, it is puzzling that the often controversial topics, such as human sexuality, are not included in the *Bibliography*.

One of the important contributions this work gives is its bioethics thesaurus. It serves as a valuable tool to organize and access the massive amount of information in bioethics. Under the carefully organized indexing subjects the entries include the citation information, controlled vocabulary keywords, bioethics accession number, and other references (when available). Abstracts appear in citations for some journal articles and all court decisions. This is a remarkable resource in bioethics and is highly recommended for collections of academic and health care institutions.
—**Eveline L. Yang**

7. **Consumer Health Information Source Book.** 6th ed. Alan M. Rees, ed. Phoenix, Ariz., Oryx Press, 2000. 323p. index. $59.50pa. ISBN 1-57356-123-1.

Rees's *Consumer Health Information Source Book* is now available in its 6th edition, a testament to its usefulness as a resource and Rees's authority on consumer health resources and librarianship. This work, written by Rees and other consumer health information professionals, is dedicated to empowering health consumers through their use of information, but it is also a bible to librarians developing collections and providing reference assistance. Rees, along with health consumers, has embraced the World Wide Web as an information resource and performs a valuable service in this edition by directing consumers toward reliable, quality consumer health information on the Web. Because readers are not likely to read this work from cover to cover, the topic of Web health information quality is addressed in several different chapters. This is an effective strategy, since readers are exposed to this issue at appropriate points in the text.

Although a myriad of health information is now available via the Internet, many consumers still prefer information from newsletters, pamphlets, books, and other printed resources. Chapters provide a mix of advice for information seekers, essays on consumer health trends, topical subject guides, and select lists of recommended resources with evaluative and descriptive reviews. A "best of" list includes recommended and highly recommended resources listed in other chapters, for those who want to identify the most essential resources quickly. Rees reviews books and pamphlets in English on over 50 medical subjects, and recommends pamphlets in Spanish on nearly as many topics. An entire chapter is devoted to alternative and complementary healing resources. One chapter is devoted to clearinghouses, information centers, hotlines, and toll-free telephone numbers. Indexes provide access to entries by author, title, and subject. This thoughtful and thorough work is an essential purchase for any library that provides assistance to health care consumers. —**Lynne M. Fox**

8.	**Doody's Rating Service 1997: A Buyer's Guide to the 250 Best Health Sciences Books.** Oak Park, Ill., Doody Publishing, 1997. 263p. illus. index. $50.00pa. ISBN 1-885234-07-4. ISSN 1074-9640.

Selecting books in the health sciences can be a formidable task. Many expensive volumes appear each year, and librarians with limited budgets need to spend their money wisely. Doody Publishing is an independent organization that provides reviews of professional and student-level health sciences materials. Doody produces three print and five electronic review products. Reviews are prepared by 140 editorial groups covering the major medical and allied health disciplines. Each group is chaired by an academic health sciences professional who appoints appropriate reviewers and evaluates all titles submitted in the assigned area. The selection of the 250 best books, including the book of the year, is made from a field of 2,900 titles submitted by approximately 200 publishers. A list of review board chairs, submitted titles, and participating publishers appears in the front of this book.

The reviews are divided into broad categories: basic sciences, clinical medicine, nursing, associated health professions, and other disciplines. Within these areas, they are alphabetically arranged by specialties—anatomy, general surgery, case management, veterinary medicine, and so on. Each review contains a full bibliographic citation, a description, a 150-word evaluation, and information about special features and the target audience. In addition to author and title indexes, four appendixes list the titles by specialty, author affiliation, target audience, and book type. Book types are defined on the last page. Videos and CD-ROMs are included.

Health sciences, academic, and special librarians will find this source to be extremely useful for collection development. Public librarians with large collections will also find it helpful because it lists many appropriate titles. The reviews are clear and to the point, and they contain all the relevant acquisition information.—**Barbara M. Bibel**

9.	Haley, Barbara A., and Brian Deevey, comps. **American Health Care in Transition: A Guide to the Literature.** Westport, Conn., Greenwood Press, 1997. 336p. index. (Bibliographies and Indexes in Medical Studies, no.14). $79.50. ISBN 0-313-27323-5.

The compilers call this book a guide rather than an annotated bibliography, although it is a list of sources and the citations are all accompanied by abstracts. According to *Books in Print PLUS* (see ARBA 94, entry 8), it is the only book in print for either compiler, although Haley has published articles in *Humanity and Society*. Neither is a librarian—Haley is an applied sociologist and Deevey is a field data capture specialist for a digital map company. Buyers of this book should know that there are no books represented in this guide, only periodicals and government documents. It would be helpful to have this stated in the introduction. The introduction also fails to state the time span of the entries covered—the earliest one that was noticed had a date of 1979, the latest a date of 1996. Periodicals cited range from health care administration journals such as *Hospitals and Health Networks* to medical and even nursing journals. The government documents included are publications of two agencies, the U.S. General Accounting Office, which audits federal spending in areas like health care, and the Agency for Health Care Policy and Research, part of the U.S. Department of Health and Human Services. At $79.50, this book is a little expensive, but recommended, especially for collections supporting public health departments teaching health care administration.—**Lambrini Papangelis**

10. Haynes, Craig. **Ethnic Minority Health: A Selected, Annotated Bibliography.** Lanham, Md., Medical Library Association and Scarecrow, 1997. 503p. index. $65.00. ISBN 0-8108-3225-9.

This work serves to point out the disparities in health between minorities in the United States, who will make up one-third of the population by the year 2000, and nonminorities. The author, head of the Medical Center Library at the University of California, San Diego, Medical Center, concentrates on four minority groups: Native Americans, including Alaska Natives; African Americans; Hispanic Americans; and Asian/Pacific Islander Americans.

The book is organized into chapters devoted to medicine, mental health, medical education, health professions, research, service delivery and access, and prevention and health promotion. Every chapter begins with general information and then treats each group separately, so it is easy to locate relevant sections. What could be either a plus or a minus is that the annotations do not appear with the citations under these topics but are grouped together by main entry in a separate chapter. There are also an author and a subject index. It would have been easier to target specific citations from the subject index if the author had used entry numbers instead of page references, but this is a minor problem.

Sixty percent of the bibliography consists of monographs, although other material, such as government documents, research reports, and conference proceedings, is included. It is important to note that journal citations are not given here. Almost all the citations were published between 1970 and 1995. A list of dissertations and theses, journals, multimedia products, and federal and state publications appear in appendixes. This is a solid bibliography that will be most useful to people without access to OCLC's WorldCat, although the nonmonographs included definitely increase the book's value.—**Hope Yelich**

11. **Health Industry QuickSource: A Complete Descriptive Reference to Health Care Information Resources.** Mary Jeanne Cilurzo, ed. Nanuet, N.Y., QuickSource Press, 1995. 1023p. $225.00pa. ISBN 1-886515-08-5. ISSN 1077-9469.

This text is a guide to the world of medical CD-ROMs, online databases, and printed periodicals. Presented in a user-friendly style, individuals involved in or who wish to know more about health care/medicine will find this text useful. One nice feature is that it provides the sources of information for more than 70 medical topics ranging from AIDS to sports medicine to women's health. The reader can look up a specific medical condition, and reference sources are provided, including addresses and telephone and fax numbers.

Throughout most of the text, hundreds of medical resources are provided and listed according to the categories of either CD-ROM, online databases, or printed periodicals. The reader simply looks up the name of the reference (e.g., *Journal of Emergency Medical Services*), and information such as number of persons subscribing, subscription cost, frequency of publication, address, and telephone contacts are provided. All material involving a computer discusses compatibility features (IBM, Macintosh) and gives a summary of the software. An extensive list of printed periodicals that may also be of use to the reader completes the text.

Overall, this reference is well presented and a valuable resource for gaining information regarding the health care field as a whole. Individuals involved in medicine (including practicing, teaching, or publishing) should find this text to be a valuable resource. [R: C&RL, Oct 95, p.661]—**Paul M. Murphy III**

12.   **Health Statistics: An Annotated Bibliographic Guide to Information Resources.** 2d ed. Frieda O. Weise, Patricia G. Hinegardner, Barbara L. Kuchan, and Phyllis S. Lansing, eds. Chicago, Medical Library Association and Lanham, Md., Scarecrow, 1997. 178p. index. $42.00. ISBN 0-8108-3056-6.

Statistics are an important part of health sciences research. Finding a source with the necessary data for a specific project can be a challenge. This new edition of a basic guide to statistical sources will be helpful. *Health Statistics* was first published in 1980 (see ARBA 81, entry 1554). The 2d edition, by 4 experienced health sciences librarians, updates the material and adds new sources, including electronic databases. Nothing was added after 1994.

The 8 chapters cover broad subject areas, such as general references, vital statistics, demographics, health resources, morbidity, and so forth. Each is subdivided into such topics as specific diseases, age or ethnic groups, and types of health personnel. Within each topic, entries are numbered and arranged alphabetically by title. Entries include title, publisher, and frequency of issue. Entries for electronic sources list dates of coverage. There is no subscription, price, or ISBN/ISSN information. Annotations describe the type and scope of data and their arrangement. Four appendixes contain a brief list of newsletters and journals, a directory of state and federal agencies, a directory of associations and foundations, and a directory of regional federal depository libraries. A short glossary of terms and an index complete the text.

This book is a good starting point for students doing research on health care policy and epidemiology. It would also be helpful for librarians doing reference and collection development work in these areas. *Health Statistics* will be a useful addition to academic health science collections and large public libraries.—**Barbara M. Bibel**

13.   **Medical and Health Care Books and Serials in Print 1998: An Index to Literature in the Health Sciences.** 27th ed. New Providence, N.J., R. R. Bowker/Reed Reference Publishing, 1998. 2v. $249.95/set. ISBN 0-8352-3992-6. ISSN 0000-085X.

This 27th edition covers books and serials related to the major health science disciplines, such as medicine, dentistry, nursing, veterinary medicine, psychology, and biomedical sciences. Titles have generally been selected for a professional or college student audience. Author and title indexes to books include 91,753 entries for titles from 5,894 publishers, plus addresses and prices. Under the titles of journals are 43 domains of information on each periodical, from its Dewey Decimal Classification to whether it is refereed.

Medical and Health Care's 3,896 pages are enclosed in 2 volumes. Volume 1 lists books and journals under subject and author indexes. Volume 2 categorizes its contents under a book title index, serial subject index, vendor listings and serials online, serial title index, and publishers' and distributors' symbols and abbreviations. Type is dark, if not large, and quite readable.—**Anthony Gottlieb**

14.   Nordquist, Joan, comp. **The Health Care Crisis in the United States: A Bibliography.** Santa Cruz, Calif., Reference and Research Services, 1997. 72p. (Contemporary Social Issues: A Bibliographic Series, v.46). $15.00pa. ISBN 0-937855-90-1.

Managed care, managed cost, mangled care, market driven care—these are the words and phrases being used to describe the current evolution of the U.S. medical system. This reference provides a comprehensive list of the most current literature on this state of affairs. More than 850 entries effectively incorporate the spectrum of thinking on health/medical care delivery. Health care delivery "classics" from the 1980s are noted, but the majority of citations are from 1990 to 1996. The entries are organized under broad topical areas, including individual sections on the major populations at risk in the care system: women, children, the elderly, the homeless, minorities, and the poor.

The advantage to this particular reference is that it includes information that would not be found in any one computer database or hardcover medical index. A range of resources are cited —the usual books and journal articles but also dissertations, congressional hearings, and Websites. In addition, the Contemporary Social Issues Series includes literature from the less mainstream publications (e.g., activist organizations and alternative presses). Overall, this book is an excellent, all-inclusive, easy-to-use, quick source for the literature on health care delivery in the 1990s. It is highly recommended, particularly for libraries serving health care students or professionals.—**Mary Ann Thompson**

15.   Palmegiano, E. M. **Health and British Magazines in the Nineteenth Century.** Lanham, Md., Scarecrow, 1998. 282p. index. $59.50. ISBN 0-8108-3486-3.

Throughout the nineteenth century, the British public was both interested in and concerned about a diverse group of health-related topics, ranging from epidemics to personal hygiene to government involvement promoting public health. Many of the major popular and medical journals of that era reflect these concerns over wellness issues, as demonstrated by the article titles relating to medical/health matters found in these publications. Using the *Wellesley Index* and *Poole's Index*, Palmegiano has selected article titles found in 48 leading British journals published between 1824 and 1900 that pertain to the public's chief health interests.

Regrettably, this novel approach to social history of medicine is seriously flawed in its implementation. The 2,604 entries in this mostly unannotated bibliography are organized chronologically under each of the 48 journal titles rather than by subject headings. This fact forces the reader to rely on the limited subject index to find articles on any given topic. This organization is the major weakness of this reference tool and greatly decreases its potential value. There is no explanation for the selection of these subject headings, and one has to question how thoroughly they have been used in compiling this index. The author, who is not a medical historian, fails to explain the inclusion/exclusion of articles from these journals: Were all health-related titles included, or were there some limiting factors applied for selection? Even the author index is of limited usefulness unless one is interested in finding articles by such public health leaders as Edwin Chadwick. There are simply too many unanswered questions about the purpose and organization of this book to justify its inclusion as a history of medicine reference work.

The approach of examining popular journal article titles to determine the public's health interests is a worthwhile venture. Unfortunately, this initial attempt does not live up to this challenge and will be of little, if any, value to history of medicine scholars. Future bibliographic surveys of a similar nature should construct their studies based on a subject approach to this important topic.—**Jonathon Erlen**

BIOGRAPHY

16. Scrivener, Laurie, and J. Suzanne Barnes, with Cecelia M. Brown and Dana Tuley-Williams. **Biographical Dictionary of Women Healers: Midwives, Nurses, and Physicians.** Westport,

Conn., Oryx Press/Greenwood Publishing Group, 2002. 340p. illus. index. $65.00. ISBN 1-57356-219-X.

This biographical dictionary is a welcome and timely addition to women's biographical resources. The biographies are of women physicians, nurses, and midwives in the United States and Canada from the 1600s to 1999. One of the unique aspects of this book is the inclusion and recognition of the contribution of lay midwives, in addition to more formally educated physicians, nurses, and midwives. Entries are signed and have references, and some photographs are presented. The biographical information includes not only education and professional histories but personal histories as well, another unique feature that makes this book fascinating. There was a small item of incorrect information in the biography of Nancy Wilson Dickey, the first woman president of the American Medical Association. Dickey's undergraduate studies were done at Stephen F. Austin State University, which is located in Nacogdoches, Texas, and not in Houston. Sadly, this type of small detail error calls into question all of the detailed facts in the book. However, the book is still recommended as a useful addition to any high school, community or junior college, undergraduate, or public library.—**Lynn M. McMain**

17. **Who's Who in Medicine and Healthcare 2000-2001.** 3d ed. New Providence, N.J., Marquis Who's Who/Reed Reference Publishing, 2000. 1220p. $249.95. ISBN 0-8379-0004-2 (classic edition); 0-8379-0005-0 (deluxe edition).

The 3d edition of this ready-reference volume (see ARBA 98, entry 1507, for a review of the 1st edition) provides biographical and career information for more than 28,000 professionals in the medical industry. Biographees were chosen based on their level of achievement in their field. The majority come from the United States, but there are health care professionals represented from more than 115 countries worldwide. The purpose of this volume, as stated in the preface, is for health care professionals to have a means of identifying achievers in the medical community as well as discovering the progress of the work of their peers. It can also be used as a source for networking for health care professionals.

Organized in alphabetic order, the volume provides biographies for those practicing medicine in the fields of dentistry, geriatrics, gynecology, internal medicine, mental health, nursing, pediatrics, public health, surgery, and more, as well as those in support positions, such as association and governmental administration, corporate management, and legal practice. Information provided for each professional listed includes: name and occupation, birth date, education, professional history, and contact information. Information for the majority of professionals listed is provided by the biographee; for those listed that did not provide their own information, the staff at Marquis Who's Who researched the data (noted with an asterisk). This work will be most useful in the medical libraries of hospitals and universities.—**Shannon Graff Hysell**

DICTIONARIES AND ENCYCLOPEDIAS

18. **Bioethics Thesaurus.** 1999 ed. Washington, D.C., Kennedy Institute of Ethics, Georgetown University Press, 1999. 84p. index. $25.00pa.

The *Bioethics Thesaurus* is a compilation of keywords used at the Kennedy Institute of Ethics, Georgetown University, for the field of bioethics. The words listed here are also used as search words for the National Library of Medicine's BIOETHICSLINE database, which is a cumulation of the citations from *Bibliography of Bioethics* (Georgetown University Press). This work contains 700 searchable terms, with extensive cross-references. Terms that are searchable on the database are in bold typeface and uppercase letters; terms in bold typeface with lowercase letters give their searchable counterpart. For example, users are directed to use *Gene Therapy* or *Genetic Intervention* when they consult *Genetic Engineering*. The thesaurus also provides information on when the term was first used in the *Bioethics Thesaurus*, what it means, what the term is used for, a comparable broader or more narrow term for that word, and related terms. Some proper nouns are also included, such as names of persons, corporate bodies, laws, court decisions, and places. The five appendixes that conclude the volume provide a sample of a BIOETHICSLINE record, the most used keywords by subject area, publication types in BIOETHICSLINE, a list of subject captions, and an outline of an approach to researching on BIOETHICSLINE. This reference work will be extremely valuable when used in conjunction with the BIOETHICSLINE database or the *Bibliography of Bioethics.*—**Shannon Graff Hysell**

19.   **Encyclopedia of Biostatistics.** Peter Armitage and Theodore Colton, eds. New York, John Wiley, 1998. 6v. illus. index. $2,400.00/set. ISBN 0-471-97576-1.

Considerable understanding of statistical methods and theory and some knowledge of biomedical sciences is needed for best utilization of this major reference work. "Biostatistics" means application of statistical methods in medical and health sciences; however, social sciences are well represented here as well.

The application of statistical methods to medical research has expanded rapidly in recent years, as has the reporting of such in many technical journals and books. The number of individuals and institutions involved with some aspect of health care has also increased dramatically. Although there have been older statistical encyclopedias, such as the *Cambridge Dictionary of Statistics in the Medical Sciences* (see ARBA 96, entry 1699), the editors decided that a new and more comprehensive work was overdue: hence, this monumental product, in which they have eminently succeeded.

A panel of international experts is responsible for subject areas, but the entries of varying length are alphabetized by title. The final volume contains long subject and author indexes for the full set. Most of the illustrations are formulas, requiring skill to decipher. Others are tables and charts, with occasional portraits of famous persons who made significant contributions to statistics as a science. Both cross-references and bibliographies are extensive.

A selected list of review articles in the encyclopedia, such as "Disease Modeling," indicates the extensive coverage of the work, and serves as a rapid index to the main components of biostatistics. A long list of acronyms, many specific to the subject, is also provided in the index volume.

Subjects include the design of studies and experiments, collection of data and analysis, descriptions and application of statistical theories, definition of terms, listings of research and scientific organizations, and historical notes. Authors and researchers can find material on many specific questions. For example, the reader can look up BMI (body mass index) being discussed in the popular press because of new standards on obesity, and discover that Quetelet's index was developed in the 1830s by a scientist working on the statistically "average man." Or one can look up the biostatistical requirements in the design of health and morbidity surveys. This set is a significant addition to the literature of biostatistics. Many of the review articles are of general interest, such as the overview on vital statistics, but this is primarily a research tool.—**Harriette M. Cluxton**

20.   **Encyclopedia of Complementary Health Practice.** Carolyn Chambers Clark, ed. New York, Springer Publishing, 1999. 635p. index. $59.95pa. ISBN 0-8261-1239-0.

Millions of dollars are spent each year on alternative/complementary health care in the United States, yet no general reference has been available to assist the health care consumer or practitioner in better understanding these options. This encyclopedia begins to fill that void. The editors, the majority of whom are nurses, have compiled an extensive amount of reliable information about this topic, and presented it in an easy-to-use format. The book is composed of four major sections. The first gives a theoretical introduction to health, healing, and complementary therapies. Part 2 provides encyclopedic entries on approximately 100 medical conditions and their suggested alternative therapies. A particular strength in this section is that only alternative practices based on research are included. A 3d section discusses "substances," and a 4th section provides a brief explanation of more than 100 complementary health care practices. A variety of practices are included, some requiring a trained practitioner, whereas others can be practiced autonomously. The reference concludes with an extensive list of bibliographic references, a directory of organizations associated with the various practices, and a subject index. The book does what it intends to do—provide an encyclopedia-type overview of a comprehensive list of alternative/complementary health practices. It is a welcome addition to the health care literature. The *Encyclopedia of Complementary Health Practice* is highly recommended for public libraries and libraries serving health care practitioners and students. [R: Choice, Jan 2000, pp. 904-905]—**Mary Ann Thompson**

21.   **Encyclopedia of Health.** 3d ed. Anne Hildyard, Claire Cross, and Clare Hill, eds. Tarrytown, N.Y., Marshall Cavendish, 2003. 14v. illus. index. $329.95/set. ISBN 0-7614-7347-5.

Containing a full range of information on hygiene, exercise, sports, diet, diseases, and medicines, and written specifically for middle and high school students, the 3d edition of the *Encyclopedia of Health* is an interesting and informative source for health and medical information. Topics are arranged alphabetically with full-color photographs, charts, and diagrams. Also included are 12 in-depth features, covering such topics as careers, cleanliness, drugs, mental health, and diseases. Volume 16 contains comprehensive alphabetic and topical indexes, a first aid manual, a chronology of health and medical events, a list of health organizations, a glossary, a pronunciation guide, and a list of "health heroes." Overall, it is an easy-to-use reference for students and adults alike.—**Denise A. Garofalo**

22.   **Encyclopedia of Immunology.** 2d ed. Peter J. Delves and Ivan M. Roitt, eds. San Diego, Calif., Academic Press, 1998. 4v. illus. index. $750.00/set. ISBN 0-12-226765-6.

Immunology has emerged as a science that is vital for understanding physiology and disease. The rapid advances in this field during the past few years have made a new edition of the *Encyclopedia of Immunology* a necessity. First published in 1992, this 2d edition contains 64 new articles. The majority of the other entries have been completely rewritten.

An international group of distinguished academic scientists make up the editorial board and the group of 1,200 contributors who have created this 4-volume encyclopedia. The 630 alphabetic entries provide the most pertinent information on the subjects that are covered. All articles are signed and all have brief bibliographies of review articles and key papers in the field. The articles range in length from one to four pages. Many have charts, diagrams, black-and-white photographs, or color plates. They cover a broad range of subjects that are of interest to biomedical researchers: the behavioral regulation of immunity; ABO blood group system; spleen; nutrition and the immune system; reptile immune system; gel electrophoresis; and Candida, infection and immunity are examples. Although the articles are written at the professional level, educated lay readers will be able to understand them. Each volume has the complete table of contents and index for the set as well as a glossary.

The *Encyclopedia of Immunology* is a fine addition to academic science and health sciences reference collections. Purchase of the print set includes a trial subscription to the online version available on the World Wide Web.—**Barbara M. Bibel**

23.   **Encyclopedia of Public Health.** Lester Breslow, ed. New York, Macmillan Reference USA/Gale Group, 2002. 4v. illus. index. $475.00/set. ISBN 0-02-865354-8.

This 4-volume encyclopedia contains more than 900 essays covering the field of public health. Its scope is broad, and among the categories represented are: agencies involved in public health, communicable and noncommunicable diseases, epidemiology, environmental health, history, philosophy and ethics, laboratory services, and others. Written by authorities in their respective fields, the set is intended for educated lay people at a high school or community college level. Yet the organization of this set is puzzling and no table of contents provides order. Entries are alphabetically arranged by their central concept, which is a logical choice, but the reason for inclusion of some subjects is a mystery. A section within each entry explaining its implications to public health would be useful.

A good contents outline establishes placement of topics within the field. Unfortunately, it is only referred to in the preface, and then hidden in the last volume. Also mentioned in the preface, but not easily located, are an annotated bibliography of important historical and modern works and an appendix that contains reprints of such documents as The Oath of Hippocrates, Universal Declaration of Human Rights, and World Scientists' Warning to Humanity. Some subjects are covered in depth while others get superficial treatment. For example, the concept *overwintering* received one paragraph of attention and ovarian cancer, which affects 12 out of 1,000 women, received the same.

Although the authors have attempted to keep medical jargon to a minimum, technical language is used and unexplained in some articles. By contrast, other entries use simplistic statements that could lead the average reader to form incorrect conclusions. There is no comparable treatise in the area of public health, so this encyclopedia fills a gap. It is a shame the material could not have been presented in a more competent manner. [R: LJ, 15 April 02, pp. 71-73]—**Susan K. Setterlund**

24.   Freudenheim, Ellen. **HealthSpeak: A Complete Dictionary of America's Health Care System.** New York, Facts on File, 1996. 310p. index. $30.00. ISBN 0-8160-3210-6.

This dictionary covers the language of health care and is not a medical/clinical dictionary. More than 2,000 terms are defined clearly and concisely, and they are referenced and cross-referenced for helping the user better understand a concept. Approximately 100 terms have longer essay definitions for clarity. The entries also include definitions for health care and health insurance organizations, economic terms related to health care, health care laws or acts, and compound terms. If an insurance company or health care provider uses a nonclinical term, it is probably in this book.

The book is arranged alphabetically, has a bibliography with more than 55 citations for further information, and contains an extensive index. The one deficiency is the font size of the index. The typeface is extremely small, making it difficult to read. There are half-a-dozen graphs that illustrate specific definitions. This book was written for the layperson and is highly recommended for all public libraries at this price. [R: RBB, 1 May 96, p. 1528]—**Betsy J. Kraus**

25.   Gay, Kathlyn. **Encyclopedia of Women's Health Issues.** Westport, Conn., Oryx Press/Greenwood Publishing Group, 2002. 300p. illus. index. $69.95. ISBN 1-57356-303-X.

According to the preface of this work, the *Encyclopedia* focuses on "social, economic, political, and ethical issues that affect policy decisions regarding women's health as well as women's physical and mental well-being" (p. vi). There are more than 200 entries, written in a readable, nonscientific style, including historical perspectives when appropriate. There are *see* references and suggestions for further reading following most entries, usually consisting of government or organizational Websites, one or more newspaper articles (usually from *The New York Times*), and books (often including the Boston Women's Health Book Collective's *Our Bodies, Ourselves for the New Century: A Book by and for Women* [Touchstone/Simon & Schuster, 1998]) or medical journal articles, all recompiled as an appendix. There are a few black-and-white photographs, useful in the case of illustrating articles about individuals or institutions. Examples include former U.S. Surgeon General Antonia Novello; birth control advocate Margaret Sanger; the Emma Goldman Clinic (the first women's health care center in the midwest); and writer and environmentalist Rachel Carson (illustrating the *Silent Spring Institute* entry). This organization was included because of its work on the possible links between environmental toxins and breast cancer. Unfortunately, its Website (http://www.silentspring.org/) is nowhere in evidence. A photograph of intrauterine devices (IUDs) might have been useful in the entry on birth control, while stock photographs of teenagers smoking, to illustrate the entry on smoking, are unnecessary. A few entries, such as "Hospital Mergers," seem peripheral to the *Encyclopedia*'s stated purpose, but the author discusses the problems that arise for women's reproductive rights when nonprofit community hospitals and religious hospitals merge. "Hospice Care" is listed because "women have been at the forefront of this kind of care" (p. 120). Appendixes include selected Websites and organization addresses. The *Encyclopedia*'s high price will probably put it out of the range of its target audience. If budgets allow, it can be considered an optional purchase for those high school and public libraries where Internet access is problematic, or where there are insufficient online databases available. [R: LJ, Dec 02, p. 106]—**Martha E. Stone**

26.   **Handbook of Health Behavior Research.** David S. Gochman, ed. New York, Plenum, 1997. 4v. index. $85.00/vol.; $275.00/set. ISBN 0-306-45443-2 (v.1); 0-306-45444-0 (v.2); 0-306-45445-9 (v.3); 0-306-45446-7 (v.4).

This is not a handbook in the traditional sense; rather, it is a state-of-the-art review presenting "a broad and representative selection of mid-1990s health behavior findings and concepts in a single work." The 4 volumes cover broad interdisciplinary fields, focusing on the health behavior of individuals, society, and providers; the demography, development, and diversity of health behavior; the professional relevance of health behavior research, and future issues. Each volume begins with an introductory chapter and ends with a chapter integrating the topics covered. There are 117 authors, many of whom are acknowledged experts in their fields, who contributed 75 chapters to this work. Each chapter ends with a list of bibliographic references.

The index is extensive, but not comprehensive, and this fact is acknowledged in the book. Most terms in the 16-page glossary cite the handbook volume and chapter in which they are defined—a useful feature, particularly because some words, such as *healmeme*, are unique to this area of study, and other words, such as *prevention*, have specific meanings in this field of research. The use of figures, tables, graphs, and other illustrations is minimal.

This is clearly an academic work, not intended for the average layperson. The style of writing is concise and pedagogic, as found in a research article. The stated objectives are fulfilled, and no other single work in the field comes close to it in terms of coverage, comprehensiveness, scholarship, and currency. It is recommended for libraries supporting medical, behavioral, and social science collections.—**Michael R. Leach**

27.   Harding, Anne S. **Milestones in Health and Medicine.** Phoenix, Ariz., Oryx Press, 2000. 267p. illus. index. $59.95. ISBN 1-57356-140-1.

Librarians are frequently asked questions about the history of medicine that requiring information on specific individuals, events, and diseases. Fortunately, there are a number of quality reference tools to answer most of these queries. Regrettably, this new volume by Harding, who is a professional journalist rather than a medical history expert, cannot be used as a reliable resource.

The compiler states that this book, although not all-inclusive, includes selected diseases, organizations, health care issues, and treatments. Specific selection criteria, however, are very vague. An examination of the entries reveals many factual errors, repetitious entries, omissions of key facts and individuals, and a simplistic approach to complicated subjects that can mislead the reader.

There are many serious problems in this reference, such as the major historical figure Galen of Pergamon, who lived from 129 to 215 B.C.E., being incorrectly listed as Claudius Galen, 129-199 B.C.E. Also, in the preface, Harding places the discoveries of aseptic techniques, anesthesia, and X rays in the same century as the breakthroughs in DNA and antibiotics rather than in the nineteenth century. Margaret Sanger, while a strong advocate for the creation of a birth control pill, never personally financed its development as this book claims. Among many other problems, huge topics such as dentistry and health insurance are all too quickly overviewed in one to two pages. Finally, while citing a number of secondary sources for her information, Harding relies heavily on a few standard reference works—thus providing no new insights on these topics.

Librarians answering patrons' history-of-medicine questions can rely on standard reference tools such as *The Cambridge World History of Human Disease* (see ARBA 95, entry 1662) and the *Companion Encyclopedia of the History of Medicine* (see ARBA 95, entry 1654). This new text contains no new material and has many factual errors and omissions. [R: BL, 1 Dec 2000, p. 752]—**Jonathon Erlen**

28.   **Health & Wellness Resource Center. http://www.gale.com/HealthRC.** [Website]. Farmington Hills, Mich., Gale. Price negotiated by site. Date reviewed: Mar 02.

The *Health & Wellness Resource Center* from the Gale Group evolved from Gale's *Health Reference Center*. This Website provides readable medical information for both the student and the lay person researching particular diseases, conditions, and treatments. This site provides access to a variety of medical reference sources, including the *Gale Encyclopedia of Medicine* (2d ed.; see entry 158), *PDR Family Guide to Nutrition and Health* (Medical Economics Data, 1995), U*X*L's *Body by Design* (see entry 110), and *The Complete Directory for People with Disabilities* (11th ed.; see ARBA 2003, entry 818), just to name a few. It also provides access to more than 400 medical journals, some 200 pamphlets, and 2,200 general interest publications that discuss health and medical topics. Alternative health topics are covered here as well and include information from *The Gale Encyclopedia of Alternative Medicine* (see entry 205) and *PDR for Herbal Medicines* (2d ed.; see entry 409), to name only two.

This Website is easy to navigate and the information is easy to retrieve. For those seeking general information on a variety of topics the best place to start is with the "Quick Start" guide. Here, users can choose to browse topics in the "Medical Encyclopedia," "Health Organization Directory," "Drug and Herb Finder," "Medical Dictionary," "Alternative Health Encyclopedia," and "Health Assessment Tools" (which gives users access to such Websites as Cancerfacts.com and Healthanswers.com). A link to "Health News" gives users access to daily news in the health and medical worlds. Users can do more specific searches by using the "Search" button or the "Advanced Search" button. An advanced search allows the user to put in keywords and tell the database where specifically to look for them (e.g., article title). Results from each search can be printed, e-mailed, or marked with "Infomark" to save the source for later reference.

This resource provides a lot of medical and health care information in one easy-to-use site. It is most appropriate for consumer health libraries and public libraries and would be a valuable addition to both.—**Shannon Graff Hysell**

29.   **The Health Care Almanac: A Resource Guide to the Medical Field.** Lorri A. Zipperer, ed. Chicago, American Medical Association, 1995. 505p. index. $24.95pa. ISBN 0-89970-748-3.

This useful guide was assembled by the reference staff of the American Medical Association (AMA) library. Similar to its predecessor, *The Healthcare Resource and Reference Guide*, it is designed to address common queries by doctors and patients about a broad range of health and medical practice-related issues. The book contains a 360-page section of alphabetized entries, an extensive segment on the AMA itself, and a section containing display copies of the Principles of Medical Ethics, the Hippocratic Oath, and the Patient Bill of Rights. The entries are carefully edited and always readable. Coverage, however, is highly idiosyncratic: Breast feeding lists an address (for La Leche League International), while smoking covers seven pages, more than half of which is a list of magazines that will not accept tobacco advertising. Physicians will find detailed advice on how to close a practice, but there is no advice for patients who wish to find a doctor. A significant number of entries are distilled from AMA publications, particularly *JAMA* and the *AM News*. There is minimal cross-referencing, but an excellent index. The AMA section provides a comprehensive history and overview of association activities from 1846 to the present. Here are described the association's legal functions, business and management services, scientific and educational affairs, policy and political advocacy, and much more. On the whole, the volume is geared more to physicians than to patients, but it should be a popular general reference item in both academic and general libraries.—**Bruce Stuart**

30. **Health Issues.** Tracy Irons-Georges, ed. Hackensack, N.J., Salem Press, 2001. 2v. illus. index. (Magill's Choice). $95.00/set. ISBN 0-89356-042-1.
       This book is not about health issues. A college librarian might conclude from the title *Health Issues*, and from the series name "Magill's Choice," that it would be similar to standard undergraduate series like Contemporary World Issues (published by ABC-CLIO). But it is not similar to them, because it does not discuss the issues. It does not even identify the issues because it does not contain issues. It contains health topics. Instead of actual issues, such as stem cell research, it has chapters with titles like "Sunburn," "Asthma," and "Obesity." Plenty of encyclopedias that discuss health topics already exist. Actually, to be fair, the asthma chapter did make one good point that "Self-treatment [of one's asthma] with nonprescription drugs should be avoided" (p. 105). That might constitute an issue. But, sunburn does not constitute an issue. Thus, this book's title is a misnomer, and the price of $95 for the two-volume set is just silly. It appears that the intended audience of this book is undergraduates. This work is not recommended.—**Lambrini Papangelis**

31. Kurian, George Thomas. **Encyclopedia of Medical Media & Communications.** Gaithersville, Md., Aspen, 1996. 985p. index. $175.00. ISBN 0-8342-0685-4.
       The title of this book is misleading in the fact that it is primarily a guide to the print medical literature. As the author states in the preface, "It serves as a roadmap to the universe of print medical literature." With that limitation in mind, the book is useful. There is a substantial section that includes some online and CD-ROM databases. The title leads one to believe that mention is made of electronic medical journals and other multimedia resources distributed through the World Wide Web. Unfortunately, this book does not include WWW-accessible medical publications.—**Diane Kovacs**

32. Lee, Kelley. **Historical Dictionary of the World Health Organization.** Lanham, Md., Scarecrow, 1998. 333p. (Historical Dictionaries of International Organizations, no.15). $62.00. ISBN 0-8108-3371-9.
       Publishers have been marking the World Health Organization's (WHO) 1998 golden anniversary with a number of publications. Scarecrow Press offers the *Historical Dictionary of the*

World Health Organization, the 15th entry in the Historical Dictionaries of International Organizations series. During its 50 years, WHO has evolved to become an important force in the health care of citizens worldwide. This required numerous committees, commissions, forums, and task forces. These groups are incorporated into a complex set of bureaus, agencies, and offices. The groups' efforts include a variety of declarations, symposiums, reports, programs, guidelines, and recommendations. Any government documents librarian can attest to the challenge of acquiring, organizing, and then locating a WHO document for a patron. This dictionary helps with those tasks by offering thoroughly researched entries; a chronology; list of acronyms; and information on units, key figures, events, and major publications. A bibliography includes major publications of WHO. The work features eight appendixes. Appendix A presents the Constitution; appendix B lists member countries and the year they joined; appendix C includes contact information; appendix D reprints organizational charts (some are poorly reproduced); appendix E lists personnel; and appendixes F through H include other documents, financial information, and cooperating organizations. International documents collections and medical libraries where international health and health policy are important will want to add this resource to their collections. [R: Choice, Dec 98, p. 667]—**Lynne M. Fox**

33.   Levchuck, Caroline M., Michele Drohan, and Jane Kelly Kosek. **Healthy Living.** Edited by Allison McNeill. Farmington Hills, Mich., U*X*L/Gale, 2000. 3v. illus. index. $95.00/set. ISBN 0-7876-3918-4.

This three-volume set is one element of U*X*L's Complete Health Resource series. The companion sets are *Sick! Diseases and Disorders, Injuries and Infections* (see entry 198) and *Body by Design: From the Digestive System to the Skeleton* (see entry 110).

Each volume is divided into five chapters. The 1st volume addresses nutrition, hygiene, sexuality, fitness, and environmental health. The second volume discusses health care systems, health careers, preventive care, over-the-counter drugs, and alternative medicine. And the third volume covers mental health, mental illness, eating disorders, and mental health therapies.

A cumulated table of contents and a glossary are repeated at the beginning of each volume. Each chapter begins with a summary, a table of contents, and a glossary of terms specific to that chapter's main subject. However, chapter tables of content are lacking page numbers, decreasing its usefulness. There are inset boxes throughout the chapters that offer interesting facts and health and safety tips relevant to the discussion. The further readings and pertinent Websites listed at the end of each chapter provide additional information, but are limited. Each volume ends with a repeated cumulated bibliography and index. The very useful index is cross-referenced and denotes illustrations associated with a subject. The text is liberally sprinkled with photographs and illustrations to visually demonstrate the main points of the text. The text itself is organized more like a textbook than an encyclopedia.

There is a definite bias toward alternative forms of health care and medication. The book devotes 12 pages to a history and discussion of homeopathy and naturopathy. More conventional physician training, both traditional medical doctor and osteopathic physician, comprises a mere four pages of text. In addition, at the beginning of the section on herbal medicine there is a one-sentence blanket statement that the "benefits of herbal medicine and their effectiveness and safety have not been proven," but the subsequent discussions of individual herbal medicines is written as if the information were verified by proven research.

Overall, *Healthy Living* presents a balanced discussion of most topics and is suitable for high school libraries, especially if a thorough discussion of alternative health care and medicine is desired. [R: BL, 1 Oct 2000, p. 372; SLJ, Nov 2000, pp. 92-94]—**Bronwyn Stewart**

34.   Levinson, David, and Laura Gaccione. **Health and Illness: A Cross-Cultural Encyclope-dia.** Santa Barbara, Calif., ABC-CLIO, 1997. 253p. illus. maps. index. (Encyclopedias of the Human Experience). $49.50. ISBN 0-87436-876-6.

Levinson, editor-in-chief of the *Encyclopedia of World Cultures* and senior editor of the *Encyclopedia of Cultural Anthropology*, has written many books on cross-cultural topics since the 1970s. He has edited and produced numerous dictionaries and encyclopedias on human experiences. Gaccione is a professional journalist and Associated Press correspondent. This book is the first of its kind in presenting global information on three different types of medical treatment—biomedicine, alternative and complementary medicine, and traditional medicine. Yet the major emphasis is on the alternative and traditional approaches. The authors reviewed journals, books, encyclopedias, magazines, and materials from organizations and gathered relevant information for this volume. They also collected ethnographic records and medical anthropology from books, articles, doctoral dissertations, reports, and so on.

The A to Z format is easy to use. The book contains unique explanations on wife beating and types of wife beating, supernatural explanations, reflexology, magnet therapy, the Saraguro health system, genital mutilation, culture-bound syndromes, ayurvedic medicine, anthrosophical medicine, and many other topics of interest. However, this book does not attempt to be comprehensive in scope. Only the best-known cultural healing systems and health issues are illustrated. A good bibliography is included.—**Polin P. Lei**

35.   **Macmillan Health Encyclopedia.** rev. ed. New York, Macmillan Reference USA/Gale Group, 1999. 9v. illus. index. $395.00/set. ISBN 0-02-865040-9.

The nine volumes of this encyclopedia each cover a different topic that was chosen to correspond to those typically included in a school health course. The volumes cover anatomy and physiology; communicable diseases; noncommunicable diseases and disorders; nutrition and fitness; emotional and mental health; sexuality and reproduction; drugs, alcohol, and tobacco; safety and environmental health; and health care systems. The last volume includes an index to the entire set, while each volume also has an index to its own contents.

Within each volume there are short entries (one to two pages) on subjects within the broader topic, arranged alphabetically. The placement of the topics within the nine volumes is somewhat arbitrary, but numerous cross-references and the index help overcome this problem. Each volume also has a glossary and a list of supplementary sources. Most of the supplementary sources are older, classic texts, although there are also lists of organizations with Websites for access to more recent information. The text covers a wide array of subjects with an emphasis on wellness and healthful living. The articles include colorful, but usually simplified, illustrations and diagrams. The language is also clear and simple, and the treatment of each subject is broad, not detailed or in-depth. The overall result is something that would be a good supplement to a junior high or high school health course.—**Carol L. Noll**

36.   Modeste, Naomi N. **Dictionary of Public Health Promotion and Education: Terms and Concepts.** Newbury Park, Calif., Sage, 1996. 161p. $39.95; $18.95pa. ISBN 0-7619-0002-0; 0-7619-0003-9pa.

Some 240 books and journal articles were used as resources to select the range of terms in the dictionary. None was written after 1994. Terms relevant to the four settings of health promotion and education (community, workplace, primary care, and school) are emphasized (foreword). The terms, listed alphabetically, reflect the process of health promotion and education rather than focusing on disease-specific terminology, unlike most medical dictionaries. Approximately 130 additional sources provide broader coverage of the field. Also, 32 health and professional organizations are listed, with addresses, where more information can be sought.

The definitions vary in length, and many are cross-referenced. A brief example follows each entry to shed further light on the term. These may be of some assistance to the novice selector. Some terms and concepts may not meet standard public health, health promotion, and health education definitions, and one should keep that in mind when accessing a specific term. User frustration may arise due to the fact that the term one is searching for may not be within the parameters selected for inclusion. No firm criteria for selection are given. Although brief, this dictionary should be useful for public, medical, and health science reference collections, but probably not as an individual purchase. [R: Choice, May 96, p. 1454]—**Judy Gay Matthews**

37.   **The Oxford Companion to the Body.** Colin Blakemore and Sheila Jennett, eds. New York, Oxford University Press, 2001. 753p. illus. index. $65.00. ISBN 0-19-852403-X.

Any publication from Oxford University Press produced in conjunction with the Physiological Society (United Kingdom) carries an expectation of quality, and *The Oxford Companion to the Body* does not disappoint. Editors Blakemore and Jennett are of outstanding ability and reputation, as are the section editors and the more than 350 contributors. Entries are alphabetically arranged and have *see, see also*, and further reading references. A detailed index incorporates commonly used synonyms, thus providing for expanded access. Lastly, a section of plates illustrate various human organ systems. Beautiful full-page photographs decorate the text intermittently and there are more than 150 illustrations, some quite historic and interesting, such as the line drawing by Christopher Wren of the base of the human brain found in the entry under the headword "Vision." The use of British spelling will be confusing for readers outside the United Kingdom. For example, to locate the entries on *estrogen* and *edema* readers must look under *oestrogens* and *oedema*. However, this does not detract from the overall superior quality of this book, which is highly recommended for secondary school, college and university, and public libraries. [R: LJ, 1 May p2, p. 92; AG, Nov 02, p. 72]—**Lynn M. McMain**

38.   Rinzler, Carol Ann. **Why Eve Doesn't Have an Adam's Apple: A Dictionary of Sex Differences.** New York, Facts on File, 1996. 200p. index. $25.95; $14.95pa. ISBN 0-8160-3352-8; 0-8160-3356-0pa.

Much has been written about the psychological and behavioral differences between men and women. In this new reference book, the author emphasizes physiological differences: For example, which sex is more likely to get heart disease, ulcers, and thumb pain? Do more men or women suffer from nightmares, cold hands, or headaches? Who is better at spatial reasoning? The entries, 232 in all, are presented in a straightforward alphabetic sequence. While most are short, some go on for a page or more, and some include tables. A nice feature is a section of "notes and references," which enables readers to see where the author found her information.

Much of that information is culled from such respected medical sources as the *Merck Manual* the Physicians' Desk Reference (56th ed.; see entry 412); and publications from such organizations as the American Cancer Society, although in a few cases (e.g., AIDS, mathematical skills) the sources are popular publications, such as *The New York Times* and *Newsweek*. There is also a handy index, providing greater access to the information embedded in each entry. The book is physically attractive, with easy-to-read typeface and a provocative cover. This is an entertaining but hardly an exhaustive treatment of the subject. Its strength is its readability and the fact that the author brought together diverse information, making it a good jumping-off point for further research, a source for term paper topics, or even an inspiration for cocktail party conversation. [R: RBB, 1 Sept 96, p. 173]—**Hope Yelich**

39.   Rognehaugh, Richard. **The Managed Health Care Dictionary.** Gaithersville, Md., Aspen, 1996. 211p. $19.95pa. ISBN 0-8342-0856-3.

Rognehaugh wants his dictionary to "emerge as the Gold Standard in comprehensive managed care terminology." He also wants it to please a widely diverse population—everyone from patients and physicians to government agencies and insurance companies. How well does he succeed? In a word, admirably: He has compiled a unique, comprehensive, up-to-date managed care dictionary with a few correctable elements.

Among the suggested improvements are making the cross-references consistent and always giving terms with the accompanying acronym (e.g., Rognehaugh gives the term *admission per thousand* but not the acronym APT). Another detriment is that medical occupations and specialties are omitted entirely. Patients often do not know an RN from an LPN. Also, some omissions were noted, which can be found in other glossaries.

One of the positive features is the inclusion of 1,100 terms, many cross-referenced; there are 23 entries on Medicare variations alone. In addition, slang and insider terms are included (e.g., *face sheet, turfing, snif,* and *unbundling*). Nearly 20 percent of the terms are acronyms; some are five unpronounceable letters long (e.g., DXNNH, RBRVS). The definitions are clear and include pros and cons as well as related terms. The terms defined are of all levels of sophistication. Also of benefit are the publisher's solid reputation and its commitment to update and revise (comments and differing perspectives are invited via e-mail, fax, and regular mail).—**Pete Prunkl**

40.   Sebastian, Anton. **A Dictionary of the History of Medicine.** Pearl River, N.Y., Parthenon, 1999. 781p. illus. $89.00. ISBN 1-85070-021-4.

This text provides a comprehensive review of terminology that relates to the history of medicine. It begins with an informative and well-written preface. The body of the text contains 781 pages that are dedicated to terminology that has been used throughout the history of medicine.

This book has been designed with an effective use of space. As in most dictionaries and encyclopedias, key words, sentences, and paragraphs are clearly identifiable. Although the illustrations in this book are primarily black and white, their clarity is outstanding. This book appears to be most appropriately suited for adult readers. Individuals interested in learning about history, medicine, or the history of medicine may find this a fascinating resource. This book will complement home, public, and medical libraries. It is a well-written and informative reference. [R: Choice, Feb 2000, p. 1082]—**Paul M. Murphy III**

41.   Slee, Vergil N., Debora A. Slee, and H. Joachim Schmidt. **Slee's Health Care Terms.** 4th ed. St. Paul, Minn., Tringa Press, 2001. 638p. $29.95pa. ISBN 1-889458-02-3.

It is rare to describe a dictionary as lively as this, and while one may not want to curl up in bed with the 4th edition of *Slee's Health Care Terms*, if any dictionary can be called a delight this one can. The history of the work is interesting; a 12-page glossary of key health care terms was drafted by one of the authors at an academic conference of physicians, hospital administrators, and trustees so the attendee's spouses could understand the health care system. However, by the end of the day no copies were left since the original glossary was "snatched up by the doctors, trustees and administrators" (p. 7).

The dictionary's purpose is to define terms in all aspects of the health care field so professionals, consumers, students, policymakers, journalists, and patients all can communicate with one another. Areas covered include health care administration and delivery, payment systems, safety, quality control, legislation and regulation, managed care, and health care planning. The dictionary does not include purely medical terms such as diseases. The definitions are clear and coherent without being overly academic; for example, college freshmen will be able to understand what stem cells are. New words and terms are included, such as *nutriceutical* or *personal digital assistant.* The dictionary also has jargon and acronyms as well as a timeline that tells what happened in health care in the United States. The authors are a physician with a Masters in public health and two lawyers with experience in health care.

The book is missing some features. Pronunciation and entomologies of the words are not given and there are no examples of usage. Perhaps this was done to keep the price reasonable and the size portable. This resource is highly recommended for all college and medical libraries. Public libraries will also want it for their health care consumers.—**Natalie Kupferberg**

42.   **World of Health.** Brigham Narins, ed. Farmington Hills, Mich., Gale, 2000. 1424p. illus. index. $99.00. ISBN 0-7876-3649-5.

The introduction to this encyclopedia states that it is intended for students or nonexperts in the field of health and medicine. The reference goes on to provide an accurate, concise, and sufficient discussion of approximately 1,400 alphabetized topics. A broad range of subjects have been included—diseases, medical therapies, alternative or complementary therapies, health professionals, broad categories of medications, health care delivery systems, and major scientists and physicians who have contributed to medicine and public health. Within the entries, individual concepts or words are printed in bold typeface to indicate their inclusion elsewhere in the reference. The encyclopedia is enhanced by illustrations and photographs. A chronology, dating from 5000 B.C.E. to 1999, traces the history of medicine. Finally, an extensive general index assists the reader in finding not only the major topical entries, but also concepts that are embedded within the entries but not given distinct coverage. This volume is recommended for high school or public libraries, or other libraries seeking a quick and easy general health and medical reference. [R: BL, July 2000, p. 2063; Choice, Sept 2000, pp. 98-100]—**Mary Ann Thompson**

DIRECTORIES

43.   **Bacon's Medical & Health Media Directory 2000.** 3d ed. Chicago, Bacon's Information, 1999. 1011p. index. $245.00pa. ISSN 1520-2674.

This directory is a comprehensive guide to medical and health media contacts and was designed as a companion media guide to *Bacon's Magazine Directory* (47th ed.; see ARBA 2000, entry 50), *Bacon's Newspaper Directory* (47th ed.; see ARBA 2000, entry 51), *Bacon's Radio Directory* (13th ed.; see ARBA 2000, entry 824), and *Bacon's TV/Cable Directory* (13th ed.; see ARBA 2000, entry 825). Bacon's database contains nearly 400,000 contacts to the U.S. and Canadian print and broadcast media. Compiled to help public relations and communications professionals reach the media with news of interest to the media and health community, the directory contains six listing sections and three special index sections—newspapers, magazines, news services and syndicates, freelance journalists, television/cable/radio, television/radio syndicates and independent producers, all media index, all personnel index, and subject specialties index. Entries include names and subject specialty, address, telephone numbers, e-mail addresses of appropriate contacts, and a URL for the organization. Magazine entries include a brief profile of the publication, frequency, and circulation numbers.

Although this directory contains useful information about various periodicals, it is not an essential resource for a library. It is clearly intended for the individual who wants to locate appropriate media contacts for the purpose of distributing health-related information to a large audience.—**Vicki J. Killion**

44.   **Canadian Health Facilities Directory.** Don Mills, Ont., Southam Information Products, 1999. 1v. (various paging). $199.00. ISBN 1-55257-021-5. ISSN 1481-4463.

The *Canadian Health Facilities Directory* is a Canadian version of the American Health Association Guide, and a companion volume to the *Canadian Medical Directory*. It complements another Canadian publication, the *Guide to Canadian Healthcare Facilities*, by giving different data and key personnel. However, the *Canadian Health Facilities Directory* is not a bilingual publication. This makes it an ideal resource for U.S. libraries, especially in Canadian border states, where this directory is useful in locating medical records of visiting Canadian patients. The directory also is helpful in identifying institutions offering specialized care centers or services. This directory provides information on hospitals, long-term care facilities, and clinics.

Information in the facility listings includes statistical and contact information supplied by the institution. Data include facts such as length of stay, beds, visits, budget, and personnel. Brief profiles of the institution indicate areas of specialty care and whether they are privately or publicly supported. Long-term care providers describe the amenities and strengths of the facility. Organization is in three sections: by facility type, geographically by province, and by city. The directory also contains a supplier list, although company representative contact names are not included in the lists.—**Lynne M. Fox**

45.   **Canadian Medical Directory 2000.** 46th ed. Don Mills, Ont., Southam, 2000. 1v. (various paging). index. $199.00 (w/CD-ROM). ISBN 1-55257-088-6. ISSN 0068-9203.

The 46th edition of the *Canadian Medical Directory* contains more than just an alphabetic listing of Canadian physicians, although that is its primary focus. Each citation contains full contact information with telephone and fax numbers (without e-mail addresses), as well as languages spoken, medical school attended, year of graduation, and honors attained. Physicians are also listed in separate indexes by languages spoken as well as alphabetically by province and by specialty. Another section lists all Canadian hospitals, but each citation only contains an address and telephone and fax numbers. Other sections include detailed contact information for provincial health units, faculties of medicine in Canadian universities (with a list of 1999 graduates), and Canadian medical and health care associations (many of which include e-mail addresses and URLs). A "Year in Review" for Canadian medicine from the *Canadian Medical Association Journal* and *CMA News* covers advances in medicine and health trends in Canada. Journal references are also included. Information about the Canadian Medical Hall of Fame is provided, as well as brief illustrated sketches of new inductees. Health science and medical school libraries in North America will want to purchase this directory annually; reference departments of large public libraries and small hospital libraries may want to purchase it on a less-frequent basis. A companion CD-ROM also accompanies the text.—**Martha E. Stone**

46.   **Clinical Performance Measurement Directory.** 2000 ed. Chicago, American Medical Association, 2000. 240p. index. $149.95pa. ISBN 1-57947-009-2.

This directory "lists information about almost 330 current and/or planned performance measurement activities of physician organizations and other groups" (p. v). The American Medical Association surveyed its federation of national and state medical societies as well as large group practices, peer review organizations, and performance measurement system vendors to gather this information. In an introduction performance measurement, process measures and outcome measures are all defined. For medical libraries, the book is mainly useful for its descriptions of what specific organizations are doing in the area of performance management.

The information for each listing includes activity topic, status and purpose, database management, and any feedback the groups give to their physicians. The book also prints a copy of the measurements activities survey sent to the organizations. With a price of $149.95, and the likelihood that most of the information will be outdated by the time it is printed, readers may wonder why the American Medical Association does not just put this information on the Website. This

work is recommended for medical libraries only if this information is necessary for their clientele.
—**Natalie Kupferberg**

47.   **Clinical Practice Guidelines Directory.** 2000 ed. Chicago, American Medical Association, 2000. 332p. $179.95pa. ISBN 1-57947-008-4.

The American Medical Association (AMA), in conjunction with medical societies and the federal government, promotes the development and implementation of clinical practice guidelines. These guidelines are strategies for patient management and provide assistance to patients, physicians, and other health care professionals in clinical decision making. The AMA recommends their use as an aid to, not a substitute for, professional judgment in addressing patient needs.

This new edition lists approximately 2,000 clinical practice guidelines developed by almost 90 physician organizations and other groups and is arranged by subject, sponsoring organization, and title. Three additional sections include guidelines currently in development, recently replaced guidelines, and recently withdrawn guidelines. A final section lists the directory information of the sponsoring organizations. The appendix offers information on an application for the Clinical Practice Guideline Recognition Program and criteria for developing practice guidelines. Each practice guideline includes the source of information (i.e., bibliographic citation) and the references cited. Ordering information and Internet availability is also indicated.

This information is intended for the medical professional and as such will be useful in hospitals and medical center libraries. The primary user is the individual physician or group practice.
—**Vicki J. Killion**

48.   **The Complete Directory for People with Chronic Illness, 2001/02.** 5th ed. Lakeville, Conn., Grey House Publishing, 2001. 1137p. index. $190.00; $165.00pa. ISBN 1-891482-64-5; 1-891482-63-7pa.

The 5th edition of *The Complete Directory for People with Chronic Illness* is the most comprehensive edition to date. It includes more entries than the previous edition as well as four new chapters on carpal tunnel syndrome, Gulf War syndrome, Raynaud's disease, and sleep disorders—bringing the total number of the most prevalent chronic illnesses covered to 84. The directory provides reliable descriptive listings of resources for each illness, including Agent Orange related injuries, diabetes, heart disease, Lyme disease, stroke, and substance abuse, among others. The listings include brief descriptions of the condition and annotations of national and state associations and organizations, libraries and resource centers, research centers, support groups and hotlines, books, newsletters, pamphlets, videotapes, and Websites. The last three chapters cover general resources, wish foundations, and death and bereavement. The information has been developed and edited with the assistance of physicians and medical personnel as well as with the associations specific to the illnesses.

The well-organized format facilitates ease of use. The illnesses are arranged in alphabetic order, and within each chapter the associations and organizations are listed alphabetically by state. An entry name index and a geographic index quickly direct users to relevant resources. This directory is an excellent resource for individuals and their families who are dealing with the stress and information requirements that accompany chronic illness. It is also an important reference work for librarians in public, academic, medical, and hospital libraries, as well as for health care and social workers.—**Rita Neri**

49.   **The Complete Directory for People with Rare Disorders, 1998/99: A Comprehensive Guide to Over 1,000 Rare Disorders....** Joy E. Bartnett, Debra L. Madden, and Robert P.

Tomaino, eds. Lakeville, Conn., Grey House Publishing, 1998. 726p. index. $190.00. ISBN 1-891482-03-3.

A rare disorder is defined as one that affects fewer than 200,000 people in the United States at any given time. Patients afflicted with such disorders, their families, and their caregivers often find that information about their condition may be as rare as the condition itself. *The Complete Directory for People with Rare Disorders* provides access to organizations with information about these diseases.

The directory has 4 sections. The 1st offers alphabetically arranged entries that describe 1,102 rare diseases. The entry has a brief explanation of the disorder, followed by a list of organizations that are concerned with it. These organizations have their own entries in the 3 sections that follow; the section on disease-specific organizations lists 445 groups, that on umbrella organizations covers 444 general groups, and that on government agencies contains entries for 74 federal agencies. A name and keyword index is the main access point. The organization entries are alphabetic within their sections. Each contains the name, address, telephone and fax numbers, e-mail address, and Website address if available. A description of the organization, list of officers, number of members and chapters, year established, and a list of publications are also provided.

The book has a number of quirks. Entries are numbered consecutively throughout rather than section by section. The index is the only cross-reference, and there are no user instructions. The only introductory material is the mission statement of the National Organization for Rare Disorders and a brief guide on how to lobby members of Congress. Some of the disorders listed here are far from rare: Chlamydia is the most common sexually transmitted infection, and the incidence of tuberculosis has risen sharply in recent years.

The 2d edition of *The Physicians Guide to Rare Diseases* (Dowden, 1995) has more information, costs less, is hardbound, and includes information on orphan drugs. *The Encyclopedia of Associations* and the directory links on MEDLINE provide listings for organizations. This directory is not a necessary purchase. [R: LJ, Dec 98, p. 86; BL, 1 Dec 98, pp. 687, 690]—**Barbara M. Bibel**

50.   Consumers' Guide to Health Plans. Washington, D.C., Center for the Study of Services, 2002. 96p. $14.95pa. ISBN 1-888124-11-3.

51.   Consumers' Guide to Hospitals. Washington, D.C., Center for the Study of Services, 2002. 359p. $19.95pa. ISBN 1-888124-12-1.

These guides are full of consumer information. In these days of ever-rising health care costs, it is important to look for the best bargain possible. The information in these guides was collected by the Center for the Study of Services, a nonprofit organization. The guides are very similar in organization and content. The *Consumers' Guide to Health Plans* covers topics such as choices for the consumer, types of plans, choosing a plan, finding a good doctor, and receiving good care. A major plus is the section that rates plans in each state, concentrating on key performance measures, ratings by doctors, and ratings by members. There is a coverage and features comparison worksheet. It explains terms related to coverage, delays, denials, service, and cost.

The *Consumers' Guide to Hospitals* gives information on 4,500 acute care hospitals nationwide. Some topics include what actually happened to patients, Joint Committee on Accreditation of Healthcare Organizations (JACHO) reviews, and key facts related to quality. Some interesting subjects listed are tips on how to make your hospital stay more pleasant, playing a role in your care, learning about your care, choosing a hospital and why, and keeping costs down. The appendixes include a copy of the Patient's Bill of Rights and a list of agencies to complain to in each state.

   This reviewer highly recommends both guides for all libraries with a reference section used by the general public. These guides are very affordable and contain valuable, up-to-date information. They are well organized and give clear explanations of terms. The use of bullets and different color headings are helpful. The only drawback is that the font is very small. The pages look crowded—more white space would help. The font size may be a problem to those patrons with a lower reading level. The guides are an excellent resource for patrons gathering information on these topics and will allow patients to take a more active part in their health care options.—**Sheila Bryant**

52.   **Consumers' Guide to Top Doctors.** Consumers' Checkbook Magazine, ed. Washington, D.C., Center for the Study of Services, 2002. 454p. $24.95pa. ISBN 1-888124-13-X.
   This very interesting and informative book furnishes a unique method of evaluating physicians in 35 medical specialty areas. The Center for the Study of Services surveyed 260,000 physicians and asked them to list two names in the designated specialty areas that they would " . . . consider most desirable for the care of a loved one." The resulting list is organized alphabetically by state subdivided into metropolitan areas, and then into medical specialties. The 50 largest metropolitan areas in the United States receive primary coverage. Individual entries list the physician's name, how many times each physician was mentioned, medical school and year of graduation, any certification, and a business address and telephone number. Sections in the front and rear of the book describe how to use the book, how the lists were put together, and other helpful information. There is also a disclaimer explaining why the number of mentions varies between specialties, and why some specialties were excluded. This book will be useful principally for public libraries in the covered metropolitan areas.—**Lynn M. McMain**

53.   **Detwiler's Directory of Health and Medical Resources 2001-2002.** 8th ed. Susan M. Detwiler, ed. Medford, N.J., Information Today, 2001. 787p. index. $195.00pa. ISBN 1-57387-119-2. ISSN 1058-2797.
   The 8th edition of *Detwiler's Directory of Health and Medical Resources* is an excellent resource to consult to contact various health science-related organizations. This edition is similar to the previous ones, yet it still has enough new information to make its purchase worthwhile. It contains a wealth of information that is well organized, concise, thorough, and easy to read. One of the most important entries in this edition is the electronic e-mail and Web page information. The directory notes how electronic information is subject to change on a regular basis. All the material included in this edition is received directly from the organization.
   The entries are arranged in alphabetic order. The introduction explains in detail how to use the directory. It is divided into four sections: "Alphabetical Profiles," "Service Index," "Subject Index," and "Acronym Index." Each section has a short explanation of what the section covers and how to use it. The profile section contains basic contact information, including, but not limited to, the organizations' name, address, telephone and fax numbers, e-mail, and URL, along with a description of the organization and services offered. The service index indicates how the organization makes its information available to the public. It is divided into more than 40 topics that may include research reports, statistics, mailing lists, databases, and videotapes, among others. The subject index provides more than 900 subjects, including private, public, and government resources. It lists the organizations' field of particular strength. Since many companies are known by their acronyms, and many organizations may have the same ones, this section helps take the guesswork out of knowing which organization is which.
   This directory is an excellent resource to consult when beginning a search for health and medical information. It does a good job of cross-referencing. Almost any level of reader can use this resource, from the layperson to the professional. This directory is recommended for any hospital

library, especially one with a consumer health section. Health science, academic, and public reference collections would also benefit from this resource.—**Sheila Bryant**

54.   **Directory of Health Care Group Purchasing Organizations, 2002.** 12th ed. Lakeville, Conn., Sedgwick Press/Grey House Publishing, 2002. 953p. index. $325.00pa. (print edition); $650.00 (online database); $750.00 (print edition and online database). ISBN 1-930956-09-6; 1-930956-08-8pa.

55.   **Directory of Health Care Group Purchasing Organizations. http://www. greyhouse.com.** [Website]. Millerton, N.Y., Grey House Publishing. $325.00pa. (print edition); $650.00 (online database); $750.00 (print edition and online database). Date reviewed: Dec 02.

The 12th edition of the *Directory of Health Care Group Purchasing Organizations*, published by Grey House Publishing, is a comprehensive resource that provides general information on over 20,000 institutions that make "volume health care purchases." Consisting of almost 1,000 pages, this directory guides the user through the vast maze of organizations listed. This edition has done a fine job of organizing the volume into a user friendly, easy-to-search resource. The directory includes a table of contents, user's guide, and user's key to assist patrons looking for information. The main body is arranged alphabetically by organization and provides profiles of companies. The majority of the companies are based in the United States but there are a few Canadian listings. The listings include a wide variety of information on the organizations, from general description and basic contact information (many with URLs and e-mail addresses) to a list of the company's member institutions. It contains more than twice the number of last year's listings.

To assist the user there are five indexes available: an index by expanded services, a geographic index, a key personnel index, an index of member institutions, and an index by organization type. This directory is also available online from the publisher. The information is searchable by organization name and state. It provides the same information as the print edition but with the convenience of an online format. Because this directory is geared to a specialized area and audience this reviewer would recommend it for large public, medical, or corporate libraries. Companies that sell health care supplies will find this text useful.—**Sheila Bryant**

56.   **Directory of Health Grants: A Reference Directory Pinpointing Health, Hospital....** Loxahatchee, Fla., Research Grant Guides, 1996. 148p. index. $59.50pa. ISBN 0-945078-12-9.

This premier edition covers 761 sources in the United States and Puerto Rico for grants in health, hospitals, and other related areas. The main body of the book is arranged alphabetically by state, with the entries/funding agency numbered consecutively. Each entry consists of the organization name; address; telephone number; subject areas of funding; ranges of grants; and any conditions for funding, such as a specific local. The appendixes treat the Foundation Center, an independent national service organization established by foundations, and the Grantmanship Center, a training organization for the nonprofit sector. The indexes are an alphabetic list by foundation name with its entry number and a subject index. There are 15 broad subject areas, which include AIDS, cancer, hospice, medical research, nursing services, and youth. The three articles cover the topics of grantseeking and proposal writing and how to do both better for more success in receiving funding. This directory is recommended for medical and hospital libraries.—**Betsy J. Kraus**

57.   **Directory of Hospital Personnel, 2002: U.S. Hospitals and Key Decision Makers.** 14th ed. Lakeville, Conn., Sedgwick Press/Grey House Publishing, 2002. 2477p. index. $275.00pa. (print edition); $545.00 (online database); $650.00 (print edition and online database). ISBN 1-930956-28-2; 1-930956-27-4pa.

58.   **Directory of Hospital Personnel. http://www.greyhouse.com.** [Website]. Millerton, N.Y., Grey House Publishing. $275.00pa. (print edition); $545.00 (online database); $650.00 (print edition and online database). Date reviewed: Dec 02.

The *Directory of Hospital Personnel 2002* is the 14th edition of a reference work that was previously published by Medical Economics/Thompson Healthcare. It includes an alphabetic listing of approximately 6,000 hospitals and more than 100,000 key hospital personnel. The hospital listings are arranged first by state, then alphabetically by city and name of hospital. The demographic information includes hospital type, number of employees, number of beds/rooms (licensed, actual, staffed, acute, operating, and so on), teaching and purchasing affiliations, satellite treatment centers, and insurance plans accepted. The names and titles of key personnel are arranged first by top administrators, then alphabetically by title and name of the most senior person. Three indexes are provided by hospital name, personnel, and bed size.

This directory is also available online from the publisher. It provides the same information as the print edition but with the convenience of online searching. The directory is searchable by hospital name and state.

The *Directory* is a valuable reference work. However, it should be noted that the listings are subject to change, despite the exhaustive research efforts of the editorial department to provide the most current information. The healthcare industry is in a constant state of flux due to downsizing, reorganization, and opportunities for personal advancement. It is recommended for corporations interested in marketing their products (corporate libraries), organizations interested in networking (including hospitals, medical centers, and nonprofit organizations), clinicians seeking patient referrals, and job-seekers (large public libraries).—**Rita Neri**

59.   **The Directory of Independent Ambulatory Care Centers, 2002/03.** Millerton, N.Y., Sedgwick Press/Grey House Publishing, 2002. 986p. index. $185.00pa. (print edition); $365.00 (online database); $450.00 (print edition and online database). ISBN 1-930956-90-8.

60.   **The Directory of Independent Ambulatory Care Centers. http://www.greyhouse.com**. [Website]. Millerton, N.Y., Grey House Publishing. $185.00pa. (print edition); $365.00 (online database); $450.00 (print edition and online database). Date reviewed: Dec 02.

This directory provides information about ambulatory health care centers not affiliated with a hospital or major medical center. It contains facilities' names and contact information, and briefly details the numbers of physicians, employees, operating rooms, and patient visits per year. The volume is organized by state, then separated into three categories—Ambulatory Centers, Ambulatory Surgical Centers, and Diagnostic Imaging Centers. Entries are arranged alphabetically within these categories. The scope is national, but some states are better represented than others. Alaska, for instance, only has six entries; a quick Web search revealed hundreds of ambulatory care centers.

A directory is only as good as the information contained within it. Telephone numbers and zip codes change and Websites become obsolete almost as soon as they appear. Nevertheless, a directory that promises accuracy of information may be promising more than it can deliver. Some misinformation found on page 164 includes a Web address that was the link to a well-known telephone directory's search page and a telephone number that was one-digit different than the telephone number provided by the center's Website. A few other Website verification attempts led to the infamous error message: "This Page Cannot Be Displayed."

This work is also available online through the publisher's Website. It provides the same information as the print edition and is searchable by center name and state.

The most probable users of this directory are marketing representatives. Therefore, it cannot be considered an essential item for a public or academic library, even if the information were more comprehensive and accurate. [R: LJ, 1 Feb 03, p. 74]—**Susan K. Setterlund**

61.   **Directory of Physicians in the United States.** 35th ed. Chicago, American Medical Association, 1996. 4v. $545.00/set. ISBN 0-89970-827-7.

62.   **Directory of Physicians in the United States.** 35th ed. [CD-ROM]. Chicago, American Medical Association, 1996. Minimum system requirements: IBM or compatible 386DX/33MHz (486DX/66MHz recommended). Double-speed CD-ROM drive. Windows 3.0. 4MB RAM (8MB recommended). 2MB hard disk space. 256-color monitor. $745.00/single user; $1,145.00/networks. ISBN 0-89970-830-7/single user; 0-89970-831-5/networks.

The 35th edition of this standard medical reference tool is produced by the American Medical Association (AMA) in both a 4-volume book and a CD-ROM format. Both formats present difficult-to-find information on more than 723,000 MDs and DOs who are AMA members, living in the United States, the Virgin Islands, Puerto Rico, some Pacific islands, or temporarily out of the United States as of May 1996. This information has been obtained directly from the practitioners and has been verified by material provided by medical schools, the American Board of Medical Specialists, and state licensing boards. The MDs listed include both members and nonmembers of the AMA.

In the traditional book format, volume 1 alphabetically lists all the names found in the other 3 volumes, giving city locations for each name. Volumes 2 through 4 are arranged geographically, by state and then by city. The biographical information for each individual contains, when available, the following items: home/business address, medical school attended and graduation date, board certification, year of licensure, type of specialty practice, and whether the practitioner has received the Physician's Recognition Award for continuing medical education. There are no listings for the doctors' telephone numbers, residency training, academic appointments, or hospital affiliations. This additional information can be found in *The Official ABMS Directory of Board Certified Medical Specialists* (see ARBA 96, entry 1704). However, that reference work only covers 487,306 practitioners, thus making the current work by far the most comprehensive for basic information about U.S. physicians.

The CD-ROM format, although quite expensive and lacking sufficient instructions for the computer challenged, does provide worthwhile additional search capacities. This format allows patrons to formulate a search strategy combining any or all of the following criteria: name, city, state, region, primary specialty, and type of physician. The search feature is the major reason to purchase this expensive software. By double-clicking on the physician's name, the system presents the same information about this individual as appears in the book format.

All academic, large public, and health-related libraries must have this key reference tool. The cost for the CD-ROM format may require many libraries to purchase only the print version. —**Jonathon Erlen**

63.   **Encyclopedia of Medical Organizations and Agencies: A Subject Guide to Organizations, Foundations, Federal and State Governmental Agencies ….** 11th ed. Jaime E. Noce, ed. Farmington Hills, Mich., Gale, 2001. 1630p. index. $285.00. ISBN 0-7876-3414-X. ISSN 0743-4510.

The *Encyclopedia of Medical Organizations and Agencies* provides contact information and a brief description on a variety of organizations, including U.S. federal and state agencies; foundations and other funding entities; research centers; medical and allied health schools; and national, international, state, and regional organizations. More than 18,500 organizations related to clinical medicine, the biomedical sciences, and the technological and socioeconomic aspects of health care are included. The entries are arranged under 69 primary topical headings (e.g., aging, death and dying, hematology and oncology) and are further subdivided by type of organization (e.g., federal government agencies, foundations and other funding organizations). There is a brief subject cross index that alphabetically lists the primary topical headings and includes *see* and *see also* references for synonyms, related terms, and more specific subjects that are not reflected by the primary headings. An alphabetic name and keyword index is also included at the end of the volume.

Typical entries include contact information plus additional information dependent on the type of organization. For example, foundations and other funding organizations may include the founding date, priorities, types of recipients, and geographic distribution. Organization entries may include the founding date, number of members, number of national and regional groups, description of purpose, publications, and previous names for the organization. While not comprehensive, especially in the international sphere (note the absence of Medicines Sans Frontieres, an organization with activities in more than 80 countries that won a 1999 Nobel Peace Prize), this work continues to be a very valuable reference source for all large reference collections, both public and academic.—**Arlene McFarlin Weismantel**

64. Gibbs, Tyson, comp. **A Guide to Ethnic Health Collections in the United States.** Westport, Conn., Greenwood Press, 1996. 139p. index. (Bibliographies and Indexes in Medical Studies, no.13). $49.95. ISBN 0-313-29740-1.

Archival repositories dealing with health care for U.S. minorities are described in varying detail in this guidebook. Organized by state jurisdiction, information is provided about the scope and contents of collections that have housed, for the most part, materials for African Americans, Native Americans, Asians, and Hispanics. Information for this guide was gleaned from respondents to a 4-page questionnaire mailed to nearly 400 institutions.

Although the index provides some access to collections according to ethnic group, the cross-references are not always dependable. Furthermore, the lack of reported resources in states such as Illinois, Wisconsin, and Minnesota suggests that a more vigorous investigative effort would have been appreciated. The uneven style and the hasty approach do not inspire scholarly confidence. This guide is not recommended.—**Mary Hemmings**

65. **Health & Medicine on the Internet.** James B. Davis, ed. Los Angeles, Calif., Health Information Press, 1997. 610p. illus. index. $19.95pa. ISBN 1-885987-03-X.

One of the benefits of the Internet is supposed to be the decrease in the need for bulky, inflexible printed sources. Now we are seeing a new wave of books on how to use the Internet. However, given the limitations of Web browsers, there may be a need, at least temporarily, for such guidebooks. This is a particularly nice one; it is both comprehensive and easy for the layperson to use. It lists Websites in the areas of health and medicine that are of interest to health consumers. There are 69 sections, which cover broad topics such as "Fitness," "Diabetes," and "Infectious Diseases." Within each topic are subtopics, including "Organizations," "Treatment," or specific conditions or aspects of conditions. Under each of these subtopics are several Websites, many with annotations giving a description of their contents and who maintains the Website. For instance, for the subtopic "Sports Medicine," eight sites are listed. Putting these terms into AOL Netfind and Netscape yielded hits in the millions. Both browsers had ways to narrow down the focus, but it took quite a while, and none of the Websites listed in this book were easily pulled up. Five of the sites listed under "Sports Medicine" were excellent sources on the topic, giving self-diagnosis help, advice on treatment, and help in finding sports medicine professionals. However, three of the sources could not be found, either because they were temporarily down or are no longer available. That, of course, is the problem with Internet directories—any printed source is instantly out of date. Still, as a starting point this book is a great help in providing access to one of the most useful areas of cyberspace, particularly because the publishers plan on putting out yearly editions. Now if they would only put it online.—**Carol L. Noll**

66. **HMO-PPO Directory, 2003: Detailed Profiles of U.S. Managed Healthcare Organizations & Key Decision Makers.** 15th ed. Millerton, N.Y., Sedgwick Press/Grey House Publishing, 2002. 578p. index. $250.00 (print edition); $495.00 (online database); $600.00 (print and online editions). ISBN 1-930956-91-6.

67. **HMO/PPO Directory. http://www.greyhouse.com.** [Website]. Millerton, N.Y., Grey House Publishing. $250.00 (print edition); $495.00 (online database); $600.00 (print and online editions). Date reviewed: Dec 02.

Now in its 15th edition, the *HMO/PPO Directory* is still the most thorough reference tool for information pertaining to managed health care organizations and personnel throughout the United States. This one volume contains profiles of more than 450 Health Maintenance Organizations (HMOs), 445 preferred providers (PPOs), as well as information on 250 miscellaneous health care constituencies. Organized and arranged alphabetically within state chapters, each listing provides a synoptic overview of each HMO and PPO. As an added bonus, the directory also provides the names, titles, telephone numbers, and e-mail addresses to nearly 13,000 health care administrators and key decision makers within the industry. Specifically provided in each entry is such data as the type of coverage and payment plans of the health care provider. Financial history, hospital affiliations, and the number of primary care and specialty physicians are easily found in each provider profile. The online edition provides the same information as the print edition but with the convenience of having the information at your fingertips. The site is searchable by health plan name and state. Accreditation status, peer review data, for-profit status, and information concerning the federal qualifications of these care providers makes the *HMO/PPO Directory* a must for both public and academic libraries seeking a one-stop-shopping directory for valuable data about the health care industry.—**Patrick Hall**

68. Janoulis, Brenda H., and Jason F. Janoulis. **State Medical Licensure Guidelines 1998: Information Manual for MD and DO Physicians in the United States of America.** Atlanta, Ga., St. Barthelemy Press, 1998. 78p. $175.00 spiralbound. ISBN 1-887617-59-0.

This directory, compiled from individual states' applications, rules, and instructions, is intended to provide a single source for finding how states' regulations for licensure differ and what requirements must be met for each. A single-page summary is provided for each state, with a list of criteria and a column for that state's requirements in that area. Examples include years of postgraduate training required, acceptable exams, documentation required, and fees. Some criteria are not included for all states. No explanation is provided for what the various criteria mean (e.g., "Copy of CV required?") . Perhaps it is assumed correctly that most applicants would know the meaning of these terms, but there might be exceptions, especially among foreign medical graduates. Assorted tables at the book's beginning may help, such as a list of abbreviations and their meanings, lists of relevant accrediting and testing organizations with their addresses, and an explanation of some examinations. A tentative test schedule for 1998 and 1999 is provided, although without locations; there is also a table of licensure processing time guidelines by state. Because licensing procedures are subject to change, a prospective applicant should verify current regulations when he or she writes for applications. This book should be most useful to those considering where to apply and what requirements will be needed. This work provides information not available elsewhere in one place and is therefore recommended for libraries serving health services professions and large public libraries.—**Marit S. Taylor**

69.   **Major Health Care Policies: 50 State Profiles, 1998.** 7th ed. By Health Policy Tracking Service. Washington, D.C., Health Policy Tracking Service, 1999. 403p. maps. $165.00pa. ISBN 1-55516-796-9.

Aided by a small army of reporters and contacts in state agencies and legislatures, Health Policy Tracking Service (HPTS) compiles data on the status of health-related legislation. This volume is a summary of 1,500 passed and pending legislative efforts in 1998 organized by state.

Each entry begins with two pages of the state's history and recent efforts in health care legislation. Blocked off for easy reading are 13 legislative categories, which include insurance, Medicaid, Children's Health Insurance Program, managed care, patient records, facilities, regulation of physician practice, prescriptive authority, and pharmaceuticals. Programs for the indigent, uninsured, and students are also discussed. Explanations are appropriate, short, and well written.

A 60-page overview puts the state initiatives in perspective. HPTS documents the growing backlash against managed care as well as the increase in state-mandated insurance benefits. Each of the book's 133 major categories is displayed visually in 8 pages of maps and charts. Comparisons between individual states and the country as a whole are easily accomplished and informative. There are nine pages of definitions and abbreviations that round out the overview. HPTS does a nice job of informing in an area where it is easy to become confused. This volume is highly recommended for university libraries.—**Pete Prunkl**

70.   **Medical and Health Information Directory.** 13th ed. Jaime E. Noce and Lynn M. Pearce, eds. Farmington Hills, Mich., Gale, 2001. 3v. index. $650.00/set. ISBN 0-7876-3479-4. ISSN 0749-9973.

A comprehensive source of contact and descriptive information on a vast array of medical and health-related organizations, agencies, and institutions, this three-volume set has always been a key reference in medical libraries and larger public and academic libraries. The format has remained consistent through the 13 editions, with volume 1 directing users to a wide variety of organizations, including: national, international, state, and regional organizations; pharmaceutical companies; consultants; federal agencies; and medical schools. Volume 2 profiles nearly 12,000 domestic and foreign publications, libraries, and other health-related information resources. Volume 3 is a compilation of programs that provide treatment or information on a wide range of medical conditions and issues. Each volume includes a consolidated alphabetic name and keyword index. Descriptive listings within each volume give the usual directory and contact information. Entries for organizations include brief descriptions, former or alternate names, founding date, number of members, purpose, and publications.

Despite the availability of much of this information on the Web, this work still provides a convenient, one-stop source of health-related information organized for quick access. Librarians at large medical and hospital libraries will want this resource on their shelves.—**Vicki J. Killion**

71.   Miner, Lynn E. **Directory of Biomedical and Health Care Grants 1999.** 13th ed. Phoenix, Ariz., Oryx Press, 1998. 1998. index. $84.50pa. ISBN 1-57356-096-0. ISSN 0883-5330.

Now in its 13th edition, this directory continues to be an invaluable guide for biomedical and health services researchers. This is as close to one-stop shopping as the grant-hungry researcher is likely to get. The volume provides concise descriptions of 3,800 health-related grant programs offered by government, foundations, corporations, and other organizations. Each entry lists the purpose of the grant program, application procedures, sponsor information, contacts, application requirements and restrictions, level of grant awards, and a brief description of a recent award. The directory is organized around four interconnected indexes: subject matter, sponsoring organizations, grants by program type, and geographic areas. The subject matter index is extensive and provides good cross-referencing. In addition to individual program entries, the volume provides a helpful guide to proposal planning and writing and a list of sponsors' Websites. Users familiar with previous editions of this work will find the list of new sponsoring organizations to be beneficial. This work remains an essential reference for health science libraries.—**Bruce Stuart**

72.   **The National Directory of Integrated Healthcare Delivery Systems.** 2d ed. Allenwood, N.J., Managed Care Information Center, 1999. 557p. index. $175.00pa. ISBN 1-882364-31-7.

This directory provides information for a number of health care delivery systems and is aimed at managed care executives and other health care professionals. A clear and concise introduction explains the contents of the directory and the methodology. It also includes the definition of an integrated health care delivery system. The user's guide assists the reader in finding the necessary information easily. The directory is divided into four major sections. The first section is a list of network profiles by state that provides basic information about the networks, including their organizational contact information, statistics, enrollment demographics, service area, mission statement, and system affiliations. There is also a comments section. The second section explains practical approaches to health care delivery success. It includes an executive report on the systems and uses a lot of graphs and tables to help explain the findings. The third and fourth sections are listings of health care associations and resources in alphabetic order.

The directory is well cross-referenced with three indexes. The first index lists the delivery systems in alphabetic order by name. The second lists the key executive personnel in the systems, while the third lists the systems' affiliated hospitals and health care facilities by name. This edition does contain a few drawbacks. Not all of the statistical information in the network profiles is available for each system and advertisements for other products from the publisher are interspersed, distracting from the contents. Overall this directory is informative, well organized, and easy to read. Although this text may only be useful to select groups of users, it would be a welcome, but not necessary, addition to the reference department of a large public, academic, or special library. —**Sheila Bryant**

73.   **The National Directory of Managed Care Organizations.** 2d ed. Allenwood, N.J., Managed Care Information Center, 1998. 863p. index. $293.50pa. ISBN 1-882364-28-7.

This directory provides detailed profiles on health maintenance organization (HMOs), preferred provider organizations (PPOs), specialty HMOs and PPOs, point of service plans (POSs), exclusive provider organizations (EPOs), peer review organizations (PROs), third party administrators (TPAs), utilization review organizations (UROs), pharmacy benefit management companies (PBMs), pharmacy networks (PNs), and provider sponsored organizations (PSOs). The database from which the directory is printed contains more than 1,800 managed care organizations, 120 pharmacy benefit management companies, and 28 PSOs operating under the Medicare+Choice program. Data were collected from the organization's administrative office, news releases, government agency inquiries, Internet searches, annual reports, industry news services and conferences, and interviews with national trade associations.

Profiles are organized alphabetically by company name within the state of origin. An alphabetic index for each type of organization is also available. An entry can contain such information as directory information, key personnel, company profile, plan statistics, enrollment demographics, coverage type, and plan benefits. Many of the entries are not complete and lack data in several categories. The information is also available on diskette (at an additional cost), providing users with the capability of customizing reports.

This directory will have a limited market. Business libraries may want to include it in the reference collection, although the major users of this information would appear to be individuals or corporations involved in managed care.—**Vicki J. Killion**

74. **The National Directory of Physician Organizations.** 2d ed. Allenwood, N.J., Managed Care Information Center, 2000. 1092p. index. $345.00pa. ISBN 1-882364-44-9.

This text provides an organized and comprehensive list of physician organizations. The contents are well organized, which makes the book user-friendly. The opening pages are dedicated to the introduction, user's guide, and advertisers' index. The six sections, which are comprehensive and well identified, include the following: "Physician Organizations Profiles," "Physician Practice Management Companies," "Management Service Organizations," "IPA Model HMOs," "Directory of Healthcare Associations," and "Directory of Healthcare Resources." The indexes include physicians' organizations, independent practice associations, physician hospital organizations, miscellaneous physician organizations, physician practice management companies, management service organizations, personnel, and affiliated/participating hospitals.

This text is a valuable resource for individuals and corporations that will benefit from a comprehensive listing of physician organizations. Contact information, provider type, and company profile are examples of the information available through this directory. This same directory is shown to be available on diskette.—**Paul M. Murphy III**

75. **National Guide to Funding in Health.** 5th ed. Elizabeth H. Rich, ed. New York, Foundation Center, 1997. 1195p. index. $150.00pa. ISBN 0-87954-710-3.

More than 4,000 foundation, corporate, or charitable entities fill the directory section of this subject-specific guide to grants. Interest, stated or demonstrated, in health programs or activities qualified international, national, or regional grant-makers for inclusion. Some may consider a narrow field of health considerations, whereas others cover a broader spectrum. Users will benefit from the delineation of interests in the entries.

Entries are arranged alphabetically by grant-maker name under geographic location. In addition to personnel and contact information, grant-maker notations include purpose and activities, fields of interest, type of support, and limitations on giving. In some entries, specific grants are noted. A new category cites any international interests of the grant-maker.

Of special interest is the refining and expansion of the grants classification system (GCS) used by the foundation. The resulting greater level of specificity produces more entry terms for identifying grant possibilities. This access expansion is reflected in the indexes to types of support, to foundation and corporate giving programs by subject, and to grants by subject.

The Foundation Center wisely provides basic information in each of its guides: how to use the volume, a glossary of terms, information about the Foundation Center, and a bibliography of pertinent journal articles and books. Users will welcome not having to search other locations for these helpful tips. Editing errors, uncharacteristic of Foundation Center publications, appear in this edition. An introductory page heading indicates that the volume covers library and information services rather than health. In addition, the heading for the state of Maryland is missing, so Maryland entries tail the Maine entries, and the running heads on Maryland pages continue to say Maine. No Maryland information, however, is omitted or incorrect. The center quickly distributed corrected pages. The errors detract little from this health funding guide's usefulness to hospital personnel, students, researchers, social workers, doctors, and care center staffs.—**Eleanor Ferrall**

76. **National Health Directory 2000.** Lynn Antosz Fantle, ed. Gaithersburg, Md., Aspen, 2000. 366p. $99.00pa. ISBN 0-8342-1865-8.

The *National Health Directory* gives detailed contact information for health-related personnel in federal, state, and local governments. It lists specific program officers in federal agencies; regional offices of federal agencies; key legislative aids for congressional committees dealing with health policy; health officials of states, counties, and major cities; and many other government officials necessary for networking, emergency management, and political action. Health issue lobbyists or political activists will find this directory an indispensable tool. Many other directories would be required to gather the information presented in this one volume. This directory should be purchased annually to keep up with frequent changes in congressional staffs and appointed officials.

The directory is arranged by chapter, starting with federal information and ending with state and local health department contact information. The directory includes contacts for Congress, federal health agencies (including regional offices), state health offices and officials, county offices and officials, and health officials in major cities. Entries include name, title, address, and phone number. E-mail addresses or agency URLs are included in some directory entries. Maps and organizational charts aid the directory user. No index is provided, although an index would have been helpful in locating specific committee, agency, or state pages more quickly.—**Lynne M. Fox**

77. Randolph, Lillian. **Physician Characteristics and Distribution in the US.** 1997-98 ed. Chicago, American Medical Association, 1997. 356p. index. $125.95pa. ISBN 0-89970-893-5. ISSN 0731-0315.

Since 1906, the Physician Masterfile has been maintained by the American Medical Association as the most comprehensive source of information about doctors of medicine in the United States. Most of this is submitted by the doctors themselves via questionnaires. Analysis of data from this file plus some census and other material became the basis of *Physician Characteristics and Distribution in the US*, published since 1963. The current edition of this extensive statistical compilation, with tables and summaries, is arranged under the following main sections of physician data: trends, characteristics, detailed descriptions, and a new section focusing on primary specialties in which physicians practice. A few new tables have been added in addition to general updating. No personal identification is given.

Medical schools and societies, specialty boards, government agencies, and other groups involved in planning and policy-making concerned with physician supply and demand or doing research on the many healthcare issues (involving doctors) so important today will find this authoritative resource useful. Everything from the counties in Alaska with no doctors, to the age and gender of pediatricians and where they practice, to the percentage of international medical graduates in internal medicine is here somewhere. The resource claims that there are now 737,764 MDs or 278 per 100,000 population, with more than 81 percent in patient care. It is an excellent reference.—**Harriette M. Cluxton**

78. Smallwood, Carol, comp. **Free or Low Cost Health Information: Sources for Printed Materials on 512 Topics.** Jefferson, N.C., McFarland, 1998. 332p. index. $39.50pa. ISBN 0-7864-0309-8.

Pamphlets are a free or inexpensive source of basic health information. Librarians in need of items for vertical files and teachers or community organizations who need to distribute educational material rely on them. Finding an appropriate source of current, accurate information is sometimes difficult. *Free or Low Cost Health Information*, compiled by a librarian, provides a list of sources for printed material on 512 health and safety topics.

The book is organized alphabetically by subject. Within each subject, the organizations are listed alphabetically by name. Each entry includes the name, address, and telephone and fax number.

A description of the organization and the types of publications that it produces and their prices follows. Information is available on a wide range of topics—adolescent health, ethics, health careers, school safety, and Tourette's syndrome are examples. The sources include government agencies (National Health Information Center), independent agencies (National Safety Council), trade and professional organizations (American Dental Association), and nonprofit organizations (National Organization for Rare Disorders). A few commercial publishers who provide low-cost materials or quantity discounts are also included. There is a fair amount of repetition among the source listings because organizations publish material on many topics. A detailed table of contents and a subject and source index make it easy to locate specific material. *Free or Low Cost Health Information* is a source that public and school librarians, teachers, and health educators will appreciate. [R: LJ, 1 Sept 98, p. 170; BL, 1 Oct 98, pp. 362-363; Choice, Dec 98, p. 668]—**Barbara M. Bibel**

79.   **Tobacco and Health Network Directory 1996.** 4th ed. Ottawa, National Clearinghouse on Tobacco & Health, 1996. 1v (unpaged). index. $20.00 looseleaf (U.S.). ISBN 1-896025-12-9.

  Tobacco-related health issues are major concerns for health professionals, policy-makers, and the general public. The intent of this looseleaf 4th edition reference work, created by the Canadian Council on Smoking and Health, is "to provide a resource which facilitates communication, collaboration, and cooperative action amongst organizations and individuals involved in the promotion of a tobacco-free Canada" (p. v). However, the information in this brief guide will also prove useful to the broader audience of antitobacco advocates and scholars.

  The nonannotated listings are divided into six color-coded sections, followed by a comprehensive index of individuals mentioned in the preceding categories. The first three segments cover key personnel of the National Strategy to Reduce Tobacco Use, the tobacco-related offices of Canada's federal government, and the national nongovernmental organizations concerned with health and welfare. The largest section presents the health-related governmental infrastructure for each Canadian province, as well as major health associations (e.g., cancer and lung societies). The fifth category presents a useful survey of international contacts involved in the antitobacco crusade, from Albania to Zambia. This reference tool will be helpful for any patron seeking material on the worldwide antitobacco movement, especially for those focusing on Canadian activities in this area.—**Jonathon Erlen**

HANDBOOKS AND YEARBOOKS

80.   **Adolescent Health Sourcebook.** Chad T. Kimball, ed. Detroit, Omnigraphics, 2002. 658p. illus. index. (Health Reference Series). $78.00. ISBN 0-7808-0248-9.

  A new addition to Omnigraphics' Health Reference Series, this volume presents holistic coverage of adolescent health issues ranging from physical, sexual, and emotional health to social concerns such as safety, education, violence, and disasters. Like others in the popular series of about 100 subject volumes, it is written in clear, nontechnical language aimed at general readers; here, especially, parents and caregivers of teenagers. The material is up-to-date, comprehensive, and mainstream, making it a convenient first-step resource for consumers wanting basic understanding (not in-depth knowledge) of health care issues facing today's youth.

  The book is arranged in 7 parts and contains 93 articles and excerpts originally published by government agencies, professional medical associations, and other nonprofit groups. Chad T. Kimball, editor of several other books in the series, selected the documents. The parts are: "Emotional and Mental Health Issues Affecting Adolescents," which discusses normal development as well as specific disorders; "Physical Health Issues Affecting Adolescents," covering common diseases and health risks like loud music, tattooing, and tanning; "Adolescent Sexual Health"; "Drug

Abuse in Adolescents"; "Social Issues and Other Parenting Concerns Affecting Adolescent Health and Safety," including driving, gangs, and the Internet; "Adolescent Education," from school failure to preparing for college; and "Additional Help and Information." The latter comprises a glossary as well as contact information for agencies, organizations, Websites, and publications. A list of references and sources for additional reading, all pertaining to topics discussed in the book, is also provided. The *Adolescent Health Sourcebook* is recommended for public libraries, community colleges, and other agencies serving health care consumers. [R: SLJ, Nov 02, p. 102]—**Madeleine Nash**

81.   Alford, Raye Lynn. **Genetics & Your Health: A Guide for the 21st Century Family.** Medford, N.J., Medford Press/Plexus Publishing, 1999. 267p. index. $29.95; $19.95pa. ISBN 0-9666748-2-0; 0-9666748-1-2pa.

The goal of this book is to explain genetics and its current and future applications to personal health in a language that is accessible to the average reader. The book is written by a highly qualified genetic scientist. Short chapters with illustrations discuss basic and more complex topics such as patterns of human inheritance and ethical, legal, and social implications. Individual chapters explain cloning and the Human Genome Project, and a well-balanced discussion of the promises and pitfalls of gene therapy is also included.

For the reader seeking specific disease information or professional help, the various genetic professionals are clearly explained. A directory of organizations and Internet sites, a chart of the most common genetic diseases, and a glossary are also included. A bibliographic listing of additional reading is probably at too advanced a level for the average person, but a listing of children's books on genetics is a unique addition.

Although written for the lay public, a high school or better reading level is required to understand the content. The book does make a contribution to the dissemination of rather complex health information and would be appropriate for public libraries or health libraries serving the public.—**Mary Ann Thompson**

82.   **Attention Deficit Disorder Sourcebook.** Dawn D. Matthews, ed. Detroit, Omnigraphics, 2002. 470p. index. (Health Reference Series). $78.00. ISBN 0-7808-0624-7.

One of the most useful titles in Omnigraphics' Health Reference Series, the *Attention Deficit Disorder Sourcebook* pulls together information from governmental and organizational sources, some of which cannot easily be located electronically. The book uses the abbreviation AD/HD (attention deficit/hyperactivity disorder) throughout. It should be noted that this book covers both childhood and adult AD/HD. It is divided into major sections covering diagnosis and treatment, help for parents and teachers, facts for specific populations (e.g., gifted children, teenagers, college students), and adults with AD/HD. Various chapters cover topics including well-known individuals with AD/HD (from http://schwablearning.org); resolving differences between teachers and parents (from an ERIC/EECE Newsletter); unproven treatments (from http://www.chadd.org); and the ramifications of the "no child left behind" educational plan (from the Website of the U.S. Department of Education). Chapters with information derived from books and articles include "Substance Abusers and AD/HD"; "Vision Therapy: Is it an Effective Treatment for AD/HD?"; and "Adult AD/HD and Social Skills." The section titled "Medication Management of Children and Adults with AD/HD" is quite comprehensive and also includes information about unproven and alternative treatments. There is a glossary, a list of support groups with full contact information, hotlines, a list of AD/HD Websites, an annotated bibliography, and an index. This book is recommended for all school libraries and the reference or consumer health sections of public libraries.—**Martha E. Stone**

83. **Biostatistics in Clinical Trials.** Carol K. Redmond and Theodore Colton, eds. New York, John Wiley, 2001. 501p. index. (The Wiley Reference Series in Biostatistics). $336.50. ISBN 0-471-82211-6.

Currently in medical research there is an increased emphasis on clinical trial experimental design. Research must meet this gold standard of research methodology to be an accepted addition to the body of medical knowledge and practice. *Biostatistics in Clinical Trials* provides an encyclopedic reference to information on the design and conduct of clinical trials. Novice to experienced researchers can benefit from the clear, well-referenced, signed articles. Additional research would be needed to establish the expertise of contributors, since the list provided in the volume lacks detail. Authors address specific aspects of clinical trials and also provide historical overviews of the development of clinical trial research. Articles include topics such as randomization, trial phases, ethics, drug approval and regulation, and evidence based medicine-related concepts. A minor shortcoming is found in the article on software, which fails to include bibliographic management software, an essential tool for large trials. The articles are arranged alphabetically by topic and include cross-references to related topics. A list of acronyms and abbreviations is much appreciated, since the field is overburdened with shorthand references. Black-and-white tables and graphs are well done, and a spot check of formulas revealed no obvious errors. A detailed index completes the book.

There have been a few introductory texts addressing the methodology of clinical trials in recent years, but these do not provide the kind of quick reference information compiled in *Biostatistics in Clinical Trials*. This work will be welcome at the researcher's workstation or in the library reference collection.—**Lynne M. Fox**

84. **Caregiving Sourcebook.** Joyce Brennfleck Shannon, ed. Detroit, Omnigraphics, 2001. 601p. index. (Health Reference Series). $78.00. ISBN 0-7808-0331-0.

"Caregiver" is a relatively new term for a role that used to be taken entirely for granted. There are an estimated 27 million individuals in the United States who care for ill or disabled friends or family members, many doing so at great cost to their own career, health, and personal lives. Perhaps attaching a name to this role is the first step in getting these people the help they need.

Like others in this series, this sourcebook is a compilation of government and nongovernment publications, artfully arranged for easy access to specific information. The first eight articles describe the role of caregivers in all their diverse manifestations, reassuring the caregiver that their situation is both common and of increasing importance in the nation's health care system. The rest of the 29 articles get into specifics. Issues such as stress; transportation needs; home safety; help with care for patients with particular illnesses; and legal, insurance, and financial information are covered. The list of chapters on individual conditions shows the extent of the caregiver's world: "Alzheimer's," "Brain Injury," "Cancer," "Cerebral Palsy," "Multiple Sclerosis," "Parkinson's," and "Physical Disabilities."

As with most of the Omnigraphics sourcebooks, much of the valuable information is in the appendixes at the end of the volume—several hundred government and nongovernment organizations are listed, along with addresses, telephone numbers, and the all-important Website addresses. These entries are arranged under topics, such as particular diseases, or under geographic headings for many state and regional agencies. One section that is especially valuable is a listing of sources for hard-to-find home health and safety equipment.—**Carol L. Noll**

85. **Code of Medical Ethics: Current Opinions with Annotations.** 1996-1997 ed. By the Council on Ethical and Judicial Affairs. Chicago, American Medical Association, 1996. 191p. index. $34.95pa. ISBN 0-89970-807-2.

Medical ethics is an area of fast-paced and complex change. As the book states, "[T]he AMA Principles of Medical Ethics and the Current Opinions of the Council on Ethical and Judicial Affairs have emerged as an important source of guidance for responsible professional medical behavior." The Code of Medical Ethics is only one component of the American Medical Association's Code of Ethics. The others include the Principles of Medical Ethics, Fundamental Elements of the Patient-Physician Relationship, and the Reports of the Council on Ethical and Judicial Affairs. As such, the code alone has limited use.

The code is divided into 9 major sections, including an introduction and opinions in various subissue areas, for example, social policy issues, interprofessional relations, fees and charges, and so forth. Each section in this text provides a position statement with annotated references to journals, court cases, and other appropriate information sources. These are indexed alphabetically, by case and by article title.

For general use, this book is limited because it must be placed in context with the other components of the Code of Ethics. One must also remember that this work is intended to be a statement of the American Medical Association's position, which is certainly important, but does not make for a general reference of broad-based ethical opinion or works. The work's primary value is for practicing physicians and libraries that serve physicians, medical schools, or teaching hospitals.
—**Luiz Alberto Cardoso**

86. **The Complete Family Guide to Healthy Living.** By Stephen Carroll. Tony Smith, ed. New York, Dorling Kindersley, 1995. 320p. illus. index. $24.95; $15.95pa. ISBN 0-7894-0114-2; 0-7894-0120-7pa.

This book is beautifully laid out and illustrated with both diagrams and photographs. It is organized into chapters that focus on function, not on specific anatomic or physiological systems. The emphasis is on health and fitness, not on disease. Diet, fitness, disease prevention, stress, and weight control are the focus of the major sections of the book. However, some chapters do address common diseases, such as cancer, back pain, and heart disease. First aid, injury prevention, and safety are also covered.

The many photographs enhance the presentation of the material in this book. The illustrations of the exercises recommended, the foods discussed, and the lifestyle suggested complement the text well. Diagrams of anatomy, graphs, and diagrams and photographs of medical procedures are accurate and informative. Additional photographs set the mood and add a dimension: A depressed woman, a man in pain, or a distressed child contrast dramatically with the relaxed and confident people portrayed when interventions are discussed.

The book focuses on things people can do without medical intervention to improve and maintain their health. Yet the guide does not ignore the need for appropriate medical advice, and it provides plenty of examples of occasions when one should seek medical help, such as prenatal care, injury rehabilitation, heart attack treatment, and cancer diagnosis and treatment. There is a pertinent and clear section devoted to genetic testing. This book is a useful guide for everyone. [R: SLJ, April 96, p. 168]—**Margretta Reed Seashore**

87. **Consumer Issues in Health Care Sourcebook.** Bellenir Karen, ed. Detroit, Omnigraphics, 1999. 618p. index. (Health Reference Series, v.35). $78.00. ISBN 0-7808-0221-7.

In this era of managed health care, it is critical that consumers keep themselves well informed about health issues that affect them. To meet the demand for more information, many books have been published to guide consumers in making good decisions about their health care. This sourcebook is another in the Health Reference Series published by Omnigraphics aimed at educating the layperson.

The book is arranged in seven broad categories covering the gamut of health care issues: health care fundamentals, physicians and hospitals, medications, cautions for health care consumers, managing common health risks in the home, caring for chronically or terminally ill patients and making end-of-life decisions, and a section on resources. Within each part, there are chapters that thoroughly cover the aspects within that section. For example, in the section on physicians and hospitals, there are chapters that describe the types of health care providers, how to check up on a doctor, how to talk to doctors, questions to ask prior to surgery, hospital hints, and a guide to mental health services. Most of the chapters contain sources of additional information. The indexing is excellent.

Among the many other books on this topic, *Health Care Choices for Today's Consumer: Guide to Quality and Cost* by Marc Miller (John Wiley, 1997) has similar coverage to this book. The layout and organization of the information in Miller's book is more pleasing to the eye than the volume at hand, and thus more readable. Aside from the difference in style, the information itself is essentially the same in both books. Both public and academic libraries will want to have a copy of either or both of these fine books in their collection for readers who are interested in self-education on health issues. [R: BL, 1 Dec 98, p. 698; RUSQ, Spring 99, p. 299] —**Elaine F. Jurries**

88.   **CQ Researcher** on Controversies in Medicine and Science. Washington, D.C., Congressional Quarterly, 2001. 247p. illus. index. $29.95. ISBN 1-56802-671-4.

This compilation explores cutting-edge health issues and diseases, health care delivery, and health care policy issues as well as the controversies surrounding them. Each chapter reads like an extensive thematic series in a quality newspaper. The chapters also resemble encyclopedic entries in that the reader is introduced to the topic, but stimulated to do further research in the select, but excellent, resources suggested at the end. Subjects discussed include Alzheimer's disease; obesity; childhood depression; asthma; vaccines; managed care; and health policy for embryo and genome research, global AIDS, and computer use in medicine. Reliable sources and topical experts are cited within the body of the chapters. Each chapter has consistent organization: a general introduction, controversial questions and a range of responses, historical background and chronology of the issue, the current and future status of the problem, and a one-page point/counter-point discussion written by experts in the area. Each chapter concludes with a quality, concise bibliography of popular and professional literature and a directory of recommended agencies or organizations. Helpful tables and graphs are interspersed. The book is written in a style that is accessible to high school students, the general public, and college students, and is a balanced, quality presentation of the issues addressed.—**Mary Ann Thompson**

89.   **Dun & Bradstreet/Gale Group Industry Handbook: Insurance and Health & Medical Services.** Jennifer Zielinski and Mary Alampi, eds. Farmington Hills, Mich., Gale, 2000. 660p. index. $135.00. ISBN 0-7876-3620-7. ISSN 1521-6640.

The *Dun & Bradstreet/Gale Group Industry Handbook: Insurance and Health & Medical Services* provides diverse information not usually compiled in other resources. A foreword introduces the general history and organization of each of the two industries. Each of the 10 chapters for the 2 industries begins with an overview of the chapter contents. In one chapter, industry statistics based on the 1992 Economic Census data are presented. These statistics include data on carriers, insurance categories, and health facilities. Another chapter tracks merger and acquisition activity from 1997 through 1999, by company, for each industry. Another chapter presents 1998 ranking data on numerous companies by sales or employment figures. Tables chart key ratios and norms by industry segments from 1994 through 1998 in another chapter. Additional value is provided in this handbook by including chapters with directories for each industry's companies, trade information resources, trade shows, consultants, and associations. SICs are still used to classify industries since much of the data presented in this volume were collected and classified under that system. A conversion table is presented as an appendix for the convenience of those now using NAICS.

Three indexes organize access to the data in the handbook: a master index, a geographic index, and a company index by SIC. Although this type of resource can become quickly dated, the information provided within the handbook would take hours to compile from other resources. Researchers would need to consult a variety of corporate and government data sources to acquire the same information. Prose portions of the handbook include shallow treatments of industry trends and current challenges in the industries, but provide a service by compiling information from many other resources such as almanacs, the media, and trade journals. This handbook provides a variety of valuable information in a convenient and organized format. [R: LJ, 1 April 2000, pp. 88-90] —**Lynne M. Fox**

90.   **Dun & Bradstreet/Gale Industry Reference Handbooks: Health and Medical Services.** Stacy A. McConnell and Linda D. Hall, eds. Farmington Hills, Mich., Gale, 1999. 1134p. index. $99.00pa. ISBN 0-7876-3003-9.

This specific handbook, one of a series of such handbooks published by Gale Research, provides detailed information in 10 chapters on several aspects of health care services. Five chapters cover companies, consultants, associations, trade information sources, and trade shows associated with the industry. Another three chapters discuss statistics and economic indicators regarding employment, finances, performance, rankings, and so on. Two more chapters provide an industry overview, covering recent history of the health care industry, current issues and concerns, mergers and acquisitions, and future trends. Information is gathered from a variety of well-known and respected resources, including Dun & Bradstreet and several Gale reference resources. A comprehensive master index contains entries organized by personal name, company or organization name, SIC industry name, and terms. This index is followed by a two-table appendix on converting SIC codes to the newer NAICS codes, and vice versa.

Listings include the name of the organization, description, and contact information (telephone and fax numbers, addresses, and e-mail and Web addresses). There is also specific information related to the type of organization such as events related to trade shows, geographical area served by a consultant, or publications distributed by an association. The industry statistics and indicators, arranged by SIC number, include industry financial norms and ratios (solvency, efficiency, and profitability) for the years 1995-1997; and number of establishments, employees, payroll, revenues, and type of ownership for the years 1987-1998. Some entries in the tables are empty due to the unavailability of data. There are also two tables ranking companies by sales and employment.

The information in this resource is useful to patients and consumers, medical professionals and health care providers, policy-makers, educators, vendors and suppliers, and researchers. It is recommended for business, medical, and health care libraries, as well as large public libraries. [R: Choice, Oct 99, pp. 308-310]—**Michael R. Leach**

91.   **Emergency Medical Services Sourcebook.** Jenni Lynn Colson, ed. Detroit, Omnigraphics, 2002. 472p. index. (Health Reference Series). $78.00. ISBN 0-7808-0420-1.

This recent addition to the Health Reference Series could easily be retitled "Everything You Wanted To Know About Emergencies and Emergency Care." Written primarily for the layperson, the book covers a comprehensive list of topics in an easy-to-read and easy-to-use format. The 60 chapters are reproduced from various reputable sources, including professional journals, texts, or Internet sites. The reader will find answers to such questions as when to use and when not to use the emergency department and the emergency medical system (EMS); how 911 and emergency rooms work and why a patient may have to wait for care; and what the legal and ethical rights surrounding this level of medical care are. Suggestions for preparing a home for a full range of emergencies or disasters, as well as how to prevent emergencies and injuries are included. Two multichapter sections discuss the unique aspects of emergency care for children and older persons. Although the book is directed toward the consumer, a few chapters are more appropriate for the health care professional or hospital administrator. The book concludes with a glossary of frequently used emergency terms and abbreviations and a resource directory of professional organizations and state EMS offices. This reference can provide the consumer with answers to most questions about emergency care in the United States, or it will direct them to a resource where the answer can be found.—**Mary Ann Thompson**

92.   Ferguson, Tom. **Health Online: How to Find Health Information, Support Groups, and Self-Help Communities in Cyberspace.** Reading, Mass., Addison-Wesley Publishing, 1996. 308p. index. $17.00pa. ISBN 0-201-40989-5.

The information age has created a large number of options for those seeking medical information and other forms of health assistance without relying on the traditional doctor visit. This volume, written by one of the United States' leading self-help proponents, is intended to introduce both the computer novice, as well as the computer expert, to the ever-expanding world of online self-help medical resources. Special attention is given to online self-help communities that can provide information and support for individuals suffering health crises, as the author claims that the old standbys of families, friends, and caring physicians no longer exist, in many cases, in the modern United States.

This reference guide is divided into three major parts. The first section, intended for beginning computer users, explains the ease of going online, the use of e-mail, and some of the basics of functioning online. The second segment presents in-depth information to help readers choose a commercial computer network for accessing online health resources (e.g., America Online, CompuServe, Prodigy). The last division lists and briefly describes some of the health-related Internet mailing lists, newsgroups, FAQ sites, computer bulletin boards, and Gopher and World Wide Web sites available to the public.

Libraries should be very cautious about acquiring this book. It is extremely anti-medical establishment in its orientation. The author fails to warn readers about the false information provided by some online health sites that could seriously mislead patrons. He also ignores the values that are the basis for the doctor/patient relationship. Libraries interested in providing reference tools discussing online health resources should purchase less biased reference works on this topic, such as *Dr. Tom Linden's Guide to Online Medicine* (see ARBA 96, entry 1709).—**Jonathon Erlen**

93.   **Health and Healthcare in the United States 1999: County and Metro Area Data.** Richard K. Thomas, ed. Lanham, Md., Bernan Associates, 1999. 437p. maps. $135.00pa. (with CD-ROM). ISBN 0-89059-188-1. ISSN 1526-1573.

Drawing from information from the National Center for Health Statistics, the Health Care Financing Administration, and the Bureau of the Census, this work represents a compilation of health and health care statistics. More than 80 statistical tables are represented for some 3,000 U.S. counties and 329 metropolitan areas. The statistical tables are arranged by state and county and by metropolitan area.

In the state and county data section and the metropolitan area data section, the statistical items are grouped under population characteristics, vital statistics, health care resources, and Medicare. Much information, such as number of physicians, dental offices, podiatry offices, Medicare statistics, population projections, births and deaths, and deaths caused by a wide variety of diseases or accidents, can be found. The year that reflects a particular type of statistic varies. For example, some statistics reflect 1998, whereas others reflect 1997, 1996, or 1995.

At the end of the work, maps for each of the states of the union can be found. The maps depict the county and metropolitan statistical areas that are listed within the tables. A CD-ROM is included that represents an electronic version of the printed publication. This resource is highly recommended for all medical, college, university, and large public libraries.—**George H. Bell**

94.   **Health & Medical Year Book 1997.** New York, Collier Newfield, 1997. 336p. illus. index. $33.90. ISBN 1-57161-119-3.

"Feature Articles" at the beginning of this yearbook are mostly by freelance writers in the style of the popular magazines to which they contribute. Subjects vary, but among the outstanding ones are "Learning to Mourn" and the true story "M.D. to Be." These essays reflect current health-related interests and are eminently readable. "Spotlight on Health" contains short discussions on more specific topics, often with practical tips on how to handle these health problems. Examples are "Heartburn and Beyond" and "How to Give Medicine to Children." Liberal use of sidebars and simple illustrations enliven this section.

The section on health and medical news is arranged alphabetically by broad subject and summarizes 1996-1997 news coverage of developments in health and medical care, such as genetic engineering, government policies and programs, and public health concerns. Newly approved drugs and devices and major sources for help and information are listed. Reviews of noteworthy new books of general health interest and brief notes on contributors complete the volume. The index covers 1997, 1996, and 1995 editions of the yearbook, which extends its usefulness as a reference in health science libraries. Its readability, coverage, and general attractiveness make this book a wonderful place for the health care consumer to browse and learn.—**Harriette M. Cluxton**

95.   **Health Care Almanac: Every Person's Guide to the Thoughtful and Practical Sides of Medicine.** 2d ed. Chicago, American Medical Association, 1998. 546p. index. $27.95pa. ISBN 0-89970-900-1.

The American Medical Association's *Health Care Almanac*, now in its 2d edition, contains a plethora of disparate but useful listings for both health consumers and professionals. One will find it a useful guide for finding an association address, checking the credential process for an allied health profession, locating a copy of the Hippocratic oath, finding a definition for a condition, checking a description for a treatment or therapy, or determining whether the *Journal of the American Medical Association* (JAMA) published a theme issue on a topic. All of these questions can be answered by this reasonably priced, informative resource. Articles reprinted from JAMA often form the basis of entries, providing advice for health professionals, especially physicians.

Most of this almanac is arranged alphabetically by topic and features a thorough index. Articles are brief, but typically include references to additional resources. When appropriate, Website addresses are included. Appendixes include history and organizational information about the American Medical Association. This valuable resource will be an asset in any library. It provides an essential starting point for general health reference questions.—**Lynne M. Fox**

96.   **Health Care Software Sourcebook 1997.** Lynn Antosz, ed. Gaithersville, Md., Aspen, 1997. 467p. index. $89.00pa. ISBN 0-8342-0904-7.

The *Health Care Software Sourcebook* is intended for the medical information systems manager. Although the book does not claim to be comprehensive, it provides thorough coverage of medical information systems related software. The editor is careful to include information about software that can be integrated with a World Wide Web user access system as well as older access technologies. Such details are included in the descriptions with each entry.

The structure of the book makes it easy to look up subjects by category. The information in each entry describes the purpose, hardware requirements, and other pertinent details about the software. In addition, there are vendor, application, and product name indexes available. Another nice feature is the vendor directory, which lists vendor contact information. This book is strongly recommended for anyone working with medical information systems.—**Diane Kovacs**

97.   **Health Care State Rankings 2000: Health Care in the 50 United States.** 8th ed. Kathleen O'Leary Morgan and Scott Morgan, eds. Lawrence, Kans., Morgan Quinto Press, 2000. 512p. index. $52.95pa. ISBN 0-7401-0001-7. ISSN 1065-1403.

Health Care State Rankings 2000 is a convenient compilation of health measures that allows users to compare states' performances. Chapters group tables by theme, including births and reproductive health, deaths, facilities, finance, disease incidence, providers, and physical fitness. Thumb index markings allow quick access to sections and a subject index provides direct access to tables. The health measures are expressed in rates, percentages, and whole numbers. Many tables provide a national total or rate for reference. Each table provides an alphabetic list by state and a ranking list. Most tables are created from 1998 data, but some tables related to health care expenditures are quite old and date from the early 1990s. Each table cites its source. Sources are diverse and statistics are culled from a wide variety of organizations. These sources include many government agencies, such as the National Center for Health Statistics or the Health Care Financing Administration, as well as nongovernmental groups, such as the National Association of Attorneys General, the American Cancer Society, and the American Medical Society. A source list is provided at the end of the volume.

The editors use 21 positive and negative health factors provided in tables included in the volume to calculate a "Healthiest State Chart." There is little narrative provided with this chart, so readers must draw their own conclusions as to why, for example, Colorado jumped from 24th place in 1999 to 12th place in 2000. Health measures included are selective, so that while the number of colon cancer deaths is ranked, use of colonoscopy and other tests for early diagnosis are not given. Statistics for racial or ethnic groups are limited to whites and blacks. States with high Native American, Hispanic, or Asian populations will not find tables addressing health measures for those groups. *Health Care State Rankings* is a useful resource for quick access to general health care data.—**Lynne M. Fox**

98.   **The Healthcare Industry Market Yearbook.** 2d ed. Allenwood, N.J., Managed Care Information Center, 1999. 717p. index. $195.00pa. ISBN 1-882364-29-5.

Like its predecessor, this yearbook is crammed with information, data, lists, anecdotes, projections, and evaluations of firms in the health care industry. But, unfortunately, as a reference tool it is not a useful resource. This 2d edition of *The Healthcare Industry Market Yearbook* covers the following topics in 717 pages: looking ahead in managed care, health care industry trends, succeeding in the managed care industry, quality outcomes and cost efficiency, IS/IT prevalence in the managed care industry, spotlight on the market, stock index, market partnerships, acquisitions, contracts awarded, consolidations, and 13 more highly detailed topics. The coverage is idiosyncratic and poorly organized. For example, 58 pages are devoted to some 350 acquisitions, followed two chapters later by a 15-page chapter on "consolidations" listing another 40 acquisitions. The 35 pages devoted to contracts lists 1 contract between a private firm and the Department of Defense, one of the largest purchasers of health care services in the United States. There is a chapter on market developments indexed by company name, which permits readers to find information in an otherwise helter-skelter presentation. However, data sources are not recorded and there is no way to determine either the veracity or completeness of the information recorded. The index was obviously created by a software program with no human oversight.—**Bruce Stuart**

99.   **Health Matters!** William M. Kane, ed. Danbury, Conn., Grolier, 2002. 8v. illus. index. $409.00/set. ISBN 0-7172-5575-1.

This eight-volume combination health encyclopedia and health class text is aimed at the middle school and high school audience. The language and reading level is fairly simple and will be easily comprehended by most students. Each of the eight volumes covers a different health-related topic, which include "Addiction"; "Sexuality and Pregnancy"; "Physical Activity"; "Weight and Eating Disorders"; "HIV, AIDS and STDs"; and "Diseases and Disabling Conditions."

Each volume starts off with a several page introduction titled "Healthy Living: Teen Choices and Actions," followed by a test for the readers to assess their own behavior relating to health issues. An alphabetic encyclopedia follows, with one to several paragraph entries on terminology, health statistics, and historical facts relating to the topic of the volume. There are numerous tables, illustrations, and cross-references to other volumes. Several appendixes to each volume relate the issue to teen life through stories of teens whose lives have been affected by health problems and question-and-answer essays on difficult topics and choices. The editor also includes glossaries and lists of hot lines, Internet sites, and organizations relating to each volume's topic.

Although this set is well written, well researched, and attractively presented, the mixture of factual information with persuasive essays and arguments may turn older, more sophisticated teens off. Teenagers have a very sensitive radar to adult preaching and may tend to doubt the factual nature of information if it is presented with a clearly stated point of view. This is always a danger when presenting such information to the young. The best teachers can present the facts and let them speak for themselves. The right balance between education and advocacy is difficult to achieve. In *Health Matters!* this balance may be satisfactory for the middle school audience but not necessarily for older readers.—**Carol L. Noll**

100. **Health on File.** 2d ed. New York, Facts on File, 2002. 1v. (various paging). illus. index. $185.00 looseleaf w/binder. ISBN 0-8160-4345-0.

Like other Facts on File offerings, this publication is a collection of looseleaf illustrated pages that can be reproduced for handouts, lecture illustrations, or student use in research papers. A reproduction certificate is included, giving the legal restrictions on use. There are 10 chapters, each covering a topic treated in the typical middle school or high school health course: "Mental Health," "Family and Social Health," "Growth and Development," "Food and Nutrition," "Personal Health Choices," "Substance Abuse," "Diseases and Disorders," "Consumer Health," "Accidents and Safety," and "Environmental Health." Each chapter contains 15 to 30, 1-page handouts, illustrated with charts and graphs, cartoons, diagrams, anatomical drawings, and just about any other visual aid readers can think of. All are black-and-white and are easily modified for use in lectures and tests. An appendix gives sources (usually government publications or scholarly journals) for many of the pages.

This edition is a revision of a 1995 edition. Information is updated to reflect new research, particularly in the areas of adolescent sexual behavior, sexually transmitted diseases, smoking, and alcohol abuse. Pages have been added on newly important topics, such as sports-related concussions, mad cow disease, and school violence. Although this publication will be most useful to health teachers, it would also come in handy in biology and physical education courses.—**Carol L. Noll**

101.   **Hutchinson Trends in Science: Medicine and Health Science.** Catherine Thompson, ed. Chicago, Fitzroy Dearborn, 2001. 275p. illus. index. $45.00. ISBN 1-57958-360-1.

This book is more than a presentation of highlights that have transformed health sciences during the twentieth century. In part 1, a well-written overview by Jon Turney from University College, London, shows the advances that have taken place in the approach to diagnosis, treatment, and prevention of diseases. Turney insightfully discusses the politics of medicine and medical treatment, and ends his essay by noting some ethical and physiological obstacles that must be faced in the future. Following this essay is a selective chronology of medical events from 1900 to 2000 and biographical sketches of physicians, biochemists, Noble Prize winners, and so on who were prominent in the history and development of medicine.

Part 2 contains a directory of selected international organizations and Websites, an eclectic bibliography of suggested readings, and a glossary that clearly and concisely defines terms in lay language. A useful appendix displays common medical abbreviations, acronyms, medical prefixes, suffixes, and other tidbits of information. Although not as ethnocentric in its scope as most books sold to a U.S. market (British people and events are well represented and British spelling predominates), one shortcoming of this work is that it overlooks contributions made anywhere other than the North American and European continents. [R: LJ, Jan 02, p. 84]—**Susan K. Setterlund**

102.   Inlander, Charles B., and Michael A. Donio. **Medicare Made Easy.** rev. ed. Allentown, Pa., People's Medical Society; distr., Chicago, Independent Publishers Group, 1997. 339p. index. $18.95pa. ISBN 1-882606-67-1.

The title of this book says it all. The guide helps the consumer to understand, access, and work through the conundrum that is Medicare. The authors take the reader step-by-step through Medicare eligibility, coverage (what it pays for and what it does not), the appeals process, rights of the insured, and supplemental insurance policies. Terms and concepts that may be misunderstood are printed in bold typeface and then defined in a glossary in the appendix. A particularly helpful component is the inclusion of samples of all the Medicare forms with accompanying explanations. An extensive appendix includes directories of individual state Medicare intermediaries, insurance offices, and peer review organizations, as well as durable power of attorney and living will forms and the patient's bill of rights.

The book is written in a simple, easy-to-read style and is printed in a large font, sensitive to the vision needs of the majority of the potential readers. Although written for the consumer, the book would be helpful for health care providers who also struggle with Medicare rules and regulations. This book is an absolute must for public libraries and for any library serving a population over the age of 65.—**Mary Ann Thompson**

103.   **International Handbook of Public Health.** Klaus Hurrelmann and Ulrich Laaser, eds. Westport, Conn., Greenwood Press, 1996. 474p. index. $99.50. ISBN 0-313-29500-X.

Despite its title, this work is not a handbook in the sense of a "concise, ready-reference book." It is not a reference book, but a monograph containing a section on public health theory, training, and research; country reports on Australia, Brazil, Canada, China, France, Germany, Israel, Italy, Japan, Korea, Malaysia, Mexico, the Philippines, Poland, Russia, South Africa, Tanzania, Thailand, the United Kingdom, and the United States; and a directory of public health organizations around the world. The preface states that the work is arranged to allow easy comparisons between countries, but this is not necessarily the case. When comparing the outlines of the chapters on France and Mexico, for example, the France chapter had sections the Mexico chapter did not and vice versa. In addition, although the individual chapters have statistical tables describing their own countries, the book does not contain any international tables that would allow comparisons of epidemiologic statistics, such as primary cause of death or infant mortality rates across different countries. In fact, much of the factual information is given in the body of the text instead of in tabulated form. This may be the reason for an error found in the country report of the Philippines, which gives the infant mortality rate for the country as 57.0 percent. This would mean that over half of the babies born there die as infants; the World Factbook online (www.odci.gov/cia/publications/nsolo/factbook/rp.htm#People) states the infant mortality rate for the Philippines in 1996 as 35.9 deaths per 1000 live births, or 3.59 percent. Finally, even though the chapters have different authors, this book has a remarkable tendency to contain words and phrases not common in the English language, or at least not in *Webster's Third New International Dictionary* (New York: Merriam-Webster, 1993) or the 2d edition of the *Oxford English Dictionary* (see ARBA 90, entry 1006). Some examples are "autoaggressive," "inhibitional," "bioecopsychosocial," "sociopedagogue," "intersectorality," "aerodigestive," "hospitalocentrism," "sensiblization," "microcensus," "supermortality," "sick funds," "macrospective," "microspective," and "antipromotion," among others.

The work, however, does have its good points, such as the honesty demonstrated by certain chapter authors when admitting that physicians in Poland do not attach importance to educating their patients about the prevention of diseases that are major causes of deaths, or that the resources for mental health care in Mexico serve only patients who have a serious disease, are in acute crisis, or are chronically ill. However, at $99.50, the price is expensive for a monograph.—**Lambrini Papangelis**

104.   **Issue Briefs: 1997 Annual Edition.** Washington, D.C., Health Policy Tracking Service, 1997. 1v. (unpaged). $450.00 spiralbound.

This reference documents major health legislation considered by various U.S. state legislative bodies during calendar year 1997. More than 30 issues are covered, ranging from access to various types of health care providers to physician-assisted suicide and uninsured children. Many of the policies deal with managed care. Each issue is addressed in a separate section that begins with background information, including a brief definition and legislative history. Key issues surrounding the topic and activity current to 1997 are included. Some of the listings include a section on the pros and cons of the particular issue. Each section then concludes with a table of each state's legislative activity on that policy, including bill numbers and status.

Considering the high cost of this reference, it is not overly user-friendly. It has no index, no page numbers, and no running heads, making it difficult to locate particular sections. The sections are compiled in alphabetic order by title of the issue and are separated by colored paper. A table of contents lists the alphabetized sections. Although the reference provides an interesting account of the history of health legislation in one fairly active year (due to managed care), the book would be of true interest to a fairly specialist audience. *Issue Briefs* is recommended for state libraries, libraries serving state legislatures, and for professional health organizations that have lobbyists. —**Mary Ann Thompson**

105.   **Major State Health Care Policies: Fifty State Profiles, 1997.** 6th ed. Washington, D.C., Health Policy Tracking Service, 1998. 294p. $147.00pa. ISBN 1-55516-819-1.

Health Policy Tracking Service (HPTS) correspondents in each state watch state legislatures, executive speeches, studies, press reports, and other subjects related to health policy efforts, and contribute this information to HPTS's online service. This volume summarizes what occurred in 1997 and matters expected to be considered in 1998.

Tables in the front check off topics such as various insurance reforms in all states, and maps show current interests in such activities as genetic testing. But most of the book is a series of 50 state profiles, each providing a narrative followed by brief statements on the current status of health related bills, in categories such as finance (managed care and insurance), Medicaid, providers, behavioral health, and pharmaceuticals. Because HPTS followed 13,085 bills in 1997, with all their variations, the number of concise factual statements here is tremendous. The overall view of any state's health care policy situation is clearly evident and may readily be compared with other states. Staffs involved in developing major health care policies and getting them adopted, those who must work under these directives, and researchers on health care trends in general or in specific subjects (such as parity—equal insurance coverage of mental illnesses) will appreciate this easily accessible collection of very current data.—**Harriette M. Cluxton**

106.   **Making Wise Medical Decisions: How to Get the Information You Need.** Lexington, Mass., Resources for Rehabilitation, 1998. 224p. index. $39.95pa. ISBN 0-929718-21-6.

This volume provides an overly generalized guide for health care consumers. The book has 11 chapters and 2 appendixes. Each chapter follows a standard format—questions to ask the health care providers, publications relevant to the topic, and organizations providing additional information or assistance. Chapter 1 directs health care consumers to appropriate information sources, including the library as a resource. Chapter 2 helps individuals locate suitable health care, listing questions to ask a potential health care provider and organizations to verify credentials. Additional chapters address understanding medical tests, how to work with a hospital, resources for comprehending pharmaceutical issues, and sections on health care for special populations (e.g., children, elderly, chronic conditions). Chapter 10 discusses somewhat controversial issues in health care—mammograms, prostate care, hysterectomies—defining the controversy and supplying resources to help individuals make the best personal decision. The appendixes provide an additional list of organizations and a list of publications from the publisher of this work titled "Resources for Rehabilitation."

Although not comprehensive for all diseases and illnesses, this handbook provides a general starting point for conscientious health care consumers. It cannot, however, replace a good reference on individual diseases and health concerns.—**Susan D. Strickland**

107.   **The Managed Care Yearbook.** 4th ed. Allenwood, N.J., Managed Care Information Center, 1998. 478p. index. $275.00pa. ISBN 1-882364-26-0.

Managed care executives can learn a great deal about the growth and development of their quickly expanding industry (as of 1998), the changes caused by the continuing shift of employer-sponsored health care plans into managed care plans, Medicare managed care, and how to combat the public's "anti-managed care sentiment" in this volume. Trends in the industry, market news, legislation, controlling costs, improving quality and humanizing relationships, and executive compensations are among the subjects covered. There are lists of advertisers as well.

A detailed table of contents makes location of topics fairly easy, but the text is often like a series of headlines, without continuity or bibliographic data. An appendix called "Sources" is merely a directory of health plan organizations and industry-sponsored study centers. Publications are listed in an appendix called "Managed Care Resources." A list of acronyms and a "Managed Care Glossary" are of some general interest, as are some of the case studies. This is an excellent update for those interested in the changing business aspects of managed care.—**Harriette M. Cluxton**

108.   **Medical Ethics: Codes, Opinions, and Statements.** Baruch A. Brody, Mark A. Rothstein, Laurence B. McCullough, and Mary Anne Bobinski, eds. Washington, D.C., BNA Books, 2000. 1074p. index. $255.00pa. ISBN 1-57018-100-4.

Currently accepted standards for ethical practices in the American medical profession are defined and discussed in the numerous codes, statements, and opinions published by a wide variety of medical societies. This significant reference guide makes many of these myriad publications easily accessible for the first time. Intended for physicians and other health care providers, health policy makers, medical ethicists, ad lawyers working in the medical/legal arena, this volume is an indispensable tool for anyone trying to understand the complex world of medical ethics.

This book is divided into 26 chapters, each containing the major ethics writings of an American medical society, such as the American Medical Association, the American College of Surgeons, and the American Academy of Pediatrics. Although not all-inclusive, this compilation provides the most thorough coverage currently available and the editors promise to expand coverage in future editions. Each chapter contains a specific medical society's code of ethics, official opinions about specific medical ethics issues, and commentary about these opinions published in major medical journals. The topics covered by these documents span the breadth of medical ethics, from abortion to fetal research to withholding life support. The documents in this book are current as of December 31, 1998, and will be updated in future editions. An extensive keyword index makes this volume easy to use. Within the next year the editors will produce a companion volume providing extensive commentaries on the documents in this current work that should greatly increase its usefulness.

This reference work to the official ethical standards of America's medial societies is an invaluable tool for anyone working in the area of medical ethics, from practicing health care workers to lawyers to health policy makers. All health science, academic, and large public libraries need to include this book in their reference collections.—**Jonathon Erlen**

109.   **The Medical Library Association Consumer Health Reference Service Handbook.** By Donald A. Barclay and Deborah D. Halsted. New York, Neal-Schuman, 2001. 197p. index. $59.95pa. ISBN 1-55570-418-2.

Intended as a primer on consumer-health librarianship for librarians and others who help the general public locate health information, the authors hope that this books helps in two ways: librarians improve their ability to provide sound information and that they develop better consumer-health information services. To achieve the first objective, the book covers standard resources for answering questions, the health reference interview, and briefly discusses the legal implications of providing health information to consumers. Topics such as creating an effective and useful Website, promoting resources through outreach, and collaborating with other health agencies and health care providers will help in developing better services. An enclosed CD-ROM includes templates to help develop these tools.

The 1st part of the book is divided into 3 chapters of essential information for librarians providing consumer health services. Chapter 1 describes the basic medical terminology readers would typically encounter when helping consumers. The 2d chapter provides brief descriptive summaries on some of the major health problems facing consumers and chapter 3 discusses complementary and alternative medicine.

The 2d part of the book starts with a chapter devoted to the best Websites for consumer health. The authors have selected these sites based on three possible types of content (originality, links to other resources, and online services) and one or more of the following characteristics: quantity, uniqueness, quality, and navigability (good Web design). Brief annotations describe the site, its content, and special features accompany the Website URL. A chapter discussing ways to select quality books and publications and a bibliography are also included.

The 3d part of the book discusses methods that can be used to establish consumer health information services, including extensive criteria for evaluating resources, creating effective print publications, and designing useful Websites. The CD-ROM provides a list of recommended sites that readers can use to build their own lists and a model consumer health Website with 18 pages, 3 PDF (protected document format) files, and 5 images.

The authors have created an easy-to-read, easy-to-understand, and easy-to-utilize guide to the challenging problem of providing accurate and authoritative answers to consumers seeking critical health information. Any librarian—school, public, or academic—assisting users in finding health information will find this book an effective professional tool.—**Vicki J. Killion**

110.   Nagel, Rob. **Body by Design: From the Digestive System to the Skeleton.** Edited by Betz Des Chenes. Farmington Hills, Mich., U*X*L/Gale, 2000. 2v. illus. index. $79.00/set. ISBN 0-7876-3897-8.

Body by Design is described by the publishers as a "medical reference product designed to inform and educate readers about the human body," and is considered "comprehensive, but not necessarily definitive" (p. xiii). Distributed in the United States by Gale Group, it is one of several new titles produced out of London by U*X*L, an imprint of Gale. Another introductory note points out that it "is only one component of the three-part U*X*L Complete Health Resource" (p. x). The two other titles are *Sick! Diseases and Disorders, Injuries and Infections* (see entry 198) and *Healthy Living* (see entry 33).

The medical information found in *Body by Design* can be found in many other books, but not in two volumes that are attractively designed and written for students or nonprofessional users. A check of the last five years of ARBA disclosed three well-reviewed atlases of anatomy (see ARBA 99, entry 1415; ARBA 98, entry 1499; and ARBA 96, entry 1694) that would certainly provide better details on anatomical design. However, this title is designed to supplement organ and structure design with three additional narratives (physiology or "Workings," diseases or "Ailments," and keeping healthy or prevention). Each of the 12 chapters (one for each of the 11 organ systems and a final chapter on special senses) describes an organ system. Volume 1 covers cardiovascular, digestive, endocrine, integumentary, lymphatic, and muscular systems, and volume 2 is devoted to the nervous, reproductive, reparatory, skeletal, and urinary systems plus the chapter on special senses.

Each chapter also includes illustrations; photographs; "words to know"; assorted historical, biographical, and informational inserts (e.g., in the respiratory system section there are sidebars on the composition of air, breathing underwater, how fish and plants breathe); and a section of book references and Websites. The first and second volumes include the same overview section and a general, medical "Words to Know" section. Both volumes conclude with the same general (and short) bibliography and Website listing as well as the same index.

The volumes are replete with reference data, although the specificity and value of the information will depend completely on the nature of the question. The "ailments" in the section on the lymphatic system include AIDS/HIV (with data through 1997), allergies, autoimmune diseases, lymphadenitis, lymphoma, and tonsillitis. Each category is described in less than a few hundred words regardless of complexity. For example, autoimmune disease includes only Graves' disease, multiple sclerosis, and lupus. The index provides a brief entry on the common cold but not the common cold sore, and carpal tunnel syndrome is referenced but not bursitis or tendonitis. All in all, school and public libraries may purchase this set, but may not find the work of major reference value except as the two volumes provide a basic overview of the human body. [R: BL, 1 Oct 2000, p. 372; BR, Nov/Dec 2000, pp. 77-78; SLJ, Nov 2000, p. 94]—**Laurel Grotzinger**

111.   **The Patient's Guide to Medical Tests.** By the Faculty Members of The Yale University School of Medicine. New York, Houghton Mifflin, 1997. 620p. illus. index. $40.00. ISBN 0-395-76536-6.

It is refreshing to note that Barrett Zaret, a prolific writer and editor of many books and journal articles on cardiology, edited a timely collaborative reference text on diagnostic tests for patients. There are many books published in this category, but this guide is a good source for patients.

There are 29 chapters, and each chapter is on a special subject that is written by a Yale faculty member who is an expert in the area. Medical testing is important and is a part of the diagnostic procedure. Required medical tests assist in the decision-making process. However, many medical tests are costly and unknown to patients, who are hesitant to ask for explanations. Thus, this book is useful and necessary to provide relevant answers to patients and other health professionals on screening guidelines, blood tests, cancer screening, fasting for the glucose tolerance test, and many other medical tests.

There are 2 parts in this book. The 1st part is the general overview that includes patients' rights and informed consent, tests for people without symptoms, diagnostic imaging, and an overview of diagnostic laboratory testing. Part 2 contains 25 chapters on specific tests relating to various anatomical parts and systems such as, the heart, vascular, respiratory, digestive, endocrine, reproductive, renal, musculoskeletal, immune, blood, skin, nervous, genetic, vision, and others. Uncommon medical tests that are not included in this source are searchable in other laboratory tests and handbooks. An added bonus of this tool is the appendix that covers tests that patients can do at home. There are essential illustrations to further explain the medical terminology. Each test is presented in a standard format that includes general information, where it is done, when is the result ready, other names, purpose, how it works, preparation, test procedure, after the test, and factors affecting the test. Each chapter in part 2 begins with a clinical case study that leads to the tests and the outcome. The index is well done and easy to use.

This reference tool was presented to several medical students and practicing physicians for locating tests of their choice. They have also found this book invaluable. Every library that provides consumers' or patient care information should acquire this copy to provide practical and reliable answers on medical tests. [R: LJ, Aug 97, p. 80; RUSQ, Summer 98, pp. 375-376]—**Polin P. Lei**

112.   Peck, Brian. **The Baby Boomer Body Book: The Complete Health Reference for Our Generation.** Naperville, Ill., Sourcebooks, 2001. 447p. illus. index. $21.95pa. ISBN 1-57071-715-X.

The baby boomer generation, those born between 1946 and 1964, make up one-third of the American population and are now into the age when so many health problems begin to show up. As a baby boomer himself and a physician, the author presents a single-source, easy-to-read health book prepared in collaboration with several of his colleagues who are experts in various specializations. Divided into four main sections—problems common to men and women, men's issues, women's issues, and preparation for the future—the book has chapters that cover almost every health problem that boomers are likely to encounter, all with eye-catching titles like "Where Did I Leave My Keys?" for memory problems and "Did Someone Turn Up the Heat" for menopause. The text is followed by a fairly extensive glossary with brief definitions; a bibliography of more than 70 titles; and a simple, mostly one-word index.

Each chapter gives information on a particular disease or problem, including a description, causes, symptoms, and treatments—usually the standard medical treatment, but occasionally including alternative or non-pharmacological treatments. Scientific or medical terms, which are printed in italics, are briefly described in the text and also found in the glossary. Many chapters are followed by information on additional resources (mostly organizations) and include Websites. In order to make it more useful as a reference work the author has written each chapter to stand alone so that someone interested only in skin problems, for example, can read that chapter without having to check preceding chapters. What makes these chapters different from similar health books is not only its reader-friendly style but the use of real, sometimes humorous, case studies with which the reader can easily identify.

The value of the book is enhanced by such features as slightly larger print with bold headings, the use of various shades of color, and the black-and-white drawings and photographs. It should prove popular not only with baby boomers, but others, either old or young, who want straightforward information on health issues in a readable but lively style. Public libraries will find it particularly useful, but academic and special libraries that have health or health-related programs will also want to include it in their collections.—**Lucille Whalen**

113. **Physician Marketplace Statistics 1997-98: Profiles for Detailed Specialties, Selected States and Practice Arrangements.** Martin L. Gonzalez and Puling Zhang, eds. Chicago, American Medical Association, 1998. 157p. $399.00pa. ISBN 0-89970-911-7.

This annual survey provides statistics on practice time (by weeks/year and hours/week), patient encounters, office visit fees, professional expenses, physician net income, and percentage of revenue by source (Medicare, Medicaid, private insurers, and managed care). The report's 125 tables and 37 figures are divided by category, with an introduction that includes definitions and a summary of the questions used to elicit the responses. Variables are divided into 26 medical specialties, 6 geographic regions, and the number of physicians in the practice.

This reference provides a useful yearly overview of physician practice patterns, but there are two areas that are missing. It would be helpful to add a section comparing the current year's key indicators with past data to more readily identify trends. The survey provides the total number of administrative, secretarial, and clerical employees but does not include clinical support staff such as nurses, physician assistants, and others. With managed care changing how medicine is practiced, data on the use of physician extenders are of key interest. —**Adrienne Antink Bien**

114. **Physician Socioeconomic Statistics.** 1999-2000 ed. Puling Zhang and Sara L. Thran, eds. Chicago, American Medical Association, 1999. 269p. $495.00pa.; $625.00 (CD-ROM); $795.00/set. ISBN 0-89970-947-5; 0-89970-975-3 (w/CD-ROM).

Since the early 1980s the American Medical Association's Center for Health Policy Research has been monitoring the socioeconomic status of physicians. Data are collected via an annual survey and Medicare payment data according to CPT code from the Federal Health Care Financing Administration. *Physician Socioeconomic Statistics* represents a merger between two previous publications: *Physician Marketplace Statistics* (1997-98 ed.; see entry 113) and *Socioeconomic Characteristics of Medical Practice* (1997 ed.; see entry 122).

Nonfederal physicians providing patient care (not medical residents) are included in the survey. Responses from over 3,600 physicians were tabulated for some survey questions, and in the case of questions related to specialties, from a few hundred physicians. The 1999-2000 publication includes data from the 1998 survey (which covers 1997 earnings and activities). A summary essay highlights changes from 1996 to 1997 and general trends. An essay and tables present Medicare payment data arranged by CPT code. Information about survey design, methodology, analysis, and definitions is included in appendixes. There is not a subject index, but a detailed list of tables is included in the table of contents. While this is not convenient for ready-reference, it does allow the user to identify key tables.

Questions from the survey are included in the first chapter. The bulk of the volume is devoted to tables reporting the data collected from the survey, with an overview of all physicians first and then separated by 12 practice specialties. This volume is filled with useful data often requested by healthcare industry workers, researchers, and administrators. A CD-ROM can also be obtained that contains the data presented in this volume. —**Lynne M. Fox**

115. Plunkett, Jack W. **Plunkett's Health Care Industry Almanac 2001-2002.** 4th ed. Houston, Tex., Plunkett Research, 2000. 770p. index. $199.99pa. (w/CD-ROM). ISBN 1-891775-17-0.

This 770-page, 4th edition of Plunkett's almanac is a source of valuable information for researchers and students of all types. It provides an overview of the vast health care industry, including charts and statistical data, in easy-to-understand language. As with any printed almanac, however, financial data and statistical analyses are obsolete once they appear on the page. Nevertheless, having relatively current (through the end of 2000), in-depth analyses of growth in the "Health Care 500," health care occupations, technology updates, and outlooks for Medicare and managed care helps decision-makers, job-seekers, and prospective patients find some of the answers they need.

The book brings into focus sales, profits, and product lines of the fastest growing firms in U.S. health care and ranks them from 1-500. The firms are divided by NAIC industry codes and include an index of headquarters locations by state and country (subsidiaries). Chapter 5 focuses on new treatments for major diseases. Chapter 6 focuses on health occupations by type and includes education requirements and median salaries.

Indexes appear on pages 741-770, including one of special interest called "Hot Spots for Advancement of Women and Minorities." The content of the almanac is also available on CD-ROM, a copy of which is found on the inside front cover of the print version. Installation of the CD-ROM requires a key number obtainable by calling the telephone number listed on the front of the disc. This resource is recommended for reference collections in public and academic libraries. —**Laura J. Bender**

116. **Portrait of Health in the United States.** Daniel Melnick and Beatrice Rouse, eds. Lanham, Md., Bernan Associates, 2001. 376p. $147.00pa. ISBN 0-89059-189-X.

The number of federal resources for health statistics, both print and on the Internet, are increasing almost daily, thus challenging librarians and their patrons to locate needed information. This new reference tool is a significant attempt to present an overview picture of American health problems and trends in the late 1990s using a wide variety of federal statistical sources. It includes instructions on how to use these resources for those seeking additional information. The editors intend their work to meet a wide variety of information needs for health care workers, public health professionals, health policy researchers, and others interested in this country's physical and mental health issues.

One large section examines some of the major causes of current health problems, such as alcohol and drug abuse, air pollution, hunger, lack of prenatal care, and lifestyle issues. Another segment presents data on rates and outcomes of specific diseases and other health concerns (i.e., cancer, AIDS, injuries, and mental illnesses). Statistics explaining the costs of the American health care system are provided in a separate chapter, including coverage of insured versus non-insured; the availability of health care professionals; and the use of hospital, Hospice, and nursing home facilities. A final statistical section describes the economic costs of bad health in the United States today in terms of lost productivity and actual costs for caring for America's sick or injured cohort. The book's last chapter is a very valuable guide to print and Internet health statistical resources that readers can use to search for more health-related statistics. Each statistical section includes brief textual discussions, along with numerous worthwhile charts, graphs, and tables that are the most important part of this guide. This reference work is a valuable new tool for all public, academic, and health care librarians, as well as for individuals attempting to locate statistical information on America's late 1990s health care trends and issues. [R: LJ, 1 Mar 02, p. 88; Choice, Feb 02, p. 1030]—**Jonathon Erlen**

117. **Preventive Care Sourcebook 1997-1998.** Betty Ankrapp, ed. Gaithersville, Md., Aspen, 1997. 280p. index. $89.00pa. ISBN 0-8342-0880-6.

Much of the information in this sourcebook is available in other health-related publications, usually directed to health care consumers. However, this large compilation has been selected and arranged as a desk reference for executives and directors charged with planning and implementing programs for health promotion, patient education, prevention and management of diseases and injuries, and so forth. Improving the health of all people in the United States is a national initiative, through prevention, of the U.S. Department of Health and Human Services. Today's managed care and cost containment depend heavily on effective preventive care. This book provides an extensive overview of existing resources.

Each chapter, such as "Substance Abuse," is preceded by a chart listing for-profit and non-profit organizations, products and services offered, and the page where contact information and a description appear. "Additional Resources" has only contact information. The "Federal Agencies" chapter is fully annotated. Some organizations appear under many different headings with exactly the same wording. This repetition is especially noticeable for publishers of patient educational materials, such as Channing L. Bete Company, Inc., of "scriptography" fame, with 17 listings. State offices and ethnic resources are separately listed. The sourcebook provides subject and organization indexes.

The book is available on disk, and annual updates are planned. Administrators of various health programs should appreciate this excellent sourcebook.—**Harriette M. Cluxton**

118.   **Rehabilitation Sourcebook.** Dawn D. Matthews, ed. Detroit, Omnigraphics, 2000. 531p. index. (Health Reference Series). $78.00. ISBN 0-7808-0236-5.

Each year an estimated 38 million Americans experience conditions that limit their daily activities through chronic physical health disorders, injuries, and impairments. This volume contains information about the most common conditions causing the need for rehabilitation and the different types of rehabilitation services available to treat these conditions. The book is divided into seven different sections: Rehabilitation Basics, Types of Rehabilitation Therapy, Assistive and Adaptive Devices, Role of Family During Rehabilitation, Financial Considerations, Common Disorders and Specific Issues in Rehabilitation, and Additional Help and Information (with glossaries of terms). The bibliographies, sources of information, and the question-and-answer section are helpful. This is an excellent resource for public library reference and health collections despite its cost. The sourcebook compares favorably with *The Complete Directory for People with Disabilities* (11th ed.; see ARBA 2003, entry 818). The publication also includes medical information that is not included in the aforementioned directory.—**Theresa Maggio**

119.   Segen, Joseph C., and Josie Wade. **The Patient's Guide to Medical Tests: Everything You Need to Know About the Tests Your Doctor Prescribes.** 2d ed. New York, Facts on File, 2002. 418p. index. (Facts on File Library of Health and Living). $44.00. ISBN 0-8160-4651-4.

The tests a doctor orders for a patient can be one of the most puzzling and scariest aspects of a medical visit. And in today's managed-care environment, doctors rarely have time for detailed explanations of the reasons for a test, the possible interpretations of results, and alternatives for further testing. A source such as this handbook for the layperson can fill in the important information so that the patient can make informed decisions on what tests to undergo, how to prepare for them, and how confident to be in the results.

Although the 1st edition of this book was only published 5 years ago (see ARBA 99, entry 1455), frequent updates are necessary in this field. Many tests have been improved, some have been retired and replaced with more accurate ones, and new tests have been introduced. All are covered here, along with new information on areas of increased interest, such as Alzheimer's disease, bioterrorism, improved tests in clinical cardiology, and new forms of diagnostic imaging.

There are more than 1,000 alphabetically arranged entries in this book, each around a half a page long. Included are descriptions of each test and what it measures, what preparation the patient needs to make (such as fasting or intake of a contrast medium), the procedure the patient will undergo, and a reference or "normal" range for the results. A range is also given for the cost of the procedure and comments on precautions in interpretation and factors that could interfere with accurate results. A glossary and index help make the text more accessible. One element that is lacking is references to other sources for more in-depth information. A list of other texts, or better yet, Websites, would have been helpful, both in leading the patient to more in-depth information and in helping with updating information in such a fast-changing field.—**Carol L. Noll**

120.   Sendor, Virginia F., and Patrice M. O'Connor. **Hospice and Palliative Care: Questions and Answers.** Lanham, Md., Scarecrow Press, 1997. 250p. index. $36.00. ISBN 0-8108-3308-5.
    According to the authors of this work, hospice is a "coordinated interdisciplinary program of life-affirming compassionate care and supportive services for terminally ill individuals, their families, and significant others." Interestingly, the patient and family are treated as a whole and are to be cared for together. Hospice, when provided by a Medicare-certified program, is paid for entirely by Medicare. Over 340,000 terminally ill persons and their families were served by hospice programs in 1994. The hospice movement is growing, and if a library does not have a reference book on it, this is a good one to select. This work is poised between the academic and the popular to deem appropriate for almost all kinds of libraries. Chapters are devoted to hospice and AIDS, advance directives (orders not to resuscitate, health care proxies, living wills, and durable power of attorney), and answers to questions that deal with the end of life. In addition to being useful, this book is interesting in its treatment of concepts such as total pain (mental, physical, spiritual, social, legal, or financial), migration home syndrome (adult children returning home to be cared for in their last days), and anticipatory grief (grief that begins before the patient has died).
    The authors could not be more qualified. Sendor is the founder of the Long Island Foundation for Hospice Care and Research and the former executive director of Life-Care Hospice, and O'Connor, a nurse, is a palliative care consultant and the former director of the hospice at St. Luke's/Roosevelt Hospital Center in New York City. Highly recommended for public, academic, hospital, and personal libraries.—**Lambrini Papangelis**

121.   Shannon, Joyce Brennfleck. **Medical Tests Sourcebook.** Detroit, Omnigraphics, 1999. 691p. illus. index. (Health Reference Series). $78.00. ISBN 0-7808-0243-8.
    Written for the medical consumer as part of the Health Reference Series, this volume has a wide scope that makes it useful, although its lack of depth in many instances leaves the reader wanting to know more. The book covers basic health information, such as periodic health exams; general screening tests; "at-home" tests, such as tests for diabetes, HIV, and pregnancy; and payment for medical tests, especially through Medicare and Medicaid. The book divides medical tests into several general categories: X-ray and radiology; electrical (ECG, EEG); blood and other body fluids and tissues; scope; lung; genetics, pregnancy, and newborn; and sexually transmitted diseases. Each section is further divided into types of tests within the category and specific tests. Most sections include background information about the history and development of the test, a description, and preparation for the test if important. Black-and-white illustrations, usually of test images, help to explain some of the tests. Most chapters include references for further reading and information and the addresses and telephone numbers for any groups that deal with the medical problem. Additional chapters include information about the Hill-Burton Free Care Program, computer diagnosis and telemedicine, resources for additional help, and a glossary. An extensive topical index aids the reader.

As a whole, the volume is fairly user-friendly despite its tendency to fall into medical terminology without explanation or glossary entries. Many of the entries, especially the introductory materials, are written in a question-and-answer format. Most individual test entries explain what the test shows and how the test is done. Very little information is provided to aid the patient in interpreting test results (i.e., what each of the numbers in a blood test mean—what is normal, low, or high), with cholesterol numbers being the one exception. Many sections dealing with specific tests include a bibliographic reference for the information at the beginning of the section, but this information is provided on an inconsistent basis. Taken as a whole, this volume can be a valuable reference guide despite some inconsistencies in presentation.—**Janet Hilbun**

122.   **Socioeconomic Characteristics of Medical Practice 1997.** Martin L. Gonzalez, ed. Chicago, American Medical Association, 1997. 177p. $159.95pa.; $209.95pa. (with disk). ISBN 0-89970-865-X; 0-89970-866-8 (with disk).

This compilation of data from the American Medical Association (AMA) contains information collected from actively practicing physicians who responded to the Center for Health Policy Research Socioeconomic Monitoring System's 1996 survey. An appendix presents the design, a questionnaire summary, and the statistical methods used. Detailed statistics include age profiles of physicians, utilization and fees for visits, and expenses and income. Many of the data are also included in the 1997 survey report, also conducted by the Center for Health Policy Research and published by the AMA.

Four summary articles will interest practicing physicians and those advising physicians finishing training. The first summarizes the data on contractual arrangements with managed care organizations, pointing out that 75 percent of Americans are receiving health care coverage through some kind of managed care mechanism. Data are presented by specialty, detailing type of managed care plan, participation by payer, and reviews by plan type and capitation. The second article addresses practice size by type of employer and distribution of physicians by employer type. These data include academic as well as other kinds of practices. The relationship of size of practice to such variables as efficiency, cost, and productivity is discussed. The next article discusses trends in physician income from 1985 to 1995. Trends in medical liability claims from 1985 to 1995 are the topic of the last article. The decrease in the annual rate of liability claims, the percentage of physicians with claims, and the liability premiums are noted. The articles place the data presented in the context of other published information.—**Margretta Reed Seashore**

123.   **Source Book in Bioethics.** Albert R. Jonsen, Robert M. Veatch, and LeRoy Walters, eds. Washington, D.C., Georgetown University Press, 1998. 510p. index. $95.00. ISBN 0-87840-683-2.

The study of bioethics began in the early 1970s; today it is an important field of academic study. It is concerned with the moral dimensions of the life sciences and health care. Many of the original troublesome topics have evolved into accepted concepts; policies and procedures have been established by research and health care institutions to respect these resolutions. Many documents relating to bioethics have been produced by government bodies, courts, and legislatures. Although most reports and laws are "in the public domain," it is often difficult to locate them in the original form as opposed to book or journal discussions. Recognizing this, the editors have collected many of the most significant documents and reprinted them in full, or occasionally in shortened form. They are arranged under four general headings representing the major fields of concentration of bioethics, thus providing a history of sorts through the major documents produced. These include the ethics of research with human subjects, the ethics of death and dying, ethical issues in human genetics, and those arising from human reproductive technologies and arrangements. Thoughtful editorial comments precede each part and introduce specific documents. Often notes and references have been added.

The final portion of the book considers ethical issues in the changing health care scene. The old Hippocratic oath can no longer fully govern the relationships between doctors, patients, and other laypersons. Changes in attitudes, advances in research, questions and rights, informed consent, transplantation and donation of organs, and so on have been part of the movement toward concepts of social ethics.

As a historical survey of bioethics, this book should be very valuable as a text and as a reference source for investigating the ethical issues surrounding such particular health-related topics as the right to die or to reject treatments, surrogate birth, and so on, and how society has tried to meet them.—**Harriette M. Cluxton**

124. **Statistical Record of Health and Medicine.** 2d ed. Arsen J. Darnay, ed. Detroit, Gale, 1998. 1029p. index. $115.00. ISBN 0-7876-0093-8. ISSN 1078-6961.

With 11 chapters, more than 1,000 pages, 950 tables, and topics ranging from hospital truck driver salaries to the risk of blood clots from sitting in cramped airline seats, this compendium is fascinating, frustrating, and highly idiosyncratic. For example, chapter 2, entitled "Health Status of Americans," contains 274 tables organized under 35 headings. The first heading, "Aging," contains a single 3-line quotation from *Time* magazine indicating that 1 in 5 Americans over the age of 60 regularly take pain pills, and many have side effects. There are just two entries in the one-page section devoted to cerebrovascular disease—both quotations from *Time* magazine. By contrast, there are 45 tables and 64 pages devoted to sexually transmitted diseases (STDs). In chapter 8, which is on medical professions, 82 pages are devoted to occupational compensation in health services facilities, including wages for accountants, janitors, key entry operators, warehouse specialists, and 25 other occupations.

Huge chunks of the book are lifted directly from government sources: 218 pages of data on health care establishments from a 1992 economic census report, 70 pages on hospital procedures from a single National Center for Health Statistics publication, and the 64 pages on STDs from a September 1996 U.S. Public Health Service report. Outside of governmental publications, there is a heavy reliance on newspaper and magazine articles. No indication is given that the information taken from these secondary sources has been checked or verified. Yet the most frustrating feature of this volume is its uneven content. Obviously, with a title like *Statistical Record of Health and Medicine*, the editor needed to be selective in the choice of topics and depth of coverage. However, the reader is given no clue as to what those editorial guidelines may be. The book contains an excellent keyword index, but this addition cannot save an otherwise flawed effort.—**Bruce Stuart**

125. **Stress-Related Disorders Sourcebook.** Joyce Brennfleck Shannon, ed. Detroit, Omnigraphics, 2002. 587p. index. (Health Reference Series). $78.00. ISBN 0-7808-0560-7.

A recent entry in Omnigraphics' Health Reference Series, the *Stress-Related Disorders Sourcebook* collates information about the many facets of physical and emotional stress from a variety of reliable science and health journals as well as U.S. government publications. As with other volumes in the Health Reference Series, medical consultation services were provided to the editor by a board-certified physician.

Several early chapters are devoted to establishing a definition of stress and its origins. Of particular interest to readers in the post-2001 environment are chapters on post traumatic stress disorders, coping with grief, stress in the workplace, and the role of spirituality in stress reduction. Well written for a general readership, the *Stress-Related Disorders Sourcebook* is a useful addition to the health reference literature.—**Alan Asher**

126. **Traveler's Health Sourcebook.** Joyce Brennfleck Shannon, ed. Detroit, Omnigraphics, 2000. 635p. maps. index. (Health Reference Series). $78.00. ISBN 0-7808-0384-1.

This is a new offering in the Health Reference Series produced by Omnigraphics. The volume is primarily a compilation of materials produced by other sources, some private, but most from federal government agencies. The dates on these materials range from 1994 to 2000, but the majority are current, from 1998 to 2000. *Traveler's Health Sourcebook* is divided into 10 parts and those are further subdivided into 61 chapters.

The text provides information on health and safety aspects of travel and recreation, both in the United States and internationally. Broad topics include the health and safety issues of transportation, camping and wilderness areas, and international travel. Particularly beneficial is the fifth part on travelers with special needs. Chapters in this part include pertinent information for pregnant travelers, those traveling with children, diabetic travelers, travelers with AIDS, and the physically disabled traveler. There is an exceptionally valuable chapter listing travel agencies providing specialized travel arrangements for the physically disabled. Additionally, the seventh part on geographical health information, the eighth part on worldwide disease risks, and the ninth part on disease risks outside of the United States all have a great deal of useful information about diseases and specific health risks, organized by geographical area, country, and disease. This book is recommended for any public library, any travel collection, and especially any collection for the physically disabled.—**Lynn M. McMain**

127. **U.S. Medical Licensure Statistics and Requirements by State.** 1998-1999 ed. Chicago, American Medical Association, 1998. 118p. $79.95pa. ISBN 0-89970-924-9.

An AMA serial that has undergone many name changes, this work was first presented in the 1970s under the title *Medical Licensure Statistics*. In 1974, the series was renamed *Physician Distribution and Medical Licensure in the U.S.* By 1982 this title was changed again to *U.S. Medical Licensure Statistics, 1980-1981, and Licensure Requirements, 1982*. In 1989, it was called *U.S. Medical Licensure Statistics and Licensure Requirements*. From 1990 to 1997, the title was *U.S. Medical Licensure Statistics and Current Licensure Requirements*. Now in 1998 it has become *U.S. Medical Licensure Statistics and Requirements by State*. Whatever name is applied, this is an essential information source for the medical profession. The data collected are from a master file that has data coming in from the medical schools, hospitals, medical societies, national board of medical examiners, state licensing boards, Surgeon General of the U.S. Government, American Board of Medical Specialties (ABMS), Drug Enforcement Administration, and other federal agencies and physicians.

There are 7 parts in this series. Part 1 is on licensure policies and regulations of state medical boards that includes CME policies and "telemedicine" practice. Part 2 is on 1996 statistics of state medical board licensure activities. Part 3 is on medical licensing examination and organizations and includes United States Medical Licensing Examination (USMLE), computer-based testing (CBT), computer-based case simulations (CCS), Federation of State Medical Boards of the United States (FSMB), National Board of Medical Examiner (NBME), the FSMB Federation Licensing Examination (FLEX), and Special Purpose Examination (SPEX). Part 4 is on information for international medical graduates such as the Educational Commission for Foreign Medial Graduates (ECFMG). Part 5 is on federal and national programs and activities such as the Air Force, Army, and Navy. Part 6 is on quality assurance organizations and programs. Part 7 is on other organizations and programs. New features included for this issue are a glossary, contact information, Internet addresses, e-mail addresses, and fax numbers. There is no need to elaborate on the importance of this publication. It is a must for medical education.—**Polin P. Lei**

128.   Wellner, Alison Stein. **Best of Health: Demographics of Health Care Consumers.** 2d ed. Ithaca, N.Y., New Strategist, 2000. 494p. index. $89.95. ISBN 1-885070-32-2.

This book is much more than what its title implies. The author has extracted and summarized vast amounts of data about health care and the health care consumer in the United States from reliable sources, such as the United States government and the University of Chicago's National Opinion Research Center (NORC). The data are presented within easily understood tables and graphs in 12 topical chapters. Each chapter begins with a brief, simple textual summary of the data. The author synthesizes the data, but also integrates research from reputable health care journal articles. Each chapter concludes with a summary of future health care trends and an appendix of more in-depth statistical tables. A wide range of health care topics are presented in the chapters, from basic health care demographics to spending and economics, self care and alternative therapies, chronic and disability care, mental health issues, the Internet, and the influence of diversity. A glossary and extensive bibliography are also included.

The reference is concise, clearly written, and very easy to use and understand. In the introduction, the author states that the book is primarily for planners within the health care industry. This is so, but the text could readily be used by all levels of readers, from the layperson to the scholarly researcher or health care provider. It is highly recommended.—**Mary Ann Thompson**

129.   **The World Book Health & Medical Annual 2000.** Chicago, World Book, 2000. 352p. illus. index. $29.00. ISBN 0-7166-1150-3. ISSN 0890-4480.

The World Book Health & Medical Annual is a good addition for libraries that make heavy use of the *World Book Encyclopedia.* For many others it would fall into the category of nice to have but not essential. The volume has a list of what the editors have chosen as the eight major health stories of the year and a health update section that reports last year's major developments in health and medicine. A section entitled "Spotlight on the Millennium" makes an attempt to summarize the last 1000 years in medicine and offers projections about the future. Four other sections are entitled "A Healthy You," "A Healthy Family," "Consumer Health," and "Medical and Safety Alerts." A directory of health information centers rounds out the book.

The section on health updates does a good job of summarizing major findings of the year in such areas as health and nutrition, diseases, and managed care. It would have been a lot more useful if the signed articles had included references. A section on medicine in the year 1000 makes for interesting reading although readers may wonder how many concerned parents, even then, would rush their sick child to the local monastery when they awakened with a stomachache. A review of medical discoveries from the year 1100 through the twentieth century explains the great moments in medicine (smallpox inoculation, the germ theory of disease) but does not indicate that modern medicine still has many problems. It is unclear why the editors selected the topics for the other sections.

Just as in the *World Book Encyclopedia* the writing is clear and detailed without being too technical, and is interesting to read. There is also some good practical advice in the "Healthy You," "Healthy Family," and "Consumer Health and Medical and Safety Alerts" sections. Although the writing is not elementary, the slant seems to be for high school students. Lower-level undergraduates may find this useful, but advanced students will need broader coverage than this volume provides.—**Natalie Kupferberg**

130.   **Worldwide Health Sourcebook.** Joyce Brennfleck Shannon, ed. Detroit, Omnigraphics, 2001. 614p. index. (Health Reference Series). $78.00. ISBN 0-7808-0330-2.

Like the other books in this series, this sourcebook consists mostly of reprints from government publications—in this case the Centers for Disease Control, the National Cancer Institute, and various United Nations agencies. Also included are a few articles by nongovernment organizations and individual researchers. Unlike others in the Health Reference Series, however, this volume is not of particular interest to individual patients. Rather, this book is a look at the health of the world as a whole and has information vital to understanding the effects of health and health policies on issues of development, economics, war, and peace.

Some of the vital areas included are disease, mental health, children and women's health, aging, and environmental health. Articles on emerging diseases and statistical comparisons of the occurrence of infectious diseases, cancer, and other health problems by country, continent, and developed versus developing countries are particularly interesting. As in the rest of this series, a comprehensive index, a glossary of terms, a bibliography, and a directory of relevant organizations (including Website and e-mail addresses) add to the value of this collection.

Few libraries can afford to keep a comprehensive collection of government pamphlets and other publications —and it is often hard to find full-text copies of such sources online. This series serves as a handy way for libraries to provide access to this wealth of readable, reliable information. —**Carol L. Noll**

131. Yount, Lisa. **Patients' Rights in the Age of Managed Health Care.** New York, Facts on File, 2001. 280p. index. (Library in a Book). $45.00. ISBN 0-8160-4258-6.

Patients' Rights in the Age of Managed Health Care is a useful research guide and invaluable resource for those in the health care field, patients and their families, students, and the general public. The book covers such topics as historical information on America's health care system; laws and court cases affecting health care; a chronology of medical, legislative, judicial, and public events that affect health care; biographical profiles of key individuals in the field; a glossary of related medical, legal, and other terms; a guide to research on health care issues; an extensive annotated bibliography of books, periodicals, online publications, and other sources of information on health care; an annotated list of organizations; and appendixes and an index. The section on organizations and agencies is very good and includes Website information. There are similar books available, such as *The Rights of Patients: Basic ACLU Guide to Patients' Rights* (2d ed.; Humana, 1992), but this publication is the most up-to-date. [R: VOYA, June 02, pp. 145-146]—**Theresa Maggio**

INDEXES

132. **Health Reference Series Cumulative Index 1999.** Edward J. Prucha, Anne Holmes, and Robert Rudnick, eds. Detroit, Omnigraphics, 2000. 989p. (Health Reference Series). $78.00. ISBN 0-7808-0382-5.

The Health Reference Series from Omnigraphics began in 1990 and as of the time of this review includes over 50 books. The volumes in this series are well known in the library reference field and are often consulted in many public libraries. The information provided in the volumes is intended to be comprehensive and provide a basic overview to patients, families, and caregivers in the general public; it is not designed for medical professionals. This latest volume is simply a comprehensive index of the first 42 volumes in the series. The indexes include a name index, organization index, and a publication index. There is also a list of acronyms and abbreviations used throughout the series. Because this index provides references to so many books it is necessary to read the preface in order to understand the layout of the entries and the abbreviations for the books. The entries themselves are easy to understand. This volume will be most helpful in libraries that have a relatively complete collection of the Health Reference Series. [R: Choice, Nov 2000, p. 510]—**Shannon Graff Hysell**

2 Medical Education and Careers

DIRECTORIES

133. **Continuing Medical Education Directory 1996-1997.** Chicago, American Medical Association, 1996. 254p. $49.95pa. ISBN 0-89970-838-2.

The American Medical Association has published a highly informative guide and directory regarding accredited continuing medical education (CME). The reference is comprehensive, seeming to cover everything about CME that would need to be known by a practicing physician or an organization planning to offer such programs. Every format for continuing education is described in detail, from individual journal reading to conferences to the newer technologies of teleconferencing and computer-assisted learning. Accreditation guidelines and application procedures for each type of CME are included. The specific continuing education requirements of specialty medical organizations and individual states are noted. In addition, the index provides a directory of state medical societies and a directory of currently accredited providers. An emphasis on ethics and possible ethical conflicts related to CME is evident throughout the book. Although some sections of the text will be outdated, potential users of this type of reference are encouraged to obtain this edition. The introduction to the text notes that this is the final hard copy; future versions will be available on the Internet. Because of the depth and detail provided, it would seem to be easier to read this information in book form rather than on the computer. The directory is highly recommended for individual physicians, providers of CME, and medical school libraries.—**Mary Ann Thompson**

134. **Directory of Schools for Alternative and Complementary Health Care.** Karen Rappaport, ed. Phoenix, Ariz., Oryx Press, 1998. 250p. index. $49.50pa. ISBN 1-57356-110-X.

Although interest in alternative and complementary health care has been increasing for some time, the establishment of the Office of Alternative Medicine within the National Institutes of Health in 1992 has, probably more than any other factor, increased the interest of not only young people, but also those making a career change, in seeking careers in alternative medicine. This directory provides information on some 675 schools and colleges in the United States and Canada that offer training for careers in many areas of alternative health care, including acupuncture, biofeedback, herbal medicine, and homeopathy. Essays on some of the better-known fields, written by experienced practitioners, and a subject index precede the directory part of the book.

Directory information is arranged by state in the United States and by province in Canada and includes such typical items as name and address of the institution, administrative staff, average enrollment, accreditation and approval or licensing board, admission requirements, and cost, although not all institutions provided the complete information requested. Particularly important for this type of directory is the list of national organizations and accrediting agencies that follows the directory information. It does not, however, include state agencies, which usually set the standards for state licensing in these areas. Both the editor's introduction and the essays on particular fields, however, caution prospective students to investigate the qualifications for practitioners in the locale where they intend to practice. Other sections of the directory that enhance its usefulness are a brief bibliography, the indexes by name of school and by specialization, a list of abbreviations used, and a glossary.

Although the editor states that the directory information was taken mainly from questionnaires sent to schools, with a smaller portion coming from professional organizations, there is no indication of the criteria used for selecting the schools except that medical schools and schools offering programs in the expressive arts, transpersonal psychology, and psychospiritual fields were excluded. Because not all schools were included, it would be helpful to know if a particular school was omitted because it did not respond to the questionnaire or for reasons that had to do with the quality of the school. Nevertheless, because of the uniqueness of the subject field, the ease of access to directory information, and the added material included, this directory should be valuable to public and academic libraries, particularly on the community college level where many students are seeking career information that might lead them from an AA degree into an area of health care that is becoming increasingly popular. [R: BL, July 98, p. 1904; Choice, Oct 98, p. 294]—**Lucille Whalen**

135.   **Graduate Medical Education Directory 1999/2000.** 84th ed. Chicago, American Medical Association, 1999. 1286p. $64.95pa. ISBN 0-89970-984-2.

The 84th edition of this directory lists programs accredited by the Accreditation Council for Graduate Medical Education (ACGME). The goal of this directory is to provide medical students with a list of accredited graduate medical education (GME) programs in the United States. With this information, medical students can make the important decision on which program they will select for their residency training. This source is commonly used by the state licensing boards, specialty societies, and hospitals to verify the authenticity of programs presented by physicians who wish to apply for licensure, certification, or hospital privileges. This directory is updated annually and is a unique medical education resource that is now online at http://www.rsna.org/REG/launchpad/ama-freida.html.

The American Medical Association Fellowship and Residency Electronic Interactive Database Access system is an extensive database that enables users to search by primary and secondary criteria for fellowship and residency programs in North America. The difference between the print and nonprint product is that the online product is interactive and gives additional information, such as city and county population counts, hospital benefits, the areas cost of living statistics, and much more. However, the print version is a must-purchase for medical facilities and libraries. In this directory there are 5 sections. Section 1 lists general information and policies and procedures of the ACGME, including information for international medical graduates. Section 2 is on essentials of accredited residencies in graduate medical education (e.g., institutional and program requirements). Section 3 presents accredited graduate medical education programs, such as pediatrics, oncology, and so on. Section 4 describes new and withdrawn programs. Section 5 is on graduate medical education teaching institutions. There are also several appendixes. Appendix A reports on combined specialty programs, such as internal medicine and emergency medicine. Appendix B lists medical specialty board certification requirements. Appendix C is on medical licensure information. Appendix D lists medial schools in the United States. And finally, appendix E is a graduate medical education glossary. This directory is ultimately a renounced product from the AMA to assist any medical school student to choose his or her future role in medicine.—**Polin P. Lei**

136.   **Health Professions Career and Education Directory 2000-2001.** Chicago, American Medical Association, 2000. 548p. $60.00pa. ISBN 1-57947-063-7.

The most recent edition of this directory has again changed its name. The previous two editions were entitled *Health Professions Education Directory.* This 28th edition has added 5 new professions and 280 new programs to list over 5,800 educational programs providing entry-level educational preparation for 52 health occupations.

The directory is still divided into four sections, but the order of the sections has changed from previous editions. The 1st section now covers occupations and educational programs, providing job and career descriptions, entry-level educational requirements and educational programs available. The 2d section covers institutions sponsoring accredited programs and is organized alphabetically by state, city, institution, and programs. The 3d section supplies information on 16 of the 17 agencies that accredit educational programs for the listed occupations. The American Physical Therapy Association did not agree to participate and is absent from this list. The 4th section furnishes information collected on the 1999 AMA Annual Surveys of Health Education Programs. Features of this section include statistics on trends in health profession education, program enrollments, graduates, and attrition.

This informative, always valuable resource is highly recommended for career centers in public libraries as well as secondary school, community college and university libraries.—**Lynn M. McMain**

137.   Nagy, Andrea, and Paula Bilstein. **The Best Medical Schools.** 1998 ed. New York, Random House, 1997. 332p. index. $20.00pa. ISBN 0-679-77782-2. ISSN 1067-2176.

Guides to medical schools are popular in many libraries, and many are available with different emphases. This one is unique in that it involves input from more than 6,000 students, who rate their schools on such areas as curriculum, teaching, and student life. Two pages are included for each school, including information on admissions selection factors and financial aid. A sidebar for each school provides Gourman report ratings, application information, tuition and fees, average grade point average and Medical College Admission Test (MCAT) scores, statistical figures on the makeup of the student body, and other practical information. Both medical and osteopathic colleges are included.

Introductory chapters discuss general application guidelines, studying for the MCAT, and how to write an admissions essay. There is also relatively brief information on opportunities for women and minorities and a listing of schools with postbaccalaureate programs for adult students changing careers. Other chapters discuss financing medical school and successful interviewing skills. Another medical school guide, *Barron's Guide to Medical and Dental Schools* (9th ed.; see ARBA 2001, entry 235), includes dental schools, a sample MCAT test, and more supplementary information. *The Association of American Medical Colleges' Medical School Admission Requirements* (49th ed.; AAMC, 1998) contains official information supplied by the colleges. Because of its unique student input, *The Best Medical Schools* is a worthwhile purchase for public, academic, and medical libraries, even if they have other such guides.—**Marit S. Taylor**

138.   **NLN Guide to Undergraduate RN Education.** 5th ed. Delroy Louden and Dawnette Jones, eds. New York, NLN Press, 1997. 295p. $19.95pa. ISBN 0-88737-737-8.

This guidebook provides pertinent information about nursing and nursing educational programs that lead to registered nurse (RN) licenses. The book is divided into 3 parts. The 1st part describes the profession of nursing, educational requirements, and various professional roles of the nurse. The 2d part is a directory of schools of nursing in the United States. The 3d part includes a brief glossary of terms commonly used in nursing. Unlike the earlier editions, this revised edition for the first time includes the information about the National League for Nursing (NLN) accredited nursing programs as well as the schools that offer nursing programs for nonregistered nurse students.

For those who are not familiar with, or are interested in the nursing profession, the first part of this book is of great relevance. It addresses the different educational requirements and responsibilities for a RN and a licensed practical nurse (LPN). Also included are information about the various career choices and benefits in the nursing field. The section on the 1,508 degree programs is divided into 4 areas: Associate Degree Program, Baccalaureate Degree Programs, Diploma Programs, and Baccalaureate Degree Programs Designed Exclusively for RNs. Under each program, the school information is then organized by state. The information provided in the entries is succinct and pertinent, such as the number of enrollment; affiliation; degrees offered; and availability of weekend, evening, and distance education programs. Those who are interested in further information are referred to the name of the contact person, school address, and telephone number. For anyone considering nursing as a profession, this guidebook is a valuable source of information. This directory is recommended for reference collections in public and academic libraries. **—Eveline L. Yang**

139. **Peterson's Guide to Nursing Programs.** 7th ed. Lawrenceville, N.J., Peterson's Guides, 2001. 631p. illus. index. $26.95pa. ISBN 0-7689-0556-7. ISSN 1073-7820.

Previously, and more accurately, titled *Peterson's Guide to Nursing Programs: Baccalaureate and Graduate Nursing Education in the U.S. and Canada* (see ARBA 96, entry 356), this 7th edition maintains the quality associated with the Peterson name. *Peterson's Guide to Nursing Programs* is published in cooperation with the American Association of Colleges of Nursing. The section titled "The Nursing School Advisor" is full of essays on interesting topics such as "RNs Returning to School: Choosing a Nursing Program" and "What You Need to Know About Distance Learning in Nursing Education." This edition keeps the very useful quick reference section, followed by profiles of individual programs alphabetically arranged by state or province.

The indexes are particularly accommodating, with guidance to baccalaureate programs, master's programs, concentrations within master's programs, and doctoral and postdoctoral programs. There are also indexes for distance learning programs, continuing education programs, and the more than 700 institutions listed. Altogether, this guide remains a valuable resource for any career collection in high school, community college, university, or public libraries, and in any of the aforementioned school counseling services.**—Lynn M. McMain**

140. **Peterson's U.S. & Canadian Medical Schools 1997: 400 Accredited M.D. and Combined Medical Degree Programs.** Princeton, N.J., Peterson's Guides, 1997. 209p. index. $24.95pa. ISBN 1-56079-631-6. ISSN 1089-3342.

Peterson's U.S. & Canadian Medical Schools is a thorough and helpful guide for prospective medical college applicants. Its modest price makes it an affordable addition to most public and academic library collections. However, libraries that have the Association of American Medical Colleges's *Medical School Admission Requirements* (53d ed., 2003) will find that the Peterson's guide is redundant.

The guide under review includes the usual background information in chapters on professional trends, selecting and applying to medical colleges, testing, accreditation, and financing of costly medical educations. One-page profiles of medical colleges in the United States and Canada make up the majority of the publication. Profiles supply information on the institutional setting, student services, campus facilities, medical college personnel and programs, teaching methods, enrollment, expenses and financial aids, and contact information. Listings of information on number of applicants to size of entering class is inconsistent between profiles. Some listings provide percentage of students receiving their top choice for residency.

The information provided in this publication is valuable to prospective medical students. The guide is recommended for libraries without the Association of American Medical Colleges's guide or where demand requires both guides.—**Lynne M. Fox**

141. **RSP Funding for Nursing Students and Nurses 1998-2000.** By Gail Ann Schlachter and R. David Weber. San Carlos, Calif., Reference Service Press, 1998. 163p. index. $25.00 spiralbound. ISBN 0-918276-74-8.

This is an excellent source of funding information for student nurses and nurses. It is not just scholarships for nursing students. The coverage is for regular credit courses, continuing education classes, research, seminars, workshops, conference attendance, and a category titled creative activities. The funding sources include grants, loans, awards, forgivable loans, fellowships, scholarships, and traineeships. The text of the book is divided by the above categories instead of alphabetically to give it ease of use—no more flipping between the index and text for entries. Each entry includes the book entry number; official name of the funds; the name, address, phone, e-mail and Website of the sponsoring organization; purpose; eligibility; amount of funds; time period of funding; special features; limitations; number awarded; and the deadline for applying. The book does not cover programs that exclude U.S. citizens and residents or funding offered only by a school for their program. There are five indexes in the book: sponsoring organization, residency, tenability, nursing specialty, and calendar. The indexes make the book's information more accessible if one is looking for funding from a specific organization, for geographical areas, or for deadline date. This is an excellent tool, especially for the working nurse, since it provides all types of funding information not related directly to college credit classes. This volume is recommended for all hospital libraries and other libraries that serve nursing clientele.—**Betsy J. Kraus**

142. **Scholarships and Loans for Nursing Education 1997-1998.** New York, NLN Press, 1997. index. $16.95pa. ISBN 0-88737-730-0.

The previous title for this annual was *Scholarships and Loans for Beginning Education in Nursing* (1972-1983). Updated yearly, this reference tool attempts to identify as many funding sources as possible and to be comprehensive. The present edition has been increased from 124 pages to 141 pages, with the "Special Awards, Postdoctoral Study, and Research Grants" section expanded.

This book includes "all types of scholarships, awards, grants, fellowships, and loans for nursing education and nursing and health science research." Public, private, Canadian, governmental, academic, and profit or nonprofit funding agencies are listed for those wishing to apply for financial assistance in pursing a nursing career. The programs are listed alphabetically. Each agency entry is annotated, with contact information listed. There are numeric codes that categorize the funding level, with "1" being "Beginning RN Study" to "7" being "Special Grants, Research, Traineeships, or Postdoctoral Work" to a special category for minority students. Codes are placed next to each heading to determine the level of appropriateness for the financial seekers.

The appendix is a listing of addresses of the State Boards of Nursing. The index is grouped by the numeric codes mentioned above, the NLN Constituent Leagues for Nursing, and nursing specialties. The readers can consult the index for a quick rundown of all the programs listed in the chapters. This book is a great reference source for those who seeking funding for their nursing education. To catch up with the recent advances in information technology, it would be ideal if NLN inserted e-mail addresses for contact and Website addresses for each funding organization. This little paperback, with solid information, can be easily carried around and is highly recommended for inclusion in any nursing library or health science library.—**Polin P. Lei**

143.   Stoll, Malaika. **The Complete Book of Medical Schools 2001.** New York, Princeton Review/Random House, 2000. 392p. maps. index. $20.00pa. ISBN 0-375-76153-5. ISSN 1067-2176.

The Complete Book of Medical Schools 2001 is the latest yearly edition of what The Princeton Review has previously titled, *Student Access Guide to the Best Medical Schools* (1996 ed.; see ARBA 96, entry1705) and *The Best Medical Schools* (see entry 137). The most significant change from previous editions is the replacement of "Best" with "Complete" in the title and the exclusion of the Annual Nationwide Medical Student Survey results chapter.

Among the individual chapter titles are: "How to Use This Book," "So You Want to Be a Doctor…," "Advice for the 'Nontraditional' Applicant," "Financing Medical School," "The Interview," "Allopathic Profiles," "Osteopathic Profiles," and "Post-Baccalaureate Pre-Medical Programs." The profiles' chapters furnish valuable information on aspects of individual medical schools, such as academics, admissions policies, student body characteristics, costs, and financial aid. There are an alphabetic and a regional index to schools and 12 handy blank pages at the end of the volume for notes.

The primary audience for this affordable book is college students interested in medical school. Additionally, both secondary school and community college career counselors will find this book very helpful. This book is recommended for individuals interested in information on individual medical schools as well as secondary school, community college, and university libraries with career collections.—**Lynn M. McMain**

HANDBOOKS AND YEARBOOKS

144.   **Annual Guide to Graduate Nursing Education 1997.** Delroy Louden and Dawnette Jones, eds. New York, NLN Press, 1997. 132p. $27.95pa. ISBN 0-88737-749-1.

This guide has been a useful annual general reference tool for nursing students who seek higher education opportunities in the United States since 1995. The information collected is based on data collected by NLN Press from more than 300 master's and doctoral programs across the nation. Any data changes after November 1996 will not be reflected in this source. The publication is divided into 5 sections. Section 1 is the executive summary and contains tables of emerging infections. Sections 2 and 3 are the "Master's Degree Programs" and the "Doctoral Degree Programs." The programs are arranged alphabetically by state. The information about each program includes the name of school, address, director, telephone number, NLN accreditation, number of graduates in 1996, enrollments in 1996, length of study, program options, master of science in nursing (MSN) for nonregistered nurses with a degree in another field, tuition, and areas of study with specialization. Section 4 is on research projects funded by the National Institute of Nursing Research, with topics varying from wound healing to cancer. This is a good stop to locate institutions and contact persons for funding. Section 5 covers states that recognize clinical nurse specialists in advanced practice. This section lists the statute or regulation citation, requirements for recognition, and prescriptive authority. For the next update, perhaps it would be helpful if the Website of each institution offering programs is included so that readers can perform Net navigating as well. This publication is a must in academic nursing libraries.—**Polin P. Lei**

145.   **Exploring Health Care Careers.** 2d ed. Andrew Morkes, Carol Yehling, and Anne Paterson, eds. Chicago, Ferguson, 2002. 2v. index. $89.95/set. ISBN 0-89434-311-4.

Including over 100 careers in the health sciences, each with its own chapter, there is a plethora of information on each career listed in this 2-volume set. The chapters have multiple sections:

defining the job, describing educational and personal skill requirements, providing certification and licensing requirements, future outlook, and potential salary earnings. The unique and impressive aspect of each chapter is the "What is it like to be a . . .?" section. This section includes an interview with a person actually practicing in the profiled career, providing a perspective that goes beyond mundane data by adding a realistic and experience-based discussion of each job. Every chapter has a bibliography and a list of professional organizations with contact information. The second volume ends with three indexes: a Guide for Occupational Exploration index, an Occupational Information Network-Standard Occupational Classification (O*NET-SOC) index, and a standard job title index. This two-volume set will be a great addition to any public library, secondary school library, or a career counselor's bookshelf.—**Lynn M. McMain**

146.　Field, Shelly. **Career Opportunities in Health Care.** 2d ed. New York, Facts on File, 2002. 243p. index. $44.50. ISBN 0-8160-4816-9.

This guide provides a good starting place for researching careers in the health industry. The 80 brief, easy-to-understand commentaries span those requiring little formal education (e.g., medical clerk, food service worker) to those that require advanced degrees (e.g., physicians, dentists). Each two-page entry furnishes a career profile, description of work, employment and advancement prospects, salaries, needed education and training, and suggested skills and personality types that would encourage success.

Career information was acquired from a variety of sources—college catalogs, books, magazines, and media programs. Some information was elicited through questionnaires and interviews of those working in the fields. The author also acknowledges friends and business acquaintances for providing data. Although potentially accurate, this causes the guide to pale by comparison to the authoritative details provided by the U.S. Department of Labor's *Occupational Outlook Handbook* (OOH; 2000-2001 ed., see ARBA 2001, entry 197). The OOH also has broader coverage, supplying information on more than 250 careers in many diverse fields.

A few details are overlooked or misrepresented. Many occupations within the health care industry require state licensure. This important requirement is often noted (dental hygienist, pharmacist, physical therapist), but inexplicably excluded in the case of optometrists and registered nurses. It also seems that the employment prospects for nurses should be considered "excellent" rather than "good" given the current documented national nursing shortage and increased hiring and education initiatives.

This guide deserves a place on a guidance or career counselor's shelf. It is a good source for the beginning stages of research, but not reliable or comprehensive enough to use for a final career decision.—**Susan K. Setterlund**

147.　Ludmerer, Kenneth M. **Time to Heal: American Medical Education from the Turn of the Century to the Era of Managed Care.** New York, Oxford University Press, 1999. 514p. index. $29.95. ISBN 0-19-511837-5.

Many important question concerning the growth of American medicine in the twentieth century are examined in-depth in this thought provoking, densely written book by Kenneth Ludmerer, one of the nation's leading medical historians and a practicing physician. Picking up on the evolution of American medical education where his left off in his 1985 widely acclaimed text, *Learning to Heal*, the author, using unparalleled access to the archives of one-quarter of America's medical schools, details many of the key factors that fostered the growth of American medical education.

From the rapid public acceptance of the Flexner Report though World War II, America's medical schools have quickly surpassed their European counterparts. Ludmerer clearly describes the growth of these American institutions where faculty time was equitably divided between teaching medical students, doing limited research, and providing medical care for the sickest and poorest groups of patients. These medical schools gained the public's trust, and subsequently the public's financial supports by turning out an ever increasing supply of high-quality physicians, making medical discoveries that were shared with the community doctors, thus improving the public's health and providing the bulk of the nation's charity health care.

Ludmerer spends almost half of the book examining how medical schools lost the American public's trust and their former close ties to their university communities. He also examines how they encountered an erosion of their learning environments for both medical students and house staff and seemed to be moving backwards toward the proprietary medical school model of the late nineteenth century when the financial interests of the faculty superseded all other institutional goals. He describes a complex collection of external and internal conditions that have led to this drastic reduction in the quality of American medical education including the decline of American cities, a new adversarial relationship with both federal and state governments, and competition between community and teaching hospitals. The loss of the physicians' moral authority in society and the harsh realities created by managed care in the past 15 years that severely limits the faculty's time for teaching and the students' access to patients are also discussed.

Ludmerer ends with a challenge to all parties interested in correcting the current weaknesses in American medical education. He calls on medical school administrators and faculty to sacrifice part of their financial gains and resume a leadership role in protecting both quality medical education and the public's access to the best medical care. American health centers must focus more on chronic diseases and produce the types of physicians demanded by the public. Medical education must learn from history that to regain the public's trust and support, medical schools have to provide top-quality education, produce medical research that meets the public's rather than the scientists' interests, and ensure that they will fight for the American public's right to the best, most affordable form of health care.

This book sends a powerful message to medical educators, health care leaders, and the general public. Health care and public libraries will find this work an indispensable reference source for questions concerning the history and current status of the American medical educational system.—**Jonathon Erlen**

148.   Lyons, Dianne J. B. **Planning Your Career in Alternative Medicine: A Guide to Degree and Certificate Programs in Alternative Health Care.** Garden City Park, N.Y., Avery Publishing, 1997. 423p. index. $19.95pa. ISBN 0-89529-802-3.

As an introductory guide and selective directory to higher education opportunities in the varied fields of alternative medicine, this work provides the reader with some good basic descriptions of concepts, programs, curricula, sources, and resources. Fields of interest include aromatherapy, Ayurveda, biofeedback, chiropractic, energy healing, environmental medicine, guided imagery, herbal medicine, holistic health care fields, homeopathy, hypnotherapy, integrative medicine, iridology, massage therapy and bodywork, natrapathy, naturopathy, nutrition, polarity therapy, reflexology, traditional Chinese medicine, Vedic psychology, veterinary massage, and yoga. Basic descriptions and overviews are provided for each of these areas, followed by a listing of schools and programs. It is this latter listing that comprises most of the volume. Appendixes include listings and descriptions of accrediting agencies and councils, licensing and certification requirements, professional associations and membership organizations, self-study resources, and conventional medical schools offering courses in alternative medicine.

In an introductory section, the author explains the criteria for inclusion of various schools, but not for all. In some cases, accreditation is a criterion; in others, return of a survey questionnaire. In still other cases, no indication of criteria is given at all. This results in a work of somewhat uneven quality, leaving the reader seeking sound information on shaky ground. A listing of "Top

Schools and Programs," based upon a mail questionnaire sent to practitioners, provides no indication of the population sampled or the number of questionnaires returned. Listings of associations are also limited, and can be supplemented by the most current edition of the *Encyclopedia of Associations* (Gale).

Some public and school libraries might find this volume useful. However, it should be complemented by a variety of other reference tools—dictionaries, encyclopedias, directories—that can provide more substantial information for those contemplating a career in alternative medicine. Although this volume provides some good basic information, it seems too arbitrary and selective in its approach to be able to provide a true picture of the variety of career options.—**Edmund F. Santa Vicca**

3   Medicine

GENERAL WORKS

Dictionaries and Encyclopedias

149. **The American Heritage Stedman's Medical Dictionary.** New York, Houghton Mifflin, 2002. 923p. $27.00. ISBN 0-618-25415-3.

Stedman's Medical Dictionary was originally written in 1949 by Thomas Stedman and published by Williams and Wilkins. American Heritage is the new publisher. The dictionary contains current, accurate information about medical terms for professionals and general readers in allied medical fields, law, and the insurance industry. A special feature of *Stedman's* provides a list of more than 250 selected main entries that have subentries in traditional dictionaries as an aid for users familiar with that arrangement. The work includes more than 100 line drawings, charts, and tables and a subject index to entries. All public, college, and medial libraries should purchase *American Heritage Stedman's Medical Dictionary* for their collections.—**Theresa Maggio**

150. **The Cambridge Encyclopedia of Human Paleopathology.** By Arthur C. Aufderheide, Conrado Rodríquez-Martín, and Odin Langsjoen. New York, Cambridge University Press, 1998. 478p. illus. index. $100.00. ISBN 0-521-55203-6.

Nowhere other than in the study of human diseases is it so obvious that humans are only one of a vast array of life forms on this planet. This encyclopedia is a major reference work for all those interested in the identification of disease in human remains. The scope of the encyclopedia encompasses almost every disease that produces in human tissues an anatomic pathological change large enough to be detected by the unaided eye.

The most active research areas are explored, including the following: circulatory disorders, joint diseases, infectious diseases, diseases of the viscera, metabolic diseases, endocrine disorders, hematological disorders, skeletal dysplasia, and neoplastic conditions. In addition, a dental chapter by Langsjoen is included. Each chapter consists of several sections. The chapter on infectious disease, for example, contains various articles about bacterial, viral, and fungal infections. All articles are designed as self-contained treatments of important topics in human paleopathology and are presented on a first-principle basis, including appropriate charts, detailed figures, photographs, tables, and drawings. "Natural History" sections are employed to present the disease as a succession of tissue events that gradually cause and shape the final form of the lesions. "Antiquity, History and Epidemiology" sections are included to help maximize the integration of identified pathological conditions with information about archaeological, anthropological, cultural, and other aspects of a studied ancient population. The authors intentionally omitted a glossary of basic terms in order to prevent themselves from minimizing medical vocabulary. A subject index is included.

This major reference work will meet the needs of investigators and consultants. It will aid them in identifying the nature of the disease and in its diagnosis. The suggested reading audience will be mostly physicians and anthropologists.—**Marilynn Green Hopman**

151.   Cockerham, William C., and Ferris J. Ritchey. **Dictionary of Medical Sociology.** Westport, Conn., Greenwood Press, 1997. 169p. index. $69.50. ISBN 0-313-29269-8.

Since the inception of the discipline of medical sociology over four decades ago a special terminology has evolved in this field. The authors created this small dictionary to define these terms for the broad range of health practitioners, medical economists, health insurance companies, and hospital administrators as well as sociologists working in this area. A brief introductory essay traces the origins and evolution of medical sociology, discussing some of its pioneers such as Talcott Parsons, and the struggle to combine the applied and theoretical aspects of this emerging discipline.

The definitions that comprise the main part of the text vary from one sentence to several pages in length. Cross-references appear in bold typeface. The main problems with this limited dictionary are the inclusion and exclusion of certain terms, and the lack of accuracy and depth of some of the definitions. Although the authors state their rationales for inclusion and exclusion of terms in the preface, one has to question the inclusion of such standard medical concepts as allied health, ambulatory care, chiropractic medicine, and preventive care. Why include AIDS and not tuberculosis and cancer? More troubling are the inaccuracies in some of the definitions. The incorrect date of and information about the significant 1910 Flexner Report, providing only a partial description of the laws governing homeopathy, and the failure to mention the 1957 legal case that created the legal doctrine of informed consent are examples of this. There is a useful unannotated bibliography on medical sociology and an index is provided.

Overall, there is little in this rather expensive volume that cannot be found in other dictionaries. Although academic libraries might find this work of limited use, there is little reason for a health-related library to acquire this reference text.—**Jonathon Erlen**

152.   Davis, Neil M. **Medical Abbreviations: 12,000 Conveniences at the Expense of Communications and Safety.** 8th ed. Huntington Valley, Pa., Neil M. Davis, 1997. 332p. index. $15.95pa. ISBN 0-931431-08-5.

This text consists of thousands of useful medical abbreviations and symbols. The author has designed this text in an easy-to-use fashion, and individuals involved in health care will probably find this text to be of help when documenting or translating patient reports or medical reports. Basically, if people find a medical symbol or term that does not make sense, they should try looking in this book.

This text has 6 chapters. Chapter 1 is an introduction that offers the reader options on how to use the text and warns the reader that some of the "terms" may need to be confirmed because they may not be universally acceptable. Chapter 2, "A Healthcare Controlled Vocabulary," explains how medical terms are used, and how confusion and possible errors can arise. Individuals who decide to use this text should read chapters 1 and 2 initially to understand how such errors can occur. Chapter 3, "Lettered Abbreviations and Acronyms," comprises the majority of this text and offers thousands of abbreviations and symbols that can be found in the world of medicine. Readers should remember to confirm the proper use of terms and symbols prior to using them in the event that they are not acceptable in their area of specialty. Chapter 4 introduces hundreds of symbols and numbers that the reader will find useful. Chapter 5 is essentially a pharmacology guide to the trade and generic names of select medications. Chapter 6 provides multiple laboratory values, a nice feature to have in such a text. The last few pages of the text are left blank for the user to make notes.

Overall, this work is a user-friendly and practical text from which most individuals involved in health care could probably benefit. Although this text will not help in resuscitating an acutely ill patient, it will be helpful in documenting and charting the patient's medical records and lab reports.—**Paul M. Murphy III**

153. **Delmar's English/Spanish Pocket Dictionary for Health Professionals.** By Rochelle K. Kelz. Albany, N.Y., Delmar, 1997. 516p. illus. $17.95pa. ISBN 0-8273-6171-8.

With a large Spanish-speaking population seeking health care, providers who have little knowledge of the language need assistance in communicating. This compact dictionary of medical and dental terms will help. The author, a professor who specializes in medical Spanish, has created a work that contains "tens of thousands of words and phrases" (p. vii). The emphasis of the dictionary is pragmatic, everyday usage to promote communication between health care workers and patients. Entries include common slang and vulgarisms as well as medical and scientific cognates from the Latin and Greek. Because most Spanish speakers in the United States come from Mexico, Puerto Rico, Cuba, Central America, and the Dominican Republic, regional words and phrases from these areas are featured.

The text is arranged in two columns with the entry words in bold typeface. Although the book is small, the typeface is clear and easy to read. The translations are brief, and related words or expressions are included in the same entry; for example, *development; arrested -; delayed -; speech -; -of an x-ray film; -of an idea.* A section between the English-Spanish and Spanish-English parts of the dictionary lists anatomic terms and features black-and-white drawings labeled in both languages.

This dictionary will be useful for health care workers who are studying Spanish. Some knowledge of the language is necessary to use it effectively. Those who need to communicate immediately should use a source such as *CommuniMed Multilingual Patient Assessment Manual* (Mosby Lifeline, 1994), which contains a script for obtaining a basic medical history in 20 languages. *Delmar's English/Spanish Pocket Dictionary for Health Professionals* is a welcome addition to both health sciences collections and personal libraries.—**Barbara M. Bibel**

154. **Dictionary of Medicine.** 2d ed. P. H. Collin, ed. Middlesex, Great Britain, Peter Collin, 1993; repr., Chicago, Fitzroy Dearborn, 1998. 393p. illus. $55.00. ISBN 1-57958-074-2.

First published in the United Kingdom, this plain medical dictionary defines fairly simple terms that most individuals understand or believe they understand. Using a limited vocabulary of 500 words to define each of the 12,000 main terms, this dictionary gives clear explanations of the various terminology used in the medical profession. In-depth discussion, symptomatology, and causation are rarely indicated. Each entry provides the parts of speech and multiple definitions when appropriate; some include sentences demonstrating proper usage, while others include "comments" or "quotes." The comment on emphysema states that the disease can be caused by smoking, among other causes. Quotes are obtained from reputable sources—*Lancet*, *Nursing Times*, and the *Journal of the American Medical Association*. Common acronyms and abbreviations used by doctors and in hospitals are identified with accurate reference to a definition—OP stands for Outpatient and GDC stands for General Dental Council. Common names for diseases refer to the formal medical terminology. Lou Gehrig's Disease refers to Amyotrophic Lateral Sclerosis. Few entries, such as the eye, include a detailed illustration of the organ.

Not to replace more popular medical reference books, this dictionary provides clear and simple definitions to help young adults and adults understand common medical terminology.

Originating in the United Kingdom, this title does have a bias towards British spelling and usage.
—**Susan D. Strickland**

155.   **Diseases.** rev. ed. Bryan Bunch, ed. Danbury, Conn., Grolier Educational, 2003. 8v. illus. index. $299.00/set. ISBN 0-7172-5688-X.

The study of human disease is inherently interesting. In the middle school and high school curriculum, units on human disease are included in health or science classes as a sure-fire way of capturing student interest. An encyclopedia like this is a perfect starting place for the papers and other research projects students are assigned in these courses.

The eight volumes of this set contain hundreds of entries, including diseases, symptoms, and body systems. Special attention is given to diseases of particular interest to young people—from acne to sexually transmitted diseases. This is a revision of a 1997 publication (see ARBA 98, entry 1557), which has been updated to include discussions on some of the new and emerging diseases (e.g., Ebola Virus), diseases in the news (e.g., West Nile Virus), and issues of current interest (e.g., stem cells). Entries are arranged alphabetically and include pronunciation, classification (disease, disorder, symptoms), and type (infectious, environmental, cause unknown). The text for each entry is one to three pages, giving the cause, incidence, symptoms, diagnosis, treatment options, stages, and progress of the disease, and possible prevention measures. All of this is written in a very readable style with few technical terms; it is very accessible to middle school students. The graphic arrangement too is very pleasing and well organized. A clever feature is the use of icons to denote important points, such as "call an ambulance," "avoid alcohol," and so on. There is a detailed index to the entire set included in each volume—an important feature for library and class use.

There are many Websites useful in researching medical and health topics. A few are given in the introduction to the first volume of this encyclopedia, along with some other information sources such as newsletters and books. However, most of these other sources are presented in a form most accessible to adults or medical professionals. This set of books presents information at a middle school level, making it a good first step for students researching a disease.—**Carol L. Noll**

156.   **Encyclopedia of Family Health.** Tarrytown, N.Y., Marshall Cavendish, 1998. 17v. illus. index. $499.95/set. ISBN 0-7614-0625-5.

First published in 1971 in England, Marshall Cavendish's *Encyclopedia of Family Health* is a source of basic medical and health information. The current edition, prepared with David B. Jacoby of the Johns Hopkins University School of Medicine, is aimed at U.S. readers. British spelling, usage, and vocabulary have been eliminated.

This edition continues to present simple, profusely illustrated articles on anatomy, physiology, health care, diseases, and conditions. The alphabetic entries range in length from one to three pages. Each entry has a sidebar with questions and answers that serve as an introduction to the topic. The text is written in language that is accessible to readers from middle school to adult levels. Many new illustrations and articles have been added, and older articles have been revised in varying degrees. *AIDS* has been extensively updated with the latest information on the HIV viruses and treatment options. *Cancer*, however, needs further revision. Treatments are covered superficially, and the book states that hormonal therapy has no unpleasant side effects. The first aid guide in volume 17 contains obsolete information and errors in the protocols for treating choking and performing cardiopulmonary resuscitation. New articles include "Acid Rain," "Carpal Tunnel Syndrome," "Mind-Body Therapy," and "Sick Building Syndrome." The entries dealing with alternative therapies, such as aromatherapy, are objective.

Volume 1 has a table of contents for the entire set. The other volumes have tables of contents for their own entries. The addition of cross-references to this edition makes finding related material easy. A glossary and a short list of U.S. and Canadian associations for referral complement the text. A bibliography of recent books provides further information. Most of the works are current, but the 1993 edition of *The Mayo Clinic Family Health Book* is listed instead of the 1996 edition. Alphabetic subject indexes complete the work.

Encyclopedia of Family Health serves as a starting point for students doing reports and patrons in need of basic information. Those who need greater depth can consult *The Merck Manual of Medical Information* (see entry 193). *Everything You Need to Know About Medical Emergencies* (Springhouse, 1997) provides current, accurate information on first aid. The encyclopedia's ease of use, accessibility, and illustrations make it a good, but rather expensive, addition to school and public library collections. [R: RUSQ, Summer 98, p. 376] —**Barbara M. Bibel**

157. **Encyclopedia of U.S. Biomedical Policy.** Robert H. Blank and Janna C. Merrick, eds. Westport, Conn., Greenwood Press, 1996. 363p. index. $89.50. ISBN 0-313-28641-8.

Encyclopedia of U.S. Biomedical Policy is a compendium of U.S. biomedical policy since the early 1970s. The goal of the encyclopedia is to focus on subjects that relate directly to the array of issues on the public agenda raised by the use of biomedical technologies. The focus is on public policy. The purpose of this encyclopedia is to shed light on a range of public decisions that face society. Decision-making has become more complex as an array of biomedical issues have been raised, such as human genetics and reproduction issues, prenatal and neonatal issues, biomedical issues within the life cycle, and death-related issues.

Entries are arranged alphabetically and are cross-referenced with an asterisk to related entries. The extensive index offers another means of cross-checking entries by subject. Entries vary in length. They include a mixture of legislation and court cases, as well as descriptions of key government agencies, private organizations, technologies, and issue areas. Each entry has a short, selected bibliography of key sources for further reading. Entries are authoritative. Entries include such subjects as egg donation, euthanasia, RU-486 (the abortion pill), the Human Genome Project, and HIV testing. Appendix A is a chronology of key events, court cases, and legislation and can be read as a summary of the cumulative development of policy activity in biomedicine. Appendix B provides a directory of key sources of information.

This easily accessible reference source describes court cases, legislation, public policies, technologies, issues, key government agencies, and private organizations dealing with the complex economic, cultural, social, and political context for biomedical decision-making. The resource is recommended for students and professors; policy-makers; public administrators; college, university, and special libraries; and public libraries.—**Marilynn Green Hopman**

158. **The Gale Encyclopedia of Medicine.** 2d ed. Jaqueline L. Longe and Deirdre S. Blanchfield, eds. Farmington Hills, Mich., Gale, 2002. 5v. illus. index. $525.00/set. ISBN 0-7876-5489-2.

This five-volume set is intended for the lay person needing a source with more information than consumer brochures or health education materials hold but not as comprehensive as the ones designed for medical professionals. It contains more than 1,600 articles covering disorders and conditions and tests and treatments. The volumes follow a standard format for disorders and conditions containing definitions; descriptions; causes; symptoms; diagnosis; treatment (including alternative treatments); prognosis; prevention; key terms; and bibliographies that include books, periodicals, organizations, and Websites. The key terms are in a gray shaded box and explain terms used in the text. The format for tests and treatments provides definitions, purpose, precautions, descriptions, preparation, aftercare, risks, normal/abnormal results, resources, and key terms. The volumes are arranged alphabetically with disorders and conditions and tests and treatments interfiled. Each entry is clearly written, without using medical jargon unfamiliar to the general public and illustrated (if necessary) for a better understanding of the topic. The illustrations are either drawings or photographs and are usually in color for better clarity. There is an extensive index with cross-references. The alphabetic list of organizations includes the address, telephone number, and Website for each entry. This is an excellent encyclopedia for the nonmedical person. It would be an excellent purchase for the public library, a health education library, or a medical office for patient's usage and is highly recommended. [R: Choice, May 02, p. 1564]—**Betsy J. Kraus**

159. Gilbert, Patricia. **Dictionary of Syndromes and Inherited Disorders.** 3d ed. Chicago, Fitzroy Dearborn, 2000. 373p. index. $45.00. ISBN 1-57958-226-5.

The number of syndromes in child health care is rapidly increasing and few doctors, social workers, school counselors, and parents are able to recognize the early onset of these conditions. This reference work is intended for the broad audience of health care providers, educators, and families who are forced to confront the complexity of this wide range of childhood health syndromes.

The compiler uses two criteria for selecting the 100 syndromes included in this volume: the syndrome must produce long-term or lifelong physical or mental problems, and there must be assistance available to deal with these conditions. The type of information provided for each syndrome includes alternative names, incidences, history, causation, characteristics, management implications, and future goals. There is also contact information for self-help groups that are valuable to parents trying to handle their children's health problems.

This 3d edition includes 20 additional syndromes as well as an expanded glossary. Thorough indexing directs the reader to both specific disease conditions and general health categories. These updates, along with the self-help group material, make this reference guide considerably more useful for the general public than standard syndrome dictionaries that contain briefer and much more technical coverage. [R: Choice, Sept 2000, p. 95; BL, 15 Oct 2000, p. 478]—**Jonathon Erlen**

160. Haubrich, William S. **Medical Meanings: A Glossary of Word Origins.** Philadelphia, American College of Physicians, 1997. 253p. $29.95. ISBN 0-943126-56-8.

Understanding medical terminology can be a challenge. There are several excellent, comprehensive medical dictionaries available, but they provide only brief information about the origins of the words that they define. Serious students of language will want more depth. *Medical Meanings* is a delightful supplement to the traditional dictionary.

The book has approximately 3,000 entries arranged in 2 columns per page. Arrangement is alphabetic with a few exceptions: Broad categories, such as colors, numbers, and phobias, are grouped together under one heading. The entry headings are in bold typeface, and words within the entry in languages other than modern English are in italics. Greek terms are transliterated. The introduction contains instructions for using the book, a Greek transliteration table, and an invitation to send suggestions for improving the work to the author.

What sets *Medical Meanings* apart from the traditional dictionary is the text. Neither syllabication nor pronunciation appear. The entries are short etymological essays tracing the history of the word and offering witty comments. For example, the entry for AIDS states, "Often when a medical condition is poorly understood, it is described rather than specifically named, and it is called a syndrome when its status as an entity is uncertain" (p. 7). The entry on hysterectomy, literally "cutting the uterus," leads to a discussion of Plato's belief that the uterus was an animal roaming freely within the female body and causing moodiness. The author wisely concludes, "A safe assumption is that this notion was proclaimed and promoted, in the main, by men. From this anatomic designation comes the term hysteria, a term doubtless conceived by a confirmed male chauvinist" (p. 107).

Although this is a small volume—the 28th edition of *Dorland's Illustrated Medical Dictionary* (Saunders, 1994) has 115,000 entries—it makes a unique contribution to medical reference by focusing on history and etymology rather than clinical usage. Students of linguistics will find it as useful as students of the health sciences. Those who want more than a definition will find the book enjoyable and entertaining. The work is an excellent companion to traditional dictionaries, and it belongs in health sciences collections. [R: LJ, 15 May 97, p. 72]—**Barbara M. Bibel**

161. **Human Diseases and Conditions.** Neil Izenberg, ed. Farmington Hills, Mich., Charles Scribner's Sons/Gale Group, 2000. 3v. illus. index. $245.00/set. ISBN 0-684-80543-X.

The human body and its ailments are fascinating subjects for most people. Much of the literature in this area is very technical and difficult for lay readers to understand. *Human Diseases and Conditions*, although edited by a group of physicians, is written for readers from middle school to adult level. The 3-volume set has information on 294 diseases and conditions.

An introduction provides a very basic overview of physiology, the health care system, and medical research. The alphabetical entries that follow are two to six pages long. They include a definition of the disease or condition; an explanation of what it does to the body; and information on the causes, symptoms, diagnosis, and treatment. Many articles also have short scenarios describing people who have had or currently live with the illness. Pictures of Stephen Hawking, Magic Johnson, and Jackie Joyner-Kersey accompany the entries on amyotrophic lateral sclerosis, AIDS, and asthma, respectively. References to Michael J. Fox, Muhammad Ali, and Janet Reno in the article on Parkinson's disease demonstrate that serious illness does not have to interfere with life. Articles on chronic diseases such as diabetes and cystic fibrosis explain what it is like to live with the illness. All articles have brief bibliographies and referral lists.

There are ample cross-references and a comprehensive index to lead users to the information they need. A bibliography of recent medical textbooks appears in the third volume. Several color photographs, charts, and illustrations augment the text. Sidebars in the margins provide definitions and keywords for searching other reference sources and the Internet. Fact boxes offer historical information and literary quotations about diseases. These features enliven the text.

While *Human Diseases and Conditions* is an attractive encyclopedia that is easy to use, it provides very basic information that is readily available in many other sources. It is also rather expensive. The *Harvard Medical School Family Health Guide* (Simon & Schuster, 1999) and the *American College of Physicians Complete Home Medical Guide* (DK, 1999) provide more information in a single volume at a fraction of the price. The *Gale Encyclopedia of Medicine* (2d ed.; see entry 158) is a multivolume set that covers this material in greater depth. *Human Diseases and Conditions* is an optional purchase for school and public libraries. [R: SLJ, May 2000, pp. 86-88; BL, July 2000, p. 2062; VOYA, Aug 2000, p. 212; RUSQ, Sept 2000, pp. 413-414; BR, Sept/Oct 2000, p. 66]—**Barbara M. Bibel**

162. **Human Diseases and Conditions: Behavioral Health and Disorders. Supplement 1.** Neil Izenberg and Steven A. Dowshen, eds. New York, Charles Scribner's Sons/Gale Group, 2001. 463p. illus. index. $80.00. ISBN 0-684-80643-6.

This first supplement to the three-volume *Human Diseases and Conditions* set (see entry 161) focuses on developmental, emotional, and psychological conditions and their treatments. The 98 alphabetic entries follow introductory material that defines behavioral health and explains the function of the brain and the nervous system. Each article begins with a definition of the main entry term. A brief case history illustrating the condition appears at the beginning of most articles. Further information about the signs, symptoms, and treatment options complete the article. All entries have resource lists that include organizations, books, hotlines, and Websites.

Sidebars and color boxes contain supplementary material, such as definitions of key terms, brief articles on related issues, and biographies of important contributors to the field or famous people with the disorder. Color photographs and charts enhance the text. Cross-references make it easy to locate related material. A bibliography and a cumulative index of the set supplement and complete the volume. With a variety of articles covering disorders (addiction, mental retardation, stress, suicide), social issues (homelessness, violence, divorce), and physiological topics (brain chemistry, memory, birth defects), this supplement will be very useful as a starting point for middle and high school students doing reports. Although owning the entire set will allow students to locate all of the indexed material, this volume can stand alone.—**Barbara M. Bibel**

163.   Isler, Charlotte. **The Patient's Guide to Medical Terminology.** 3d ed. Los Angeles, Calif., Health Information Press, 1997. 258p. $12.95pa. ISBN 1-885987-08-0.

Few fields are filled with as much specialized and obfuscatory terminology as medicine. Yet, in no other area is it so important that laypeople understand what specialists are telling them. This reference guide is just the tool for the patient who walks out of the doctor's office confused as to the meaning of a diagnosis, test, or treatment. It also could be invaluable in translating the medical language in billing statements or correspondence with insurance companies. The guide is divided into 3 parts. The 1st is a list of abbreviations with one-word definitions. There are more than 30 pages in this section, which contains most acronyms commonly used by medical professionals, an indication of the enormity of the problem facing the uninformed patient. Section 2 is an alphabetic list of terms, with clear, understandable definitions. A valuable feature is the inclusion of normal ranges of values for the results of diagnostic tests. The coverage is comprehensive, including pediatric to geriatric conditions, both common and obscure. The contents are particularly valuable for the myriad of tests involved in the modern management of pregnancy. Finally, at the end of the guide is a short section explaining some of the measurement units used in diagnostic results and prescriptions.

A guide such as this should be in every doctor's waiting room. More and more, patients must be the managers in managed care, and the first step is being able to speak, or at least understand, the language.—**Carol L. Noll**

164.   Kay, Margarita Artschwager. **Southwestern Medical Dictionary: Spanish-English, English-Spanish.** 2d ed. Tucson, Ariz., University of Arizona Press, 2001. 308p. illus. $17.95pa. ISBN 0-8165-0529-2.

Patients and health care providers use different vocabularies when discussing health and illness. Add the fact that the patient's first language is Spanish, and the communication gap increases. Kay, a professor emerita of nursing at the University of Arizona, wrote the 1st edition of the *Southwestern Medical Dictionary* in 1977. This new edition incorporates suggestions from users of the previous version. The dictionary will help health care providers and patients understand each other.

The *Southwestern Medical Dictionary* uses "Norteno" Spanish that is spoken in Arizona and the Mexican state of Sonora, but many of the words are part of the Chicano Spanish vocabulary. The dictionary has approximately 3,000 entries. Part 1, "Spanish-English," offers words with simple definitions and sentences illustrating their usage. The emphasis is on idiomatic usage in both languages. For example, the English expression, "You can take pills," becomes the passive construction, "Se puede tomar pastillas," in Spanish. Part 2, "English-Spanish," contains the most common lay and biomedical terms with brief Spanish definitions and English synonyms. A series of appendixes cover food-related words, kinship terms, and selected poisonous plants. The book also has basic anatomical charts labeled in both English and Spanish.

Although the *Southwestern Medical Dictionary* is a useful, portable source, it contains only 3,000 entries based on interviews that were very modest. Many terms, including common slang and the Spanish words found in the definitions provided in the English-Spanish section, do not appear. *Delmar's English/Spanish Pocket Dictionary for Health Professionals* (see entry 153) contains more than 20,000 entries comprising terms from more Spanish-speaking regions. These entries include slang, common vulgarism, and idioms. The wider scope makes it more useful for patrons.—**Barbara M. Bibel**

165. **Magill's Medical Guide.** 2d rev. ed. Tracy Irons-Georges, ed. Hackensack, N.J., Salem Press, 2002. 3v. illus. index. $325.00/set. ISBN 1-58765-003-7.

Magill's Medical Guide is a popular reference text for both health professionals and the general public. It provides the general reader with self-help guides and authoritative information, and it provides health professionals knowledge for their practice. This is a rare and valuable resource for most consumers.

This revised new three-volume edition is a key ready-reference tool in major libraries. Since its 1995 debut (see ARBA 96, entry 1700) this set has grown in size. It now contains 883 entries that describe major diseases and disorders of the human body, the basics of human anatomy and physiology, specializations in medical practice, and common medical procedures. The set also examines various diseases, both genetic and acquired, and the detailed knowledge of human bodily systems. New features include 18 revised articles; 39 newly commissioned articles; 101 new and expanded articles in a variety of new topics; updated bibliographies; and Websites, medical journals, and additional resources. The four new appendixes list journals, general bibliographies, provide a Website directory, and provide a resources list of support groups and organizations. Cross-references are available.

Since this source is encyclopedic in scope, the articles are arranged alphabetically with drawings and photographs. The index is in volume 3. This set also contains another new feature—"In the News" sidebars that evaluate recent media stories about ongoing research and experimental treatments. Critical insight of new treatment of certain medical conditions is provided. The articles range from brief 100-word definitions to 3,500-word overviews and are written by 265 writers from the fields of life science and medicine in academia. These articles are written in such a way that the general public can comprehend and use the content. [R: BL, 1 April 02, pp. 1356-1358]—**Polin P. Lei**

166. **Medical Discoveries: Medical Breakthroughs and the People Who Developed Them.** Bridget Travers and Fran Locher Freiman, eds. Detroit, U*X*L/Gale, 1997. 3v. illus. index. $79.95/set. ISBN 0-7876-0890-4.

Containing 215 entries, this 3-volume set profiles medical and dental inventions, discoveries, and practices that have advanced the health field. The individuals behind these breakthroughs are identified either within the article or in a separate entry devoted to their contributions. The set is alphabetically arranged over the 3 volumes and is written in nontechnical language. Each volume is prefaced with a timeline of medical events, a glossary of 100 terms used within the set, and a bibliography of resources for further investigation. Likewise, each volume contains a master index at the rear.

Entries vary in length from 200 to 2,500 words. Titles are boldfaced, with subheadings also in bold typeface, which assists the user in outlining the topic. Cross-references within and at the end of each entry are in bold typeface to draw the reader's attention to related information. Wide margins allow space for sidebars of related items of interest. Visual appeal is further enhanced by more than 150 black-and-white photographs. Filled boxes provide information that expands a topic. Controversial issues—such as breast implants and abortion—are noted under applicable topics without taking a position. More recent medical procedures, such as radial keratotomy, gamete intrafallopian transfer, and genetic engineering, are discussed.

Although the set covers its intended content, medical breakthroughs and the people behind them, it is not a health encyclopedia or biographical dictionary. Format and reading level are similar to other U*X*L titles. The set is recommended for school libraries in grades 5 through 10 or the children's area of public libraries. —**Elaine Ezell**

167.   Melloni, B. John, Gilbert M. Eisner, and June L. Melloni. **Melloni's Illustrated Medical Dictionary.** 4th ed. Edited by Ida G. Dox. Pearl River, N.Y., Parthenon. 2002. 764p. illus. $39.95. ISBN 1-85070-094-X.

Updated with more than 4,000 new entries and 500 line drawings, this dictionary continues to provide clear, concise definitions of current medical terminology. The integration of the illustrations and definitions not only improves comprehension of the defined term, but also aids in the retention of that information. Two colors are used in printing to highlight the illustrated definitions. Pronunciations now appear directly next to the corresponding term. The table of contents lists the full-page plates and various tables (e.g., arteries, bones, units and measures, vitamins). A brief guide to the Greek and Latin derivations of medical prefixes, suffixes, and combining forms is provided in addition to a considerable list of abbreviations. The clear, easily understood definitions and line drawings give this dictionary an audience beyond the health sciences professional or practitioner. Secondary school and public libraries, as well as medical libraries, should consider adding this book to their collections.—**Vicki J. Killion**

168.   **The Merck Manual. http://www.merckhomeedition.com.** [Website]. Merck & Company. Free. Date reviewed: Oct 02.

The Merck Manual has been a trustworthy source of information for more than a century for both medical professionals and laypersons. Now available in a full-text online version, this familiar work is made even more accessible and convenient. Users can search this source by using either a text version or an interactive version. The interactive version provides users with a "Quick Start Guide" and "A Guide for Users," both of which explain how to most effectively use this tool. The user can search *The Merck Manual* by selecting a section on the left-hand side of the screen (e.g., "Drugs," "Mental Health Disorders," "Blood Disorders") and then selecting the chapter they would like to research. There are about 10 chapters per section. Once a chapter has been selected a box of "Chapter Topics" displays the illustrations, animations, videos, and pronunciations that are available in that chapter. For instance, when researching skin disorders researchers can find photographs of dry skin disorders, an illustration of the skin layers, and a glossary of medical names for growths on the skin surface. Buttons at the top of the screen allow users to go forward and back, conduct a search, check the index, bookmark pages, and print.

This electronic resource provides all of the information of the print edition of *The Merck Manual* with the convenience of an online format. The information is updated regularly and corrections are posted. Libraries who use *The Merck Manual* regularly will want to bookmark this page for easy consultation.—**Shannon Graff Hysell**

169.   **On-line Medical Dictionary. http://cancerweb.ncl.ac.uk/omd/**. [Website]. Free. Date reviewed: Jan 03.

This free Website was designed in 1997 by Dr. Graham Dark in order to serve as a one-stop resource for those seeking definitions to medical terms. The site now contains more than 46,000 terms and new terms are added frequently. In fact, searches are logged and a list of terms that are frequently requested that are not available are listed. Users are encouraged to provide definitions of these terms, which are then carefully researched and edited by the Website's host. Terms included here come from a variety of fields related to medicine, including biochemistry, molecular biology, and chemistry. And, along with medical terms users will find acronyms, jargon, theories, institutions, and medical projects.

Medical terms can be search by clicking on the letter the term begins with or by clicking on the subject area of interest. The layout of the site is a bit confusing as the terms often run together and the user has to look through a long list. This takes away from the user-friendliness of the site. The wide spread use of cross-references (or links) throughout the site, however, make up for this inconvenience. For example, when looking up the term "obesity-related diseases" the user is given links to diabetes, stroke, heart attack, pickwickian syndrome, and gallstones, just to name a few. Also listed are the five previously listed terms and the five terms that follow "obesity-related diseases," many of which will lead the user to a greater understanding of the disease.

This site will be a useful site for librarians working the reference desk of academic and public libraries. The definitions provided are easy to understand and will often lead the user to further research.—**Shannon Graff Hysell**

170. **The Oxford Illustrated Companion to Medicine.** Stephen Lock, John M. Last, and George Dunea, eds. New York, Oxford University Press, 2001. 891p. illus. index. $60.00. ISBN 0-19-262950-6.

This guide will serve as an easy-to-use reference for those seeking basic information on the topics of the history of medicine, various diseases, medical practices in other countries, and medical and nursing specialties, just to name a few. Designed primarily for the educated lay reader, this work may also be a welcome addition in consumer health libraries and even academic medical libraries because of its interesting text and illustrative photographs.

The more than 500 entries are arranged alphabetically and run from a half page to several pages in length. The editors of this volume have changed the format some as compared to previous editions by adding sidebars that highlight key discoveries, diseases, and technologies. At times this interferes with the alphabetic organization; to remedy this there is extensive cross-referencing throughout the volume. For example, the entry on Salerno Medical School is placed within the entry on Italy, but there is a cross-reference to this when one looks under Salerno Medical School. There are four indexes located at the end of the volume to aid those using this tool for research: a topic index, a list of conditions and diseases, a people index, and a general index.

This encyclopedic work differs from many others available because of its focus on the history of medicine and the practice of medicine throughout the world. Even the photographs shown here are most often of the historical practice of medicine instead of current photographs. For its easy-to-comprehend style, this work is recommended for public and consumer health libraries, but it should be supplemented with other medical encyclopedias. [R: LJ, 1 April 02, p. 96]—**Shannon Graff Hysell**

171. **Routledge German Dictionary of Medicine, Volume 1: German-English/Deutsche-Englisch. Worterbuch Medizin Englisch.** 2d ed. By Fritz-Jurgen Nohring. New York, Routledge, 1997. 1117p. $150.00. ISBN 0-415-17130-X.

The 2d edition of this attractive, easy-to-use dictionary was necessitated by the recent plethora of new words appearing in fast-breaking fields, such as genetic engineering, molecular biology, immunology, and transplantation. In fact, 16,000 of the 92,000 entries are new. To test the dictionary's practical usefulness, this reviewer attempted to translate an article from a German cardiology journal. Looking up the words in this article, for a guy who uses his college German only occasionally, was quick and painless (the hardest part was finding umlauts on my font list). This is an excellent resource for someone needing to translate a article only available in German, a situation that this reviewer rarely runs across, but that must be much commoner in some areas of medicine.—**Anthony Gottlieb**

172.   Sharma, Rajendra. **The Family Encyclopedia of Health: The Complete Family Reference Guide to Alternative & Orthodox Medical Diagnosis, Treatment, & Preventive Healthcare.** Rockport, Mass., Element Books, 1998. 692p. illus. index. $24.95pa. ISBN 1-86204-426-0.

The Family Encyclopedia of Health is the most thorough resource to date that integrates discussion of alternative therapies within articles on common health concerns and their recommended Western medical treatments. The author is affiliated with the Hale Clinic, a British organization that promotes alternative health care practice. British and European health systems have moved more quickly than U.S. health care to accept and blend alternative therapies into mainstream medical practice. As a result, much of the advice given in this resource is not commonly accepted practice in the United States, and qualified practitioners of some of the recommended alternative modalities may be scarce in this country. Some U.S. libraries may find this work unsuitable for purchase if they strongly emphasize scientific or evidence-based medical information in their collections because only anecdotal evidence is available for many therapies discussed in this work.

However, this reference has many strengths. It is the first work on complementary or alternative care that discusses alternative practice side by side with Western medical practice, allowing the reader to evaluate the pros and cons of both therapies. As well, the multicultural approach of the work helps to ground the theories or rationales behind alternative therapies within the culture of origin. The work also explains the therapies in a clear and forthright manner that is suitable for its intended audience of health care consumers. The resource includes a contents list for a basic alternative medicine chest and recommends providers of the listed preparations. This work is generously illustrated, with diagrams of anatomy and procedures including, for example, a detailed topography of the eye used in iridology. There is an interesting glossary that includes many terms not found in medical dictionaries. The encyclopedia follows an arrangement that subdivides the book into 3 sections. Part 1 contains articles on sexuality, fertility and conception, and pregnancy and childbirth, then addresses health throughout periods of the life span. Part 2 addresses nutrition topics, diagnosis, alternative therapies, and drugs. And finally, part 3 includes a glossary, a recommended readings list, and an address list for alternative medicine information and practitioners. A thorough index provides access to the three parts of the encyclopedia by topic. [R: LJ, July 99, p. 84; Choice, Dec 99, p. 696]—**Lynne M. Fox**

173.   Spilker, Bert, comp. **Medical Dictionary in Six Languages.** New York, Raven Press, 1995. 665p. $99.00. ISBN 0-7817-0182-1.

Among the 7,500 definitions in this English dictionary are translations for common phrases and multiword terms in French, Italian, Spanish, German, and Japanese. If one knows the English term, the front part of the book is the place to begin searching; other languages are cross-referenced to the main English listings by entry number. British and American spellings are used (e.g., aetiology, etiology; anaemia, anemia), but only universally understood abbreviations are included. Oriented vertically instead of horizontally, which is the most comfortable reference mode for many people, this book will not lie flat when opened, so handling the bulk of it could hamper reference use.

Two-, three-, and four-word phrases that cannot be translated word-for-word into languages other than English are listed, which could be helpful in conversations, at seminars, during patient examinations, and in writing reports. This is a book of considerable utility, and medical transcribers, in particular, are sure to applaud it.—**Judy Gay Matthews**

174. Szycher, Michael. **Szycher's Dictionary of Medical Devices.** Lancaster, Pa., Technomic Publishing, 1995. 212p. $75.00. ISBN 1-56676-275-8.

Medical devices are among the most closely regulated of products; their names and definitions must also be closely monitored by the Food and Drug Administration (FDA). Title XXI of the Code of Federal Regulations publishes these definitions. Because they are spread over several medical specialties, they may be difficult to find. In this book, the author provides an alphabetic listing of officially defined devices in an attempt to ease this situation. However, if the searcher is unfamiliar with the device, or simply cannot recall it, finding the item may still be difficult as no cross-references have been added to the terms used by the government. When *braces* is not listed, who but sophisticated users would go directly to *limb orthosis* or *orthodontic band*?

Device is defined in the text as "any instrument, apparatus, implant, machine, contrivance, in vitro reagent, or similar or related article, including any component part or accessory" (p. 52). Such a broad definition reflects the great variety of regulated items, from tooth brush to some 26 devices listed under "cardiopulmonary bypass." Each entry gives the purpose or use of the device and its class. The text lists three classes. Class 1 devices are those that can be regulated by general controls, as they do not represent a health risk (e.g., a stethoscope). Class 2 devices require performance standards to ensure safety and effectiveness (e.g., cardiographs). Class 3 devices are the critical ones—life-supporting or -sustaining—requiring premarketing approval (e.g., pacemakers). This is not a catalog: There are no manufacturers, costs, and so forth. Specific statutes are not cited.

The author suggests using the book as a companion to his *Szycher's Dictionary of Biomaterials and Medical Devices*, also published by Technomic (see ARBA 93, entry 1639). Those interested in technology as applied to the medical field and the standards for its regulation should find this dictionary valuable, but it is not too useful for general readers, despite a possible familiarity with many medical devices and tests.—**Harriette M. Cluxton**

175. **Taber's Cyclopedic Medical Dictionary.** 19th ed. Donald Venes and others, eds. Philadelphia, F. A. Davis, 2001. 2770p. illus. $35.95. ISBN 0-8036-0654-0. ISSN 1065-1357.

The 18th edition of this classic nursing dictionary is famous for its nursing appendix and the easy-to-read definitions and graphics. For the revised 19th edition, the addition of complementary and alternative medicine terms and appendixes reflects today's health care practices and usages of information. Not only health care clinicians and students are using this dictionary for their needs, but patients are also taking information from this dictionary as a valuable source of health information.

There are more than 56,000 terms in this dictionary, with more than 2,200 new terms included. The extra value of *Taber's* is its appendixes. The expanded nursing appendix (in red thumb tab) lists 300 disease disorders, nursing interventions classification, nursing outcomes classification, nursing organizations in the United States and Canada, home health care classification, concept models and theories of nursing, and the Omaha System. The original appendixes includes sections on nutrition; integrative therapies; normal reference laboratory values; prefixes, suffixes, and combining forms; Latin and Greek nomenclature; medical abbreviations; symbols; units of measurement; phobias; manual alphabet; interpreter in three languages; medical emergencies; computer glossary; health care resource organizations; professional designations and titles in the health sciences; documentation system definitions; and standard and universal precautions.

The body of the work includes 150 new color illustrations that enhance the text of selected definitions. Selected disorder entries include cross-references to an appendix of nursing diagnoses grouped by disorder. Also, caution statements are highlighted in red underscore for readers' considerations. The table of contents lists consultants, Taber's feature finder, features and their use, illustrations, tables, abbreviations used in the text, and vocabulary. The text is completely revised and some of the terms are rewritten from scratch. Another bonus for purchasing this dictionary is that the online version is free for subscription. For more information visit http://www. Tabers19.com.

Taber's, as mentioned above, is a classic health care dictionary and readability is appropriate for the audience it serves. No library should miss this item on their reference shelves.—**Polin P. Lei**

176. Turkington, Carol, and Bonnie Ashby. **Encyclopedia of Infectious Diseases.** New York, Facts on File, 1998. 370p. index. $50.00. ISBN 0-8160-3512-1.

Finally, this broad-based encyclopedia of infectious diseases from Facts on File has arrived on the bookshelves. This is a concise guide and easy-to-read resource for the layperson. There are roughly 600 entries discussing the cause, diagnosis, symptoms, treatment, and prevention of the known infectious diseases. For other infectious disease terms, readers need to go for a medical textbook for more information. However, this book would be more interesting if there were color illustrations of cases inserted. This work claims to have the "curriculum-oriented information" that includes biology, health, anatomy, and premed courses. The glossary at the end of the book is a plus, and the bibliography, sorted by authors, would be more helpful if each citation was cross-referenced to the disease in the content. Six useful appendixes are provided—"Drugs Used to Treat Infectious Disease," "Home Disinfection," "Health Organizations," "Disease Hot Lines," "Health Publications," and "Infectious Disease-Related Websites." The Websites and drugs sections give readers a new perspective on how to use the information in a more meaningful way. Usually an encyclopedic item does not need an index, but the index in this book collects the keywords in the content to give more access points for the readers. This book is recommended for public or school libraries. Because there are not many publications of this type in the market, this reviewer thinks *Encyclopedia of Infectious Diseases* is a timely resource to supply consumers the much-needed information on infectious diseases. [R: LJ, 1 Oct 98, p. 78; BL, 15 Dec 98, p. 763]—**Polin P. Lei**

177. **Webster's New Explorer Medical Dictionary.** Darien, Conn., Federal Street Press, 1999. 764p. $8.98. ISBN 1-892859-07-6.

Webster's New Explorer Medical Dictionary is a product of Merriam-Webster's Federal Street Press. Created in 1998, Federal Street Press produces value, popularly priced, reference books. The intention of this work is to provide an affordable medical dictionary for the average consumer and, at the listed price, this book fulfills that intent.

The dictionary has over 35,000 entries, including frequently prescribed drugs and medical abbreviations commonly used in medicine but little known by laypersons. The dictionary begins with 27 pages of helpful explanatory notes, including information on cross-references, eponyms, pronunciation, abbreviations, and illustrations of usage. Additional information in some entries includes brief biographical notes, chemical symbols, and even a table of chemical elements.

This dictionary is affordable enough to be accessible to both health-conscious consumers and students —especially students in health-related educational programs. This medical dictionary is highly recommended for the above groups and for high schools, public libraries, and any consumer health collection. [R: LJ, 1 Nov 99, p. 75; Choice, Feb 2000, p. 1083]—**Lynn M. McMain**

178. Wiseman, Nigel, and Feng Ye, comps. **A Practical Dictionary of Chinese Medicine.** 2d ed. Brookline, Mass., Redwing Book Company, 1998. 945p. index. $125.00. ISBN 0-912111-54-2.

Wiseman and Ye have created an exemplary reference work characterized by its erudition, completeness, and accessibility. The compilers' preface details every aspect of the work's purpose, genesis, and scope. The stated objective was to create a dictionary that would be "useful to practitioners, students, and teachers of Chinese medicine in the English-speaking world, whether or not they have knowledge of Chinese and whether or not they are familiar with the terminology presented." The arrangement is alphabetic in order (as opposed to a thematic ordering) of English terms, with each entry followed by the original Chinese term and Pinyin transliteration. The definitions are often followed by extensive clinical information that may include specification of western medical correspondences, medication, acupuncture, and treatment. Entries are extensively cross-referenced, which is a key feature to accessing the content of this work given the unfamiliarity of many of the concepts. The entries conclude with references to sources, the vast majority of which are in Chinese. Also included are four appendixes and an index that allows access to the English entries by their Pinyin transcriptions as well as an index to medicinals and acupuncture-point names appearing in the text.

With its approximately 6,000 entries, this encyclopedic dictionary may serve as a clinical manual and would make an invaluable tool for those learning about Chinese medical concepts. It will also be of interest to translators as the compilers have extensive experience with terminological work in this area. This is a dictionary designed for specialists and can be expected to appeal to a specific audience; nevertheless, current interest in acupuncture and other forms of alternative medicine may indicate a wider audience for this title.—**Michael Weinberg**

179.   **The World Book Rush-Presbyterian-St. Luke's Medical Center Medical Encyclopedia.** Chicago, World Book, 2000. 1072p. illus. index. $50.00. ISBN 0-7166-4206-9.

What makes this book different from other medical guides or family handbooks is that it contains pertinent illustrations, either colored or graphical, that provide clear and succinct explanations. For example, the topic on automobile safety includes illustrations on how to escape from a sinking car, childproof locks, a first-aid kit, and others. These illustrations allow the readers to visualize and comprehend the meaning of automobile safety. However, this book is a one-stop health information guide for the general public and is prepared with the assistance of faculty members from the Rush Medical College at Rush-Presbyterian-St. Luke's Medical Center of Chicago. The arrangement of the topics is alphabetical. It is easy to use and the index is thorough. Even though this book calls itself a guide to good health, it does not contain a comprehensive list of drugs or clinical research information. The encyclopedia is organized in a question-and-answer format. In addition, there are useful appendixes after the A-Z entries. The appendix on charts of related symptoms can provide parents or consumers with diagnostic flowcharts. The pictorial index of symptoms links relevant symptoms or words to the anatomical parts. The age-by-age charts provide different disorders from birth to 65 and older. The appendix on health maintenance (nutrition and exercise) lists the dietary guidelines, fast food values, how to read food labels, recommended dietary allowances, recommended fiber and cholesterol levels, and choices for exercise. The last appendix is on growing older, choosing elder care, and lists health associations and agencies. This is a great book to have for school and public libraries.—**Polin P. Lei**

180.   **The World Book Rush-Presbyterian-St. Luke's Medical Center Medical Encyclopedia.** [CD-ROM]. Chicago, World Book, 2000. Minimum system requirements: Intel Pentium. 12-speed CD-ROM drive. Windows 98 or Windows 95. 32MB RAM. 100MB hard disk space. 800x600 monitor resolution (16 bit high-color). 28.8 modem. $25.00.

Like all CD-ROM encyclopedias today, this one is searchable. There are two search options through a natural language query or a full-text search in a condensed search mode. For librarians and other advanced searchers, there is also an advanced search mode.

Since CD-ROMs are a visual medium, this work contains a gallery of photos and videos. The informative photos illustrate items such as how to escape from a sinking car and how to properly apply eyedrops. The six videos included on this CD-ROM discuss asthma, the cardiovascular system, heart attacks, pneumonia, how ultrasound works, and the urinary system. They are all 30 seconds long or shorter and all have audio.

A section on safety covers automobile safety, bicycle safety, fire prevention and control, firearm safety, hiking safety, home safety, motorcycle safety, water sports safety, weather safety, and winter sports safety. The companion sections to this safety section on first aid and staying well, though, are not that good. In fact, the best thing in this encyclopedia is not any article but the symptom search feature. Another good feature is an age chart. Since physicians use the age of a patient a lot when making diagnoses, the age chart can help a layperson rule out certain worrisome conditions when confronted with a set of symptoms. In addition to the symptom search and the age chart, there is a question-and-answer section. It is good, but not as good as the symptom search. Finally, to input all of the information found into computer files there is a binder feature that eliminates the need for cutting and pasting into a word processing program. All in all, this CD-ROM is a good home medical encyclopedia, but there are better ones out there.—**Lambrini Papangelis**

Directories

181.   **Fast Help for Major Medical Conditions.** Caryn E. Anders and Lynn M. Pearce, eds. Farmington Hills, Mich., Gale, 2000. 1647p. index. (Gale Ready Reference Handbook Series). $125.00pa. ISBN 0-7876-3949-4. ISSN 1526-2723.

Reference texts that attempt to provide broad, extensive coverage of a multifaceted topic can be of tremendous help to their readership but can also often suffer from inaccurate data and out-of-date materials in the effort to present this information. This volume, part of the Gale Ready Reference Handbook series contains both the positive and negative aspects mentioned above. Although written to provide guidance for the general public, it will also be helpful to health care providers for its listings of national and state/local health care organizations and agencies, but both groups need to realize the limitations of this volume in terms of the currency of information provided.

The text is divided into 100 chapters, arranged alphabetically, covering major disease categories or medical conditions, from acne to uterine fibroids. No selection criteria are presented for these topics and one could question the exclusion of a number of important diseases. Within each of these chapters the readers are provided with an easy-to-read, multipage essay covering the description, causes and symptoms, diagnosis, treatments, prognosis, and prevention of the specific medical condition. Following the essay is an annotated list of national organizations, agencies, or research centers concerned with this health care situation. Finally, there is a state-by-state unannotated list of similar resources for the medical condition. This reference guide includes a glossary of technical terms used in the text, and a subject cross index with a thorough traditional index.

Because of the strong market forces exerted by managed care on the American medical system, many health care facilities have changed their names or disappeared over the last few years. Because of the time lag in compiling and publishing a large reference work such as this volume, many of these changes are not covered in the text, particularly in regard to state and local information. This leads to the omission of some worthwhile data (Pittsburgh AIDS Center for Treatment) and the inclusion of out-of-date facts (Shadyside Hospital's cancer center is now part of the UPMC in Pittsburgh). Although probably unavoidable, these types of errors call into question the accuracy and value of this section of this reference work. [R: BL, 1 May 2000, p. 1688; BR, Sept/Oct 2000, p. 76]—**Jonathon Erlen**

Handbooks and Yearbooks

182. **American College of Physicians Complete Home Medical Guide.** David R. Goldmann, ed. New York, DK Publishing, 1999. 1104p. illus. index. $40.00 (w/CD-ROM). ISBN 0-7894-4412-7.

This volume is a thorough guide to how the human body operates and how disease is investigated and treated. Extensive symptom flowcharts help the reader to determine the possible causes of common symptoms and recommended responses. There are succinct explanations about how disease is introduced into the body, from genetics, to infectious or contagious bacterial and viral infections, to fungal and parasitic infestations. A very complete chapter on medical tests includes an explanation of the kind of information the test reveals and a step-by-step description of the procedure. The bulk of the book consists of a summary of the ailments that affect specific body areas, such as the neurological system, the musculoskeletal system, and the digestive system. Each ailment is described, including causes, prevention, symptoms, treatment, and prognosis. Special sections cover pregnancy, birth, infancy, and childhood. Many color charts and illustrations aid comprehension and the writing is clear and easy for lay readers to understand. The index is exhaustive, but very easy to use. There are also chapters devoted to first aid and to the management of symptoms that cannot be cured. Cross-references are provided both to relevant sections of the book and to online sites. This excellent volume belongs in every public and patient library. An accompanying CD-ROM, *The Ultimate Human Body*, allows interactive examination of the body's various parts and functions, but this is strictly a lagniappe. The book stands on its own as the new standard home health guide. It is highly recommended.—**Susan B. Hagloch**

183. **The Cambridge Illustrated History of Medicine.** repr. ed. Roy Porter, ed. New York, Cambridge University Press, 2000. 400p. illus. index. (Cambridge Illustrated History). $54.95. ISBN 0-521-44211-7.

Porter's contribution to the vast array of general histories of medicine has been well reviewed and well received since it first appeared in 1996. The 10 thematic chapters are arranged in roughly chronological order. Porter himself wrote four of them: "What is Disease?," "Medical Science," "Hospitals and Surgery," and "Mental Illness." He assigned reputable scholars to the other six: "The History of Disease"; "The Rise of Medicine"; "Primary Care"; "Drug Treatment and the Rise of Pharmacology"; "Medicine, Society, and the State"; and "Looking to the Future." Each fits seamlessly into the whole. The apparatus includes a chronology from 9000 B.C.E. to 1995 C.E., a chart of the most common human diseases with the causes and vectors, bibliographic notes, suggestions for further reading, an annotated name index, and a thorough subject index.

This book will not supersede any of the standard short general histories of medicine. Despite its plethora of illustrations and sidebars, it is not to be taken lightly. It is far superior to Otto Bettmann's *Pictorial History of Medicine* (Charles C. Thomas, 1979) in scope, depth, and accuracy. In addition to the expected scientific, historical, and biographical expositions, it discusses the social, religious, economic, aesthetic, political, geographic, demographic, and philosophical aspects of medicine. It cogently and soberly facilitates interpreting modern afflictions, such as AIDS and Ebola, in the social context of past scourges, such as bubonic plague, cholera, yellow fever, tuberculosis, and typhus. It is an excellent means for high school students or college undergraduates to begin their serious study of the history of medicine.—**Eric v. d. Luft**

184. **Colds, Flu, and Other Common Ailments Sourcebook.** Chad T. Kimball, ed. Detroit, Omnigraphics, 2001. 638p. index. (Health Reference Series). $78.00. ISBN 0-7808-0435-X.

Omnigraphics' Health Reference Series provides overviews of diseases and conditions for lay readers. The new volume, *Colds, Flu, and Other Common Ailments Sourcebook*, covers a wide range of common symptoms and illnesses. Colds, influenza (flu), hemorrhoids, and dandruff are among the ailments included. Fever, nausea and vomiting, headache, and diarrhea are also covered, although they are symptoms rather than diseases. The information provided comes from publications of United States government agencies such as branches of the National Institutes of Health and the Center for Disease Control and Prevention as well as from professional organizations (American Academy of Dermatology), newsletters (Harvard Health Letter), and Websites (Healthcentral.com). Full citations appear at the beginning of each chapter.

The book has seven parts covering different groups of ailments. Each part contains several chapters. Some of the chapters are divided into sections. Each chapter or section begins with a description of the disease or condition, its symptoms, treatment, and prevention. Information comparing similar conditions, such as colds and flu, and separate chapters covering these conditions in adults and children are very useful. The editors discuss self care, alternative therapies, and when to consult a physician. Part 6, "General Information About Drugs and Medicine," offers valuable information that explains the differences between prescription and over-the-counter drugs, caveats about buying medication or looking for health information online, food/drug interactions, and choosing a physician. *Colds, Flu, and Other Common Ailments Sourcebook* is a good starting point for research on common illnesses. It will be a useful addition to public and consumer health library collections.—**Barbara M. Bibel**

185.   **Ear, Nose, and Throat Disorders Sourcebook.** Linda M. Shin and Karen Bellenir, eds. Detroit, Omnigraphics, 1998. 576p. index. (Health Reference Series, v.37). $78.00. ISBN 0-7808-0206-3.

The introduction to this reference notes that ear, nose, and throat (ENT) problems are one of the most common reasons for people to seek medical care. The editors thus establish the importance of this book, an addition to an extensive series of texts for the layperson on health care and medical problems. The book begins with a glossary of terms, descriptions of the various ENT specialists, and a directory of associated organizations. The nearly 70 chapters provide comprehensive coverage of ENT problems, from minor to serious. As appropriate, each chapter provides definitions of terms, explanations of the problems, and a discussion of the treatments available, from home care to radical surgery. The information in each chapter is reprinted from reputable sources, including government agencies and ENT specialty organizations. The chapters are referenced, and directory or Internet addresses are included for further information.

Only a few negatives deter from the overall good quality of the reference. A few chapters are more appropriate for physicians than the general public. Second, more comprehensive coverage of hearing loss should have been included. The editors note that this problem is covered in another volume in the series. Finally, explanations and illustrations of the anatomy and physiology of the system are scattered throughout the text. One introductory chapter on this topic would have been more helpful for the reader. Overall, this sourcebook is helpful for the consumer seeking information on ENT issues. It is recommended for public libraries. [R: BL, 1 Dec 98, p. 698]—**Mary Ann Thompson**

186.   **Ethnic Disease Sourcebook.** Joyce Brennfleck Shannon, ed. Detroit, Omnigraphics, 2001. 664p. index. (Health Reference Series). $78.00. ISBN 0-7808-0336-1.

It is recognized within the health care community that racial and ethnic disparities exist in risk for chronic disease and injury. This awareness has created an impetus to improve health care research and the quality of health care delivery and education to racial and ethnic groups in the United States. The *Ethnic Disease Sourcebook* is one of the latest to be published in the Health Reference Series. It consists of documents and excerpted publications from U.S. government agencies, organizations, and individuals. The work provides information about genetic and chronic diseases, the availability of genetic tests and counseling, and the impact of chronic diseases as they relate to African Americans, Asian Americans/Pacific Islanders, Hispanic Americans, Native Americans, and ethnic women.

The sourcebook is organized into 8 parts and 45 chapters, many of which contain references and additional resources. Among the topics covered are health indicators and behaviors by race and ethnicity; genetic diseases such as lupus, sickle cell anemia, and Tay-Sachs disease; chronic diseases such as diabetes and cardiovascular disease; alcohol, tobacco, and drug use; mental health; health insurance and access to health care; and healthy eating. Part 8, "Additional Help and Information," contains very useful resources on minority health, sources of health education materials, information on genetic testing laboratories in the United States, and a glossary of important terms.

Not many books have been written on this topic to date, and the *Ethnic Disease Sourcebook* is a strong addition to the list. It will be an important introductory resource for health consumers, students, health care personnel, and social scientists. It is recommended for public, academic, and large hospital libraries.—**Rita Neri**

187. **Everything You Need to Know About Diseases.** Springhouse, Pa., Springhouse Publishing, 1996. 918p. index. $24.95. ISBN 0-87434-822-6.

188. **Everything You Need to Know About Medical Tests.** Springhouse, Pa., Springhouse Publishing, 1996. 691p. illus. index. $24.95. ISBN 0-87434-823-4.

189. **Everything You Need to Know About Medical Treatments.** Springhouse, Pa., Springhouse Publishing, 1996. 628p. illus. index. $24.95. ISBN 0-87434-821-8.

This series of books on diseases, medical tests, and medical treatments is similar to H. W. Griffith's trio of books *Complete Guide to Symptoms, Illness, & Surgery* (see ARBA 86, entry 1634); *Complete Guide to Pediatric Symptoms, Illness, & Medications* (Berkley, 1989); and *Complete Guide to Medical Tests* (see ARBA 90, entry 1667). *Everything You Need to Know About Diseases* is divided into 18 chapters by type of disorder (e.g., gynecologic, eye). With 100 leading doctors and medical experts, the book answers the following questions: What causes the condition? What are the symptoms? How is it diagnosed? and, What is the treatment? It also has special tips on prevention, self-help, and advice for caregivers.

Everything You Need to Know About Medical Tests details 400-plus tests in descriptions written by more than 70 physicians. The book answers these questions: Why are the tests done? What are the risks? What happens during and after the test? What are normal results? and, What do abnormal results mean? *Everything You Need to Know About Medical Treatments* covers more than 300 medically approved therapies. The book explains why these therapies are recommended, the risks, how doctors perform them, and what happens before and after treatments. It also includes practical advice for caregivers, self-help solutions, and straight answers to medical questions by 50 doctors and medical experts.

These are excellent new titles for the consumer health market. Few doctors today have the time or inclination to give consumers the how and why on medical disorders, treatments, and so forth. These books give consumers the opportunity to make more informed medical decisions. Springhouse Publishing has done an excellent job in preparing these informative medicine texts for the public. The series is highly recommended for small, medium, and large public libraries. —**Theresa Maggio**

190. **Injury and Trauma Sourcebook.** Joyce Brennfleck Shannon, ed. Detroit, Omnigraphics, 2002. 696p. index. (Health Reference Series). $78.00. ISBN 0-7808-0421-X.

Injury and Trauma Sourcebook is edited by Joyce Shannon and published by Omnigraphics as part of their Health Reference Series. Almost 150,000 Americans die of injury each year and 19,000 are children and young people. It is the leading cause of death for children and young people. The book is divided into nine chapters: "High Toll of Injury in the U.S.," "Common Injuries," "Trauma Injuries," "Emergency Care," "Injury Prevention," "Work-related Injuries," "Transportation Injuries," "Recreation-Related Injuries/Prevention," and "Additional Help/Information." The question-and-answer format used in most chapters is very informative. The statistics throughout the book are very helpful to the patron. The index and references are recent and many Websites are listed. All public libraries would benefit from its inclusion, with the only drawback being its price. This publication is the most comprehensive work of its kind about injury and trauma. —**Theresa Maggio**

191.   Long, James W. **The Essential Guide to Chronic Illness: The Active Patient's Handbook.** New York, HarperPerennial/HarperCollins, 1997. 625p. index. $20.00pa. ISBN 0-06-273137-8.

Studies have shown that patients who understand their illness and take an active part in their treatment do better than those who passively wait for their doctor to tell them what to do. They feel more in control, helping to make crucial care decisions. This book purports to inform patients about 47 common conditions, from acne to Zollinger-Ellis syndrome. The ailments covered were chosen, the author says, based on the relative frequency of occurrence, severity of impact on the patient and the family, and the degree of difficulty of diagnosis and management.

Even using these criteria, the selection seems somewhat arbitrary. AIDS, for example, is covered, although its frequency is considerably less than that of polycystic kidney disease, which is not. Each entry details the principal features of the disease, diagnostic methods and available therapies, and further resources. Additional sections address preventive medicine, terminal illness, special considerations for the elderly patient, and drug-induced disorders. Coverage of the included diseases is thorough, but the restrictions on this coverage make this book of marginal use to public library reference collections. A better choice for reference is *The Mayo Clinic Family Health Book* (2d ed., William Morrow, 1996), but libraries needing more circulating material on diseases should consider the title under review, as it does provide good value for the price.—**Susan B. Hagloch**

192.   **The Merck Manual of Diagnosis and Therapy.** 17th ed. Mark H. Beers and Robert Berkow, eds. West Point, Pa., Merck Research Laboratories/Merck, 1999. 2833p. index. $35.00. ISBN 0-911910-10-7. ISSN 0076-6526.

This is the centennial edition of *The Merck Manual*, one of the oldest and most widely used general medical textbooks in the world. The objective of this work is to provide clinical information to physicians, medical students, interns, residents, nurses, pharmacists, and other health care professionals in a concise, complete, and accurate manner. The manual covers all aspects of general internal medicine as well as pediatrics, psychiatry, obstetrics, gynecology, dermatology, pharmacology, ophthalmology, and otolaryngology.

The centennial edition is the product of a seven-year effort to update or completely rewrite every section and includes a brief review of medical practice as reflected in *The Merck Manual* during the past 100 years. A number of topics new to this edition include hand disorders, prion diseases, death and dying, probabilities in clinical medicine, multiple chemical sensitivity, chronic fatigue syndrome, rehabilitation, smoking cessation, and drug therapy in the elderly.

The table of contents includes listings not only for the topical sections but also for editorial board members, consultants, additional reviewers, contributors, abbreviations and symbols, and the index. Thumb tabs with abbreviations and section numbers mark the sections and index. Each section begins with its own table of contents, listing chapters and subchapters. The work is thoroughly indexed, including tables and figures, with careful cross-referencing, and boldface page numbers signify major discussions of a topic within the index. Drugs are referred to by their generic name throughout the text, but a chapter is devoted to listing the trade names of commonly used drugs.

With its tissue-thin pages, *The Merck Manual* is light and easily portable. Its broad coverage, careful editing, concise style, ease of use, and affordability will ensure its continued status as one of the most widely used medical textbooks in the world among both health professionals and the sophisticated layperson. *The Merck Manual* is essential for all general and health-related reference collections.—**Arlene McFarlin Weismantel**

193.   **The Merck Manual of Medical Information.** home ed. Robert Berkow, Mark H. Beers, and Andrew J. Fletcher, eds. New York, McGraw-Hill, 1997. 1509p. illus. index. $29.95. ISBN 0-911910-87-5.

For a hundred years, *The Merck Manual* has been the doctor's bible. Finally, here is a rewriting in everyday language, a translation of the professionals' reference book to be consulted by today's increasingly literate searchers for medical information. It is in no way paternalistic, but maintains a neutral attitude, uses medical terminology, and is not a "how to" self-care manual. Almost all of the content of *The Merck Manual* is given, except for drug dosages, microscopic slide interpretations, and so on, for which the layperson must depend on the professionals.

The home edition enables the patient and family to learn about human disorders and to understand their biological bases, diagnosis, treatment, and even prognosis, as understood by practitioners of orthodox medicine. A tremendous amount of medical information has been carefully arranged into briefly introduced sections, such as blood disorders. The first chapter under each section often covers the biology of the organ, system, or type of disorder (e.g., infections). Following chapters are more specific, such as abscesses under the skin. A pattern of symptoms, diagnosis, treatment options, and outcomes are often used. Cross-references are indicated by small red symbols in the text, repeated at the bottom of the page, with the location of related topics. There are some general sections on topics such as on death and dying. Additional information often appears in sidebars. Original illustrations have been digitized and sparingly colorized, making them easy to understand. The table of contents is detailed, and the index is extensive. There are several appendixes, such as lists of common medical terms and the generic and trade names of often-prescribed drugs.

This is a definitive, authoritative, easy-to-use current medical reference for laypeople, and should be considered for all hospital libraries, consumer health centers, public libraries, and many individual collections. It is presented from the medical viewpoint and compared to books like the *Mayo Clinic Family Health Book* (Morrow, 1996), this is more concise in statement and inclusive in essential information. It is also directed toward helping the user comprehend the basic nature of diseases and disorders and what the treatments and outcomes may be. The reader should be well prepared for more intelligent interaction with his or her doctors after consulting this excellent book.—**Harriette M. Cluxton**

194.   Morton, Leslie T., and Robert J. Moore. **A Chronology of Medicine and Related Sciences.** Brookfield, Vt., Ashgate Publishing, 1997. 784p. index. $127.95. ISBN 1-85928-215-6.

Many history of medicine-related questions require only a single piece of information; in other words a date, a name, or the location of an event. This new reference tool is probably the best place to begin looking for answers to this type of question. Whereas other medical history reference works provide chronologies, biographies, or bibliographies, no other single volume better combines these aspects of the history of medicine than Morton and Moore's volume.

This reference guide is arranged chronologically, from 3,000 B.C.E. and the Edwin Smith Papyrus through 1996 and the death of Tadeus Reichstein of vitamin C and cortisone fame. Beginning in 1529, there is at least one citation per year through 1996. The following type of entries are provided for each year, when material is available: events (major discoveries; founding of journals, institutions, and societies; Nobel prize-winners); births of significant figures in medical history and a brief mention of their contribution(s); and death dates. These entries range from one to several sentences in length. For items in the first two categories, the authors include citations to journal literature providing further information, as well as citation numbers to the relevant entries in *Morton's Medical Bibliography*, 5th edition (see ARBA 93, entry 1627).

There are a couple of minor weaknesses in this volume. Although the authors wisely state that their timeline is not all-inclusive, there is no explanation for the selection criteria used. Also, there is no clear definition of what the authors mean by medically related sciences: are they including anatomy or biochemistry? Some major aspects of the social history of medicine also lack coverage; for example, Margaret Sanger's work for birth control and the 1957 *Salgo* legal case that established the doctrine of informed consent. Despite these oversights, public, academic, and health-related libraries will find this volume an indispensable reference work. —**Jonathon Erlen**

195.   **Mosby's Primary Care Medicine Rapid Reference.** [CD-ROM]. St. Louis, Mo., Mosby, 1997. Minimum system requirements (Windows version): IBM or compatible 386. CD-ROM drive (double-speed recommended). Windows 3.1. 4MB RAM. VGA or compatible video graphics card (256 colors). Mouse. Minimum system requirements (Macintosh version): 68030 or higher processor. CD-ROM drive (double-speed recommended). System 7.1. 4MB RAM. Color monitor with display resolution of 640x480 with 256 colors. Mouse. $129.95.

This CD-ROM product from Mosby is the combination of the 2d edition of *Textbook of General Medicine and Primary Care Medicine* by John Noble (Mosby, 1995), more than 50,000 Primary Care Medline abstracts, plus the 1997 edition of *Physicians GenRx*. Considering the 1996 *Textbook of Primary Care Medicine* was selling at around $90, comparatively speaking, the cost of this software sounds like a bargain. And the use of this product is quite transparent for the general public.

Rapid Access Medical Information (RAMI) software is used for the three databases. RAMI provides two button bars. One button bar is to provide access to the most commonly used features, such as Save, Print, Back, History, Picture/Table, Notes, Bookmark, Hide/Show, Split, Search, Results, Match, and Word buttons, and the other button bar is specific to the database being viewed. There is a Mega Index button for searching the index in the *Textbook* and *GenRx* at the same time. The Search button is a powerful engine that does rapid Boolean searching with the search results displaying instantaneously. Extra features include the use of the notepad, preferences, hyperlinks, three-dimensional structures, and more.

For the textbook, an additional 29 chapters are added exclusively for this CD-ROM version from "common eye examination" to "cultural issues." This database intends to offer comprehensive primary care practice for modern physicians. A Lab Values button opens the appendix document on this topic. A Chapter Heading button allows access to other chapters. Physicians GenRx shows buttons on interaction tools, drug names, keyword index, pharmacological class, therapeutic class, indications for use, imprint index, and drug topic. The content is arranged slightly different from the printed version.

The Primary Care Medline abstracts are pulled from 31 commonly read medical journals, such as *American Journal of Medicine*, *Chest*, *JAMA*, and *Science*. However, the dates of the articles range from 1988 to 1995 only. A handy user's guide comes with this product, explaining "how to" on various buttons except on how to install. For the practitioners who prefer CD-ROM products, this might be a good resource to enhance their practice. The Web version of these databases would be even more convenient for keeping the state-of-the-art information more up-to-date. —**Polin P. Lei**

196. **Pain Sourcebook.** Allan R. Cook, ed. Detroit, Omnigraphics, 1998. 667p. illus. index. (Health Reference Series, v.32). $75.00. ISBN 0-7808-0213-6.

As pain is a virtually universal experience, this book will be a valuable addition to Omnigraphics' Health Reference Series. Addressed to the layperson, it is not intended to replace professional advice and treatment. Pain is too often ignored or undertreated by physicians, although this attitude is slowly changing. The book aims to help the reader understand the types of chronic and acute pain and conventional and alternative methods for its control. There are many practical suggestions for managing pain, especially in part 7.

The text is composed of brief discussions and recent reprints and excerpts, used by permission, from such publications as the *Mayo Clinic Newsletter, FDA Consumer*, and government and association reports. These are skillfully arranged under sections with general designations, such as "Headache," with subchapters covering more specific topics, such as "Tension-type Headache." Sources of material are clearly cited. Further references are frequently included, as well as brief glossaries of medical terms.

Although some items are moderately technical (e.g., pain assessment), the text is readable, easily understood, and well indexed. This excellent volume belongs in all patient education libraries, consumer health sections of public libraries, and many personal collections.—**Harriette M. Cluxton**

197. Rozario, Diane. **The Immunization Resource Guide: Where to Find Answers to All Your Questions About Childhood Immunizations.** 2d ed. Burlington, Iowa, Patter, 1995. 60p. index. $9.95pa. ISBN 0-9643366-2-6.

Although the author of this pamphlet-length guide claims impartiality, a glance at her work reveals she is deeply suspicious and critical of all vaccines and immunizations, childhood or otherwise. Almost all of the publications of established scientific merit are listed in a chapter title "Pro-vaccination" and are accompanied by the author's critical comments. Most other chapters are antivaccination, and are composed of publications from the popular press and various religious and alternative medical publishers. These (including publications of the Natural Hygiene movement, which denies the importance of bacteria and viruses in causing disease) are treated much less critically.

Many worthwhile publications and national and international organizations are listed in this pamphlet. Most, however, are well known and accessible through many other sources, available in any basic reference library. Parents who legitimately want more information on the dangers and side effects of childhood immunizations should consult these. This publication is for those who have already made up their mind and want a listing of all antivaccination literature, no matter how dubious the source.—**Carol L. Noll**

198. **Sick! Diseases and Disorders, Injuries and Infections.** David Newton, Donna Olendorf, Christine Jeryan, and Karen Boyden, eds. Farmington Hills, Mich., U*X*L/Gale, 2000. 4v. illus. index. $115.00/set. ISBN 0-7876-3922-2.

Sick! Diseases and Disorders, Injuries and Infections is a four-volume set covering a wide range of health-related topics of interest for students from middle school to adult readers. More than 100 entries are arranged alphabetically, with information on causes, symptoms, diagnoses, tests, and treatments and prognoses. Entries include sidebars on related people and topics and words to know, as well as a list of sources for further research. The Websites and organizations after each topic will be useful to the layperson. Research and activities for classes would be helpful for the classroom teacher. It is comparable to D. W. Griffith's *Complete Guide to Symptoms, Illness, and Surgery* (Perigee, 2000) but it is more current. It would be an excellent resource for a juvenile health section for public libraries although cost could be a deterrent at a $115 for the set. [R: SLJ, Aug 2000, p. 134; BL, 1 Oct 2000, p. 372; VOYA, Oct 2000, p. 300; BR, Nov/Dec 2000, p. 71]—**Theresa Maggio**

199.   Ward, Brian. **Epidemic.** Edited by Rob DeSalle. New York, DK Publishing, 2000. 63p. illus. index. (Dorling Kindersley Eyewitness Books). $15.95. ISBN 0-7894-6296-6.
      This short work in the Dorling Kindersley Eyewitness Books series was written in association with The American Museum of Natural History. In a style that will appeal mainly to middle school and high school students, this work focuses on epidemics throughout history and discusses what their causes and cures (if any) are. The various pages discuss what an epidemic is, how it is passed along, what major epidemics occur where, specifics about some well-known epidemics (e.g., the plague, cholera, leprosy, small pox), remedies, and the continuing war against epidemics worldwide. Each topic is covered in a two-page spread, which contains photographs and illustrations, some of which are graphic, making this work more appropriate for an older audience.—**Shannon Graff Hysell**

ALTERNATIVE MEDICINE

Dictionaries and Encyclopedias

200.   **The Alternative Medicine Home Page. http://www.pitt.edu/~cbw/altm.html.** [Website]. Falk Library, Pittsburgh, Pa. Free. Date reviewed: Sept 02.
      Developed by a medical librarian at Falk Library at the University of Pittsburgh, *The Alternative Medicine Home Page*'s intent is to provide a reference point for complementary and alternative medicine (CAM) resources on the Web. The Website has minimal graphics and loads quickly. The home page clearly states the authorship, what criteria are used when selecting Websites to be included, and a disclaimer indicating that it should not and does not take the place of a physician. The brochure on identifying CAM resources linked from the home page has good information on how to identify quality CAM resources regardless of format.
      The sections are "AIDS & HIV," "Databases," "Internet Resources," "Mailing Lists and Newsgroups," "Government Resources," "Pennsylvania Resources," "Practitioners' Directories," and "Related Resources." The majority of entries in all sections are annotated. If an entry is not annotated, the purpose is clear in the name of the Website. "Databases" has a mixture of free and fee-based databases related to CAM. "Internet Resources" are organized using the vocabulary developed by the Office of Alternative Medicine, National Institutes of Health. "Government Resources" are predominantly U.S.-based with one site each from Canada and the United Kingdom. "Pennsylvania Resources" includes a mix of private practitioners and associations in Pennsylvania. "Practitioners' Directories" has links to various Websites to locate practitioners in the various modalities.
      The Website is easy to use and will be easily understood by the general public and students as well as by health care providers. The site does not purport to be a comprehensive source of CAM on the Internet, nor is it. The strength of the site lies in its attention to the quality of the sites selected, the information on how to evaluate Internet or other resources on CAM, and the thoughtful annotations to the Websites selected.—**Leslie M. Behm**

201. Chevallier, Andrew. **The Encyclopedia of Herbal Medicine.** 2d ed. New York, DK Publishing, 2000. 336p. illus. index. $40.00. ISBN 0-7894-6783-6.

Chevallier's encyclopedia profiles more than 550 key medicinal plants, systematically detailing their history, cultivation, key constituents and actions, research, and traditional and current uses. It shows how to make different types of herbal preparations and recommends safe, effective remedies for a wide range of common health problems. Most of all, the full-color illustrations throughout are an enhancement to the text. Chevallier has also published other books on herbal medicine in addition to his lectures at Middlesex University in the United Kingdom.

The contents of this text emphasize the development of herbal medicine and its cultural history, key medicinal plants, other medicinal plants from different herbal traditions, and herbal remedies for home use. Each key medicinal plant lists habitat and cultivation, key constituents, key actions, research, traditional and current uses, and self-help use, with illustrations on parts used and key preparations and their uses. Other medicinal plants are given descriptions, habitat and cultivation, parts used, constituents, history and folklore, medicinal actions, and use.

Both sections are arranged by the plant's scientific name. Users need to know the plants' classifications, or have to rely on the index to locate the right information. The home use section is great for those who wish to perform self-help healing. There are tips on how to grow medicinal plants, harvesting and processing, infusions, decoctions, capsules and powders, tinctures, and much more. The remedies for common ailments such as allergies, skin problems, and digestive disorders are prescribed. The index of herbs by ailment is a bonus for cross-referencing. In this age of self-help, it is important to seek the appropriate information for alternative medicine. Readers also need to be aware of the importance of seeking medical help when needed. This work is a great home reading reference. [R: LJ, 15 Mar 01, p. 70]—**Polin P. Lei**

202. Chevallier, Andrew. **The Encyclopedia of Medicinal Plants.** New York, DK Publishing, 1996. 336p. illus. index. $39.95. ISBN 0-7894-1067-2.

Featuring more than 550 plants that are put to therapeutic use around the world, this book introduces readers to the rich traditions and resources of herbal medicine. With a refreshing combination of folkloric and scientific material, it brings together each plant's history and tradition with research-based information about its active constituents, key actions, and potential new uses.

After a general overview of the global development of herbal medicine, the book's focus shifts to major continents, tracing traditions within each. A colorful and well-illustrated index of herbs follows. This is divided into two broad sections—"Key Medicinal Plants" (which covers 100 herbs) and "Other Medicinal Plants" (which covers more than 400 herbs). Within the sections, herbs are listed alphabetically by their scientific name, below which appear—in large typeface—their common name or names. The following information is given for each herb: name (scientific and common), habitat and cultivation, related species, key constituents, key actions, traditional and current uses (including self-help uses), parts used, and key preparations and their uses. This same type of information is offered in each section, but it is given in greater detail in the first section. Final chapters in the book are devoted to growing, harvesting, and processing herbs; making herbal remedies; and consulting an herbal practitioner. A glossary, a bibliography, a general index, and an index of ailments conclude the book.

If this book has a weakness, it is in the sheer ambition of covering the globe with a rather slippery language. Because general readers are for the most part unaware of scientific names of herbs, they may have difficulty locating specific plants. A thorough index could make up for this problem, but although this book's index does list common names, it does not always list *all* common names for an individual herb. Hence, the Chinese herb *Angelica Senensis*, commonly known as dong quai in the United States, is listed under its Latin name and under a variation of the common name that one supposes is used in the United Kingdom, dang gui. Other herbs seem simply to be excluded. Osha root (or chuchupate), a Native American remedy for cough relief, does not appear, nor does the Asian Indian digestive ajwain (or ajawan).

Another fine work on this topic is *Rodale's Illustrated Encyclopedia of Herbs* (see ARBA 88, entry 1535), which focuses more on North American and Western European herbs and traditions. The Rodale volume also emphasizes cultivation and herb lore, rather than modern herbal medicine. In fact, these two books complement one another and should not be considered substitutes.

In spite of inevitable omissions and weaknesses of this book, it is a rare find. Used in conjunction with other herbal guides, it is a worthwhile reference book. One can always hope that in subsequent editions, the author will expand the index to provide easier access to this abundant information. For collections covering this subject area, the book is highly recommended. [R: BL, 1 Dec 96, p. 629]—**Barbara Ittner**

203.   **The Complete Illustrated Encyclopedia of Alternative Healing Therapies.** C. Norman Shealy, ed. Boston, Element Books, 1999. 383p. illus. index. $29.95pa. ISBN 1-86204-662-X.

There are many encyclopedias and dictionaries on alternative medicine and healing on the market, and their large and small differences can make selecting one difficult. This is a beautifully designed, well-organized, and objective work aimed at the general reader. Its editor is the founder of the American Holistic Medical Association and a well-known American surgeon and chronic pain specialist. The book presents 54 therapies that aim to enhance self-healing and their applications to a variety of illnesses, and is the companion volume to *The Illustrated Encyclopedia of Healing Remedies* (see entry 215). It is organized into four parts: "Energy Therapies" (acupuncture, shiatsu, yoga, and therapeutic touch); "Physical Therapies" (osteopathy, therapeutic massage, and relaxation techniques); "Mind and Spirit Therapies" (music, art, and light therapies); and "Common Ailments" (anxiety, back problems, pneumonia, and diabetes). Entries are comprehensive, well written, and meaningfully illustrated, and therapy and ailment entries are cross-referenced. Therapy descriptions include history, philosophy, precautions, what to expect from a treatment, and how the therapy is viewed by conventional medicine. Entries on ailments include description, symptoms, conventional medical treatment, and cautions. A reference area at the back of the book contains a full glossary, but recommendations for further reading and address and contact information are limited. In general, this is an outstanding guide for new and more experienced readers in this field and is appropriate for all libraries.—**Madeleine Nash**

204.   **The Encyclopedia of Alternative Medicine: A Complete Family Guide to Complementary Therapies.** Jennifer Jacobs, ed. Boston, Journey Editions/Charles E. Tuttle, 1996. 320p. illus. index. $24.95pa. ISBN 1-885203-36-5.

Consumer interest in alternative medicine is at an all-time high in the United States, with the traditional medical establishment gradually, if reluctantly, recognizing and accepting its value. Publishers have responded to the public's enthusiasm for alternative medicine with a bevy of books to help consumers educate themselves. What distinguishes this volume from several others on the same subject are the format and attractive layout. The book begins with a short, clear introduction on what alternative therapies have in common and is followed by a useful section entitled "Finding the Right Therapy." Six charts of disorders list individual medical problems, such as asthma or back problems. A quick look at the chart tells the reader which alternative therapy to consider for each medical problem.

Rather than the classic A to Z format, this encyclopedia groups each of the 30 alternative or complementary treatment modalities into 7 related groupings. For example: Part 1, "Natural Healing," includes a chapter each on color therapy, homeopathy, iridology, and polarity therapy; part 7, "Eastern Therapies," has chapters on acupuncture, acupressure, shiatsu, tai chi, and Chinese herbal medicine. Because authorship is not given, the reader must assume that each chapter is written by 1 of the 30 contributors (leading practitioners, experts, authors) listed under each alternative treatment at the front of the book.

On the verso of the title page the publisher strongly disclaims: "The information and opinions contained herein, which should not be used or relied upon without consultation and advice of a physician, are those solely of the authors and not those of the publishers who disclaim any responsibility for the accuracy of such information and opinions and any responsibility for any consequences that may result from any use or reliance thereon by the reader." Despite the lack of confidence caused by reading the fine print, the reader gets a clear, easy-to-read understanding of almost all available alternative medical treatments. Most chapters include a history of the therapy, recent developments, case studies, and what conditions are best treated with the therapy. Many sidebars and lavish illustrations make the book a pleasure to read. A glossary and a list of addresses conclude the book.

Consumers of alternative health care will welcome this quick fix on their coffee tables. Public librarians will find the book useful as well and can feel confident referring patrons to it because, as the back cover states, this encyclopedia is "endorsed by a Member of the Program Advisory Council of the National Institutes of Health Office of Alternative Medicine."—**Georgia Briscoe**

205. **The Gale Encyclopedia of Alternative Medicine.** Kristine Krapp and Jacqueline L. Longe, eds. Farmington Hills, Mich., Gale, 2001. 4v. illus. index. $350.00/set. ISBN 0-7876-4999-6.

There are many popular reference tools on the subject of alternative medicine, but none is as complete as *The Gale Encyclopedia of Alternative Medicine* by Krapp and Longe. Readers have long been yearning to learn more about alternative medicine and the impact of using these treatments. To answer this demand, there were plenty of published alternative medicine resources, guides, bibliographies, online resources, or videos. However, this ambitious four-volume set is the one-stop source to answer a great deal of questions on the various aspects of alternative medicine.

Gale's products are known to be thorough, well-researched, and good reference tools. This item is no exception. This set of books includes 157 therapies, 283 diseases or conditions, 306 herbs and remedies, and 750 full-length articles. The entries for therapies have detailed descriptions of origins, benefits, precautions, preparations, and side effects. The herb and remedy entries contain detailed descriptions of general use, preparations, precautions, side effects, and interactions. The descriptions for diseases and conditions provide definitions and information on etiology, symptoms, diagnosis, treatment, allopathic treatment, expected results, and prevention. All of these categories have resources and key terms as a bonus. The contents are listed alphabetically with the boldfaced terms cross-referenced to related entries in the encyclopedia. The key terms are defined appropriately where they are used in the essay.

There are more than 350 images. Each of the first three volumes contains a color insert of 64 herbs, remedies, and supplements. The alphabetic "Organizations" section in volume 4 lists postal, e-mail, and Website addresses along with telephone numbers of unique associations and institutions that use alternative medicine for treatment. The thorough index in volume 4 adds another access point for readers. However, it would be an added bonus if each color photograph of herbs and plants were indexed for readers to locate.

This is a valuable resource for readers who are seeking information on complementary medicine and herbal remedies. The scope of this encyclopedia is comprehensive, but not definitive. Readers should use this as a supplement, not a replacement, to professional healthcare consultation. This source has been a long-awaited product for the consolidation of general alternative medicine information. [R: LJ, Aug 01, pp. 90-92]—**Polin P. Lei**

206.　Group, David W. **Encyclopedia of Mind Enhancing Foods, Drugs and Nutritional Substances.** Jefferson, N.C., McFarland, 2001. 215p. index. $45.00. ISBN 0-7864-0853-7.

This encyclopedia grew out of the author's fascination with psychotropic (mind-enhancing) agents. In it, he analyzes properties of more than 400 foods, drugs, and nutritional substances, such as aspirin, passion flower, L-dopa, LSD, honey, marijuana, Vitamin E, bioflavinoids, tryptophan, and strychnine. Entries consist of one or more descriptive paragraphs, alternative names, general usage, and caveats regarding possible interactions with other substances, as well as medical contraindications. Unfortunately, the author does not have the credentials or nutritional background to be so freely dispensing usage information about these substances, many of which have not been thoroughly researched as to toxicity levels and possible side effects. David W. Group, "a writer and researcher living in Buffalo, New York," has collected information from a variety of secondary sources, noted in the bibliography, but does not footnote within individual entries. In spite of a brief disclaimer on the title page discouraging self-diagnosis, public libraries might wish to choose a title by a more appropriately credentialed and experienced practitioner, such as Ray Sahelian, M.D., who consulted with a number of international physicians for his latest book titled *Mind Boosters: A Guide to Natural Supplements that Enhance Your Mind, Memory, and Mood* (St. Martin's Press, 2000).

Group's encyclopedia is logically organized into chapters such as "Foods," "Herbs," "Amino Acids," "Nucleic Acids," "Hormones," "Lipids," "Essential Oils," and "Entheogens" (hallucinogens), which could make it useful for health food, alternative and conventional medicine, and New Age collections as well as for personal libraries. Although the encyclopedia is fascinating reading, it would, at best, be recommended to public and academic libraries as a companion work to more clinical and better documented works, such as alternative health journalist Mark Mayell's *A Consumer's Guide to Legal, Mind-altering, and Mood-Brightening Herbs and Supplements* (Three Rivers Press, 1998) or the work mentioned above by Sahelian. [R: BL, Aug 01, pp. 2168-2169]—**Linda D. Tietjen**

207.　**The Illustrated Encyclopedia of Body-Mind Disciplines.** Nancy Allison, ed. New York, Rosen Publishing, 1999. 448p. illus. index. $79.95. ISBN 0-8239-2546-3.

The United States has been experiencing a spiritual awakening in the 1990s that involves linking mind, body, and spirit in an attempt to find greater peace of mind and physical well-being. Many of the techniques used in body-mind disciplines have been practiced for centuries in various parts of the world. *The Illustrated Encyclopedia of Body-Mind Disciplines* describes in detail more than 100 different practices that help link the physical body with the sensing, feeling, and intuitive facilities of the mind.

The book begins by giving short definitions of the techniques covered. After a short introduction to the history and theory behind body-mind disciplines, the book is divided into chapters that supply 5-to 10-page entries on very specific techniques. The chapters include topics such as alternative health models (e.g., holistic, shamanism), sensory therapy (e.g., aromatherapy, light therapy), massage, acupuncture, martial arts, meditation, and body-oriented therapies (psychodrama, rebirthing), among others. The entries are thoroughly described and include the history and theory behind the technique. Many entries include photographs, and all include resources and suggestions for further reading. The work concludes with a name/subject index.

The encyclopedia will be a valuable inclusion in any health, public, or university library. The topic is timely and the entries offer enough information to help readers grasp the idea behind the subject. [R: LJ, July 99, p. 83; BL, 1 Sept 99, pp. 180-181]—**Shannon Graff Hysell**

208.   Lawless, Julia. **The Illustrated Encyclopedia of Essential Oils: The Complete Guide to the Use of Oils in Aromatherapy and Herbalism.** Rockport, Mass., Element Books, 1995. 256p. illus. index. $18.95pa. ISBN 1-85230-721-8.

This attractive, well-organized compendium offers schools, libraries, health workers, merchants, and consumers a colorful, economic guide to the use of fragrant and stimulating oils for health treatments and stress relief. Clearly explained and generously illustrated with photographs, the work opens with a preface expressing the author's aim in upgrading the 1992 edition. A two-page users' guide explains textual divisions and lists types of information found in the botanical index. A six-page spread models the entry arrangement, including ailments, methods of application, vital safety data, Latin and common names for plants, herbal and folk traditions, uses, related species and varieties, and where to find the plants.

Part 1 introduces the concept and history of aromatherapy, along with portraits of its founder. Guidelines stress the types of oils that are toxic and hazardous, such as arnica, mustard, and wormwood, and differentiate between natural and synthetic oils. Part 2 lists specific ills—dry skin, upset stomach, sore throat—and simples that combat or alleviate each. The author highlights with italics the oils that are most effective and readily available (e.g., benzoin for arthritis). A letter code indicates method of application, as in "F" for flower water, "M" for massage, "V" for vaporization, and "N" for neat application.

The highlight of this book is part 3, an examination of each oil, which appears in alphabetic order. A fresh, inviting layout juxtaposes data on plant names, traditions, and safety data. For example, marigold is the common name for *Calendula*, which is safe to use. A photograph shows the plant in the wild; a drawing illustrates stem, flower, leaves, and root. Back matter covers general terms, botanical classification by family, and botanical indexing, which the author codes with boldfaced numbers for major entry and italics for Latin plant name. She concludes with sources and with worldwide addresses that link consumers with sellers of oils, aromatherapists, training programs, medical herbalism, and holistic treatment. This work is well worth having.—**Mary Ellen Snodgrass**

209.   Marti, James, with Andrea Hine. **The Alternative Health & Medicine Encyclopedia.** 2d ed. Detroit, Gale, 1998. 462p. index. $47.00. ISBN 0-7876-0073-3.

The author's stated objective in this 2d edition of *The Alternative Health & Medicine Encyclopedia* is to present fully the different specialized therapies that fall under the umbrella of alternative medicine. The format of the 1st edition has not changed. Chapter 1 presents a brief overview of 15 medical systems in alternative medicine, such as acupuncture, chiropractic medicine, hypnosis, and yoga. Also discussed are other specialized alternative therapies, such as music therapy and massage; unique to the 2d edition are entries for aromatherapy, flower essences, hypothermia, and ozone therapy.

Chapters 2 through 8 describe the treatment components of alternative medicine, such as diet and botanical medicines. The remaining 11 chapters discuss treatments for specific disorders. Here, for example, the reader can identify a botanical therapy for the treatment of prostate enlargement in the chapter on common male health problems.

As in the 1st edition (see ARBA 96, entry 1716) much of the emphasis is on generally accepted principles of good health practices. Curiously, the index to the 2d edition is briefer and less detailed than that of the 1st edition. Despite the author's claim that the primary source materials for this book are available in most medical libraries, there are a number of citations to various newsletters and other forms of gray literature. Although this is a useful resource for general reference collections, there is not enough additional content in the 2d edition to warrant its purchase for most libraries already owning the 1st edition.—**Michael Weinberg**

210.   Murray, Michael T. **The Pill Guide to Natural Medicines: Vitamins, Minerals, Nutritional Supplements, Herbs, and Other Natural Products.** Westminster, Md., Bantam Dell Publishing Group, 2002. 1074p. index. $6.99pa. ISBN 0-553-58194-5.

With the increase in interest and availability of natural medicines, it is important for a consumer to find authoritative information that will help separate the good from the potentially dangerous alternatives to traditional therapies. Michael Murray, a respected naturopathic doctor and author of *A Textbook of Natural Medicine*, provides profiles of many natural products currently used to prevent and cure diseases. Over 275 vitamins, nutritional supplements, and herbal remedies are featured and rated for safety and effectiveness in this paperback guide. In addition to the medications, it also provides discussions on 70 common ailments and ways that natural medicines may or may not help.

In general the book agrees with information provided by the *PDR for Herbal Medicines* (2d ed.; see entry 409) and *The Complete German Commission E Monographs: Therapeutic Guide to Herbal Medicines* (Integrative Medicine Communications, 1998). Occasionally it glosses over side effects or cautions mentioned in those conservative tomes. It supplies recommended dosages, but not the duration for the treatment. Hopefully consumers will not assume that all these medicines are to be continued indefinitely.

Murray writes in a clear, easy-to-understand style and even avoids jargon that might discourage a lay reader from further reading while discussing the methodology of clinical trials or pharmacodynamics of a substance. While the brevity of information would not satisfy a physician or pharmacist, it nevertheless is a credible reference for a common audience.—**Susan K. Setterlund**

211.   Null, Gary. **The Complete Encyclopedia of Natural Healing.** New York, Kensington Publishing, 1998. 612p. index. $35.00. ISBN 1-57566-258-2.

This hardbound encyclopedia consists of 2 alphabetically arranged sections. The 1st section is a list of medical conditions with a short essay discussing causes, symptoms, and treatments. The 2d section addresses various modalities popular among alternative medicine practitioners. The index is comprehensive and easy to use. There are no appendixes, no bibliography, no additional reading lists, and no footnotes or endnotes. Readers wanting more information must fend for themselves. The content is extremely broad and superficial. There is an abundance of anecdotal patient stories, some with questionable connections to the topic at hand. The author addresses his newest book to confused health care consumers to give them a second opinion. The introduction claims that "every natural alternative will be here for you to refer to." Not only is his stated scope impossible to achieve, but his authority to make this claim is suspect. Neither the book jacket nor the Websites give any clue to the author's educational history except to display "Ph.D." prominently on the cover. After extensive searching, this reviewer found that the author's educational credentials appear to be sadly lacking. It will be wiser to spend limited library funds for reference books in this area on works that have better documentation and authority. —**Deborah D. Nelson**

212.   Null, Gary. **The Woman's Encyclopedia of Natural Healing: The New Healing Techniques of 100 Leading Alternative Practitioners.** New York, Seven Stories Press; distr., Emeryville, Calif., Publishers Group West, 1996. 411p. index. $19.95pa. ISBN 1-888363-35-5.

This paperback volume focuses on how natural (a.k.a., alternative, unconventional, complementary) healing techniques may impact the overall outcome of various ailments that women most often experience. Topics are appropriate for all females regardless of age, race, or cultural heritage; and thus, this work provides a handy reference for all stages of life. Examples include aging, birth control, breast cancer, eating disorders, menopause, osteoporosis, PMS, and varicose veins. In all, 28 topics are explained through causes, symptoms, clinical experience, and therapeutic approaches (e.g., nutrition, exercise, massage, mind/body, and numerous homeopathic supplements).

Most of the information was obtained through interviews with approximately 100 natural healing practitioners. Some chapters include personal testimonies. All chapters include a short bibliography that lists some references in the medical literature. The author is a medical doctor specially trained in gynecologic surgery. This training, when combined with extensive experience in natural healing, provides the expertise necessary to adequately translate complex medical and scientific data into an easy-to-understand format. Any person, whether lay or health care professional, could benefit from the explanations contained within these pages. [R: LJ, Jan 97, p. 90]—**Sue Lyon Mertl**

213.   **Nutraceuticals: The Complete Encyclopedia of Supplements, Herbs, Vitamins, and Healing Foods.** Arthur J. Roberts, Mary E. O'Brien, and Genell Subak-Sharpe, eds. New York, Perigee Books/Putnam, 2001. 669p. index. $21.95pa. ISBN 0-399-52632-3.

This book is an official guide of the American Nutraceutical Association that was established in 1997 to provide information on nutraceuticals—the components of foods or dietary supplements that have healing or therapeutic properties. Besides including herbs, vitamins, and supplements, nutraceuticals are also known as designer foods, prescriptive foods, pharma foods, or medicinal foods. Since nutraceuticals, as opposed to pharmaceuticals, are not closely regulated by the Food and Drug Administration, quality varies and accurate data are hard to locate. This book is an excellent source to help consumers and health professionals ferret out facts about these increasingly popular remedies. The information is important and libraries of many types will want to have this most reasonably priced book available to their patrons.

The book is divided into four parts. Part 1 provides a very brief history, with quick reference charts by ailment and nutraceutical. Part 2 is a "Directory of Nutraceutical Remedies," alphabetically arranged by common disorder from acne to weight problems. This section is very well done, covering diagnostic steps, conventional treatments, and nutraceutical remedies for each disorder. Each remedy is further divided into sections on how it works, recommended dosages, and potential problems. Handy sidebars increase quick retrieval for topics like strategies for relief and symptoms of overdose.

Part 3, "The Top 200-Plus Nutraceuticals," is also alphabetically arranged and clearly presented. Each entry has subsections entitled "Role as a Supplement," "Evidence of Efficacy," "Sources," "Forms and Usual Dosages," "Potential Problems," and "What to Look For." A sample of entries in this section includes DHEA, Benecol, DMSO, oat bran, and ginseng. Part 4 covers nutraceuticals for male and female problems and aging. An appendix with purchasing tips, including recommended brand names, and a selective bibliography enhance the book's value. The editors are well-credentialed physicians. Disclaimers are prominent in the book, yet the information is as factual as current research allows.

There are many fine titles available that cover similar information for herbs and vitamins: *Prescription for Nutritional Healing* (see entry 385), *Encyclopedia of Nutritional Supplements* (see entry 380), *Nature's Pharmacy* (Prentice Hall Press, 1998), and *PDR for Herbal Medicine* (2d ed.; see entry 409). However, none of them cover the naturally occurring, therapeutic food chemicals known as nutraceuticals to the extent of this book. [R: BL, 1 May 01, p. 1701]—**Georgia Briscoe**

214.   Scheffer, Mechthild. **Encyclopedia of Bach Flower Therapy.** Rochester, Vt., Inner Traditions International, 2001. 343p. illus. $29.95pa. ISBN 0-89281-941-3.

Although this volume is a translation of a German work and its author is German, the original Edward Bach, who developed the theory and practice of flower therapy, was a British physician. After completing his medical studies in London and practicing there for a few years, a major illness and his later acceptance of a position at the Homeopathic Hospital in London started him on the way to his discovery of the value of flowers in healing and restoring balance to one's life. His years of research produced the now famous Bach Flower Therapy, which, although complex in both theory and practice, is basically the use of distilled flower essences to effect appropriate mental and emotional states leading to healing. The author of this work, the most outstanding proponent of the Bach theory, brings together not only Bach's basic theories but also the results of her own years of research and study, which focus on the integration of this theory into other preventive health systems.

Much of the work relies on the original words of Dr. Bach, which are italicized throughout the book. Only one section could reasonably be called an encyclopedia and that is the detailed descriptions of the 36 essential flowers, which are placed in alphabetical order. The chapters preceding and following this text cover such topics as the theoretical foundations of Bach's therapy, how to help others to apply the therapy, and differences and similarities among the flowers. Appendixes include a listing of key words with page references, a list of contacts in other countries, and a brief bibliography. The lack of a general index makes the use of the table of contents almost mandatory, but fortunately it is fairly detailed. Intended for practitioners, students, and patients, this work is considered the most comprehensive reference on the subject. The clear writing style, beautiful illustrations, and pleasant format undoubtedly enhance the message, but this is not a book for dabblers. It will be most appreciated by those interested in the subject and willing to give time and effort to its study. This *Encyclopedia* is recommended for those public and academic libraries that have collections in alternative or complementary medicine.—**Lucille Whalen**

215.   Shealy, C. Norman. **The Illustrated Encyclopedia of Healing Remedies.** Rockport, Mass., Element Books, 1998. 496p. illus. index. $49.95. ISBN 1-86204-187-3.

Ancient humans practiced healing methods on each other until they got well or died, then made a note of the recipe and passed it down through the generations. Now, due to tedious research and careful thought, we can apply natural healing therapies thousands of years old to modern circumstances. Shealy has compiled spirited historical information on eight healing methods: ayurveda, herbalism, homeopathy, aromatherapy, traditional Chinese medicine, folk remedies, flower remedies, and vitamins and minerals and how and why they work.

Part 1, "Therapies and Healing Remedy Sources," explains how the body is physically connected from the big toe to the crown, and how influences such as attitude, pollution, planetary alignment, posture, diet, occupations, and surroundings affect our health. The five elements of the universe—space (respiration), air (movement), fire (intelligence), water (blood), and earth (bones)—are present in each of us, and when these elements are in balance we are healthy. These concepts could be complicated and intense, yet Shealy's text, illustrations, scope, resources, and sidebars make this reference work easy to absorb and understand.

Part 2, "Treating Common Ailments," deals with more than 200 disorders such as addictions, obsessions, compulsions, and phobias; troublesome lungs, teeth, and livers; and problems with circulatory, digestive, musculaskeletal, immune, endocrine, and reproductive systems. *The Illustrated Encyclopedia of Healing Remedies* contains ordinary and obscure treatments and herbal recipes and instructions on how to make salves, ointments, tinctures, and decoctions. It also includes a section of common ailments in children and the elderly. What Shealy has shared with us is more than health information, it is a healthy attitude.—**Mary Pat Boian**

216. Spinella, Marcello. **The Psychopharmacology of Herbal Medicine: Plant Drugs That Alter Mind, Brain, and Behavior.** Cambridge, Mass., MIT Press, 2001. 578p. illus. index. $24.95pa. ISBN 0-262-69265-1.

Historical use of psychoactive plants can be found in practically every culture in the world. With the continuing popularity of alternative and complementary medicine, people are interested in using these natural products to treat their diseases, usually under the mistaken belief that these products are less likely to cause adverse effects. While little empirical research exists for many alternative and complementary health practices, there is a large body of research on medicinal plants. This book attempts to organize and integrate this information into a single source to assist health care practitioners in advising their patients and to provide researchers with a broad summary of data.

The first chapter provides a concise introduction to the herbal versus synthetic drug issues that have developed during the past decade of increasing interest in the use of natural products as therapeutic agents. The author also has written introductory chapters on neuroscience and pharmacology, of which a basic understanding is critical in understanding the mechanism of action psychoactive drugs and their effects on the human body. The remainder of the book is divided into chapters based on the types of effects the herbal products are purported to have: stimulants, cognitive enhancers, sedatives and anxiolytics, psychotherapeutic, analgesic and anesthetic, hallucinogenic, and an entire chapter on cannabis.

For each herbal product, an attempt is made to include historical information, active chemical components, pharmacokinetics (how the body affects the drug), mechanism of action, pharmacodynamics (how the drug affects the body), physiological effects, toxicity, and any clinical trial results. References to the primary literature are abundant (more than 100 pages) and alphabetically listed by chapter. A separate recommended reading list is also available. Focusing primarily on the effects on cognition—especially attention, learning, and memory—this book provides a summative overview of herbal psychopharmacology for the practicing health care professional and researcher. Academic and medical libraries will find this resource brings together a vast collection of data into one organized and integrated resource.—**Vicki J. Killion**

217. Stillerman, Elaine. **The Encyclopedia of Bodywork: From Acupressure to Zone Therapy.** New York, Facts on File, 1996. 320p. illus. index. $35.00. ISBN 0-8160-3187-8.

To fully appreciate this book, one must look beyond its title. Replace the word "bodywork" with "alternative (a.k.a. unconventional or complementary) medical therapies" and this volume becomes a reference for the most rapidly growing class of medical interventions in the United States. Studies indicate that 1 in 3 patients uses these therapies routinely, 7 in 10 do not inform their doctors of these practices, and most pay for these services out of their own pockets—sobering statistics for a struggling traditional health care system.

The author states that this book was written to "provide in-depth descriptions, explanations and historical backgrounds of common, esoteric, and sacred bodywork systems to people who are unfamiliar to them." In fact, the term *bodywork* is expanded to include all the "hands-on therapies, movement reeducation systems, psychological techniques and metaphysical and energetic modalities, which recognize the unity of the body/mind/spirit/emotions." Explanations of herbal therapies are limited to aromatherapy, body wraps, and moxibustion; however, short bibliographies are included.

Appendix 1 is a comprehensive resource list of names, addresses, and telephone and fax numbers for various providers, clinics, and professional associations. Appendix 2 is a repeat format for all states and provinces (in the United States and Canada) that require a license/board certification to practice massage therapy. Patient provider education is the focus—improved communication is the goal. Within these pages are clear and concise definitions that provide the critical first step.—**Sue Lyon Mertl**

218.   Tirtha, Swami Sada Shiva. **The Ayurveda Encyclopedia: Natural Secrets to Healing, Prevention, & Longevity.** Bayville, N.Y., Ayurveda Holistic Center Press; distr., Chicago, Independent Publishers Group, 1998. 669p. illus. index. $32.00. ISBN 0-9658042-2-4.

Although there is no lack of books on alternative health care, few give an overall, in-depth picture of Ayurveda, a holistic health system that originated in India and aims to provide guidance regarding food and lifestyle in order to maintain good health throughout life. This work was intended to fill the need for an authoritative, comprehensive study of the subject, one that could be used as a text for those studying this fairly complicated system. The author, an instructor at the Ayurveda Holistic Center in Bayville, New York, states that he undertook the task of writing this guide at the request of his students, but also points out that the aim of the work is to offer credible evidence to the allopathic community and government health-regulating bodies that Ayurveda can reduce health care costs by more than 50 percent, avoid side effects, and provide effective healing treatments.

In the Ayurvedic system great emphasis is placed on the relationship between the mind and the body, so it is not surprising that much of the text is devoted to this aspect of the subject. According to the author, this encyclopedia is really 3 books in 1: the 1st includes a history of Ayurveda and its basic principles; the 2d is a description of various therapies, including meditation, herbs, and exercise; and the 3d discusses the causes and natural healing remedies for more than 1,000 disorders. From the table of contents, however, one finds the material divided into 4 main sections, with section 4 being divided into chapters on each of the various body systems, such as digestive, respiratory, and nervous systems, and further subdivided into specific diseases. Following the main text are 9 appendixes, including an Ayurvedic glossary, a bibliography, and an index.

The author reminds the reader that the information presented is only a starting point for learning and should not be followed blindly. It would be difficult, however, for most readers to consider this work a starting point. Without some previous training in Ayurveda, finding information on any specific topic would be difficult and tedious. For example, interspersed throughout the text are many words from the Ayurvedic glossary and one must refer to the glossary constantly to read even a few paragraphs in many sections. Some of the terms in the index have too many references without specific page numbers. Kidney, for example, has 19 references, in addition to 6 subheadings with page numbers. Also, some statements seem questionable—that most psychological diseases are said to be healed through color therapy is one instance. Although the volume provides a great deal of helpful information and the author is obviously well educated and knowledgeable about the subject, the way the information is organized, the frequent use of Sanskrit terms, and the sometimes tedious style make it difficult for the ordinary reader. It is recommended only for those libraries having an extensive collection in alternative medicine.—**Lucille Whalen**

219.   Woodham, Anne, and David Peters. **Encyclopedia of Healing Therapies.** New York, DK Publishing, 1997. 336p. illus. index. $39.95. ISBN 0-7894-1984-X.

With this publication the authors hope to provide an analysis of the benefits claimed by various healing or complementary therapies (not necessarily alternative therapies to conventional treatments) and to provide readers with a means of identifying therapies that may improve their health.

The book begins with a questionnaire designed to allow readers to assess their general well-being. A second questionnaire is aimed at enabling readers to identify categories of complementary therapies to which they are most suited. These categories—touch and movement, medicinal therapies (including diet or other remedies), and mind and emotion therapies—correspond to headings within the section "Key Healing Therapies." The entry for each therapy includes a defini- tion, brief history, and key principles. But given the many and often gratuitous illustrations, there is only the most basic information conveyed within the several pages devoted to each therapy. Al- though each complementary therapy is assigned a rating of its effectiveness, the text is clearly bi- ased in its favor. Scant references are made to the primary literature, and no complete bibliographic citations are provided. The section entitled "Treating Ailments" lists over 200 health problems. Entries for each include a brief discussion of conventional treatment along with descrip- tions of available complimentary treatments. Specific applications of these complimentary treat- ments for the various ailments are indicated, again without supporting references.

Although this book adequately defines the major complementary therapies currently prac- ticed and provides information for individuals predisposed to their use (including guidance on choosing a practitioner), it does not present information in a substantive or objectively critical manner.—**Michael Weinberg**

Directories

220.   Owen, David J. **The Herbal Internet Companion: Herbs and Herbal Medicine Online.** Binghamton, N.Y., Haworth Press, 2002. 193p. index. $49.95; $19.95pa. ISBN 0-7890-1051-8; 0-7890-1052-6pa.

The old caveat "don't judge a book by its cover" certainly applies to this modest paperback with its somewhat garish cover and a title that might lead one to believe it is a list of commercial Websites where ginkgo biloba can be purchased online. What a surprise to find instead a compre- hensive, authoritative guide to finding the best information about herbal medicine from respected medical and educational institutions, government organizations, and nonprofit organizations around the world. The author is a librarian and he has organized the information for efficient re- trieval by focusing on 16 topics related to herbs and herbal medicine. Subjects covered include the history of herbal treatments, botany and laws, and standards and regulations. Valuable information about adverse effects and interactions of herbs is the subject of one section. Others direct the reader to consumer topics such as quackery and fraud and how to evaluate Internet herbal sites.

Each section begins with a succinct but informative overview of the subject featured. These essays serve as a point of reference to the librarian or consumer by putting the topic in the context of the field of complementary and alternative medicine. Websites are listed alphabetically by the name of the originating group or agency. URLs are provided. Entry annotations describe the type of information to be found at the site (e.g., full text, abstracts, bibliographic, pictorial). The book is footnoted and includes a short glossary and an alphabetic index.

It is obvious that the compilation of this work was a labor of love undertaken by an expert in the field of scientific librarianship. It is unique resource that will be a valuable tool in medical and public libraries as well as a guide to practitioners and consumers of herbal medicine.—**Marlene M. Kuhl**

Handbooks and Yearbooks

221.   **The Alternative Advisor: The Complete Guide to Natural Therapies & Alternative Treatments.** Alexandria, Va., Time-Life Books, 1997. 400p. $24.95. ISBN 0-7835-4907-5.

Time-Life Books has compiled an easy-to-understand, 400-page volume that should be in- cluded in the library of those wanting information concerning the differences between pharmaceu- tical drugs and natural therapies. The book is divided into two main topics: therapies and conditions. Forty alternative therapies are mentioned, including acupuncture, Ayurvedic medicine, nutrition, massage, hydrotherapy, and yoga. Illustrations are specific and uncluttered. Sidebars include such information as whether or not the therapy is covered by insurance, Medicare, or Medicaid. Also covered are origin of the remedy, what the therapy is good for, where to get it, application techniques, and what critics have to say about it. There are 75 herbs mentioned with their target ailments, preparation methods, and potential side effects listed, which will help relieve any anxiety that comes with exploring the unknown. Thirty of the more common homeopathic remedies, plus descriptions of thirty-two vitamins and minerals, help the neophyte become educated.

The 2d half of *The Alternative Advisor* describes ailments and their symptoms, including when to call a professional health provider. This section discussing conditions has easy-to-read heads at the top edge of each page, making it easy to find the topic of interest. Time-Life Books has published a book that coaches the rookie in entry-level health management, thus making it easier to talk with a doctor about possible health care alternatives. [R: LJ, Aug 97, p. 74]—**Mary Pat Boian**

222.   **Alternative Medicine Sourcebook.** Allan R. Cook, ed. Detroit, Omnigraphics, 1999. 737p. index. (Health Reference Series). $78.00. ISBN 0-7808-0200-4.

Like the other books in Omnigraphics' Health Reference Series, this work is presented in a format to help the reader understand the basics and the breadth of a particular health issue. The *Alternative Medicine Sourcebook* is designed to help the layperson understand the issues and controversies surrounding alternative and complementary medicine. It presents an overview of the major families of therapies, and includes in-depth descriptions of some of the most common practices, such as Rolfing, aromatherapy, acupuncture, homeopathy, and reflexology.

The book is divided into 9 parts: the issues of alternative medicine; alternative systems of medical practice; "bioelectromagnetics"; diet, nutrition, and lifestyle changes; herbal medicine; manual healing; mind and body control; pharmacological and biological treatments; and additional help and information. A typical essay on an alternative medicine topic includes a brief history, a description of the practice, an objective analysis of the effectiveness of the practice, and any scientific studies that have been conducted on the particular form of alternative medicine. Many of the essays also contain a list of additional references and sources of information. There are few illustrations to aid in presenting the material. A more colorful and visually appealing work with similar information is *The Encyclopedia of Alternative Medicine* (see entry 204). As a starting point to introduce readers to alternative medicine practices, this book will be a great addition to the reference collection of every type of library.—**Elaine F. Jurries**

223.   Callinan, Paul. **Family Homeopathy: A Practical Handbook for Home Treatment.** New Canaan, Conn., Keats Publishing, 1995. 343p. index. $24.95. ISBN 0-87983-687-3.

In recent years, a number of books have been published concerning the practice of homeopathy, a system of alternative medicine that uses natural remedies to treat common and chronic ailments. Add *Family Homeopathy* to this growing list. The arrangement of this book is similar to other recent works on the topic. An introductory chapter describes how homeopathy works, and scientific evidence is cited to support the effectiveness of homeopathic treatments. Some of the author's examples are quite convincing. For instance, he cites a source that claims that a 10 percent mortality rate during the European cholera epidemic of 1832 was recorded for patients treated with homeopathy, compared to a 70 percent mortality rate for patients who received traditional medical treatment.

The balance of the work consists of two major sections: a list of treatments for common problems (e.g., acne, headache, indigestion and heartburn, gout, hair loss, constipation) and a materia medica of common remedies. Added information includes a chapter on the Bach flower remedies, a home medicine kit, a resource guide of suppliers, and a short bibliography. *Family Homeopathy* is a suitable purchase for the library circulating collection, or the home library. [R: RQ, Summer 96, pp. 557-558]—**Elaine F. Jurries**

224.   Cassileth, Barrie R. **The Alternative Medicine Handbook: The Complete Reference Guide to Alternative and Complementary Therapies.** New York, W. W. Norton, 1998. 340p. illus. index. $19.95pa. ISBN 0-393-31816-8.

This is an excellent, balanced overview of the numerous alternative and complementary medical therapies that are being practiced today. The author defines "alternative" as a therapy that is used instead of Western mainstream medicine, and "complementary" as a therapy that serves a supplementary role in conventional care. Alternative therapies tend to be unproven and may or may not be harmful. Complementary therapies, usually used alongside conventional treatment, are generally noninvasive and helpful. With great objectivity, the author describes the background, goals, benefits, and risks of each therapy, neither recommending nor condemning any of them.

The book is composed of 7 parts, each part representing a broad category of alternative or complementary medicine. The 7 parts are routes to health and spiritual fulfillment, dietary and herbal remedies, using the mind for emotional relief and physical strength, alternative biological treatments, reducing pain and stress through bodywork, enhancing well-being through the senses, and restoring health with external energy forces. Within each part, 6 to 12 individual therapies are thoroughly described. The description of each therapy contains the following information: what it is, what practitioners say it does, beliefs on which it is based, research evidence to date, what it can do, and where to get it. Among the 54 therapies discussed are acupuncture, homeopathy, Native American healing, Chinese medicine, fasting and juice therapies, macrobiotics, biofeedback, biological dentistry, oxygen therapies, craniosacral therapy, rolfing, aromatherapy, humor therapy, shamanism, and therapeutic touch.

Although there are numerous alternative medicine handbooks on the market, some of which border on the fantastical, this book stands out because it is balanced, rational, and objective. It deserves a place on the reference shelf of both academic and public libraries.—**Elaine F. Jurries**

225.   **The Complete Book of Symptoms and Treatments: Your Comprehensive Guide to the Safety and Effectiveness of Alternative and Complementary Medicine for Common Ailments.** By Roland Bettschart and others. Edzard Ernst, ed. Rockport, Mass., Element Books, 1998. 953p. index. $24.95pa. ISBN 1-86204-424-4.

This book neither promotes nor condemns alternative and complementary medicine. Instead, it attempts, through description and a rating system, to provide persons considering the use of remedies or techniques from this burgeoning field of health care with information about orthodox and complementary treatment for common complaints, enabling the consumer to make responsible and objective assessments.

A panel of experts based its ratings on "available published data" about what the therapies are supposed to do, how well they work, and potential risks. The problem is that remedies and systems of medicine, such as traditional Chinese medicine (often called alternative), are backed by centuries of tradition, but not much clinical research, so there are a lot of "cautions" and "unknowns." For example, Asians and Europeans are far more experienced with phytotherapeutics (herbal remedies) than Americans, who are now spending millions on herbs, perhaps with only "biased" information on the label.

This book is basically a translation of a popular 1995 German text. The 1st part of the book describes common ailments, by type of complaint or organs affected, and summarizes the orthodox approach and alternative or complementary therapies. Each chapter concludes with tables listing specific herbal remedies, including the benefits and risks. Often the caveat is to get professional advice from one's regular physician before turning to other "experts" or trying self-treatment. In this sense "complementary" means "collaborative" or "supportive" rather than entirely different, as the older term "alternative" may suggest.

The 2d part of the book is a fascinating compendium of the many kinds of therapies used in complementary medicine, such as acupuncture and reflexology, with history, rationale, risks, and potential benefits. The total body of scientific knowledge available today is the measure for rating each therapy. Suggestions are given for choosing a reputable therapist who should offer a treatment plan and limited trial as well as personal assistance.

A 3d section discusses the diagnostic techniques used in complementary medicine, with effectiveness claims by its practitioners. This is followed by a list of professional organizations in the United Kingdom, Australia, and the United States.

As an overview of complementary medicine in its many forms and a comprehensive guide for choosing therapies, this book ranks far above other available paperbacks. It is well indexed and cross-referenced, rather scholarly in approach, and well suited for its intended users.—**Harriette M. Cluxton**

226.   **The Complete Family Guide to Natural Home Remedies.** Karen Sullivan, ed. Rockport, Mass., Element Books, 1997. 256p. illus. index. $24.95pa. ISBN 1-86204-020-6.

This book is an excellent source of information on five forms of alternative therapy: herbalism, homeopathy, flower remedies, aromatherapy, and diet and nutrition. The book is divided into four parts. "Home Therapies" discusses the five therapies and their application. It explains how the therapies work, their history, and how to prepare various remedies. "The Ailments" lists common problems and injuries grouped under 13 systems of the body (immune, circulatory, respiratory, etc.), plus one group for childhood problems and one group for childhood illnesses. "The Remedy Sources" provides detailed descriptions of 225 well-known and not so well-known substances. "Practical Matters and Useful Information" includes a section on first aid, putting together a home medicine chest, information on vitamins and minerals, a one-page bibliography of related books, a listing of organizations, a glossary, and a subject index.

Parts 2 and 3 make up the bulk of the book. Each ailment listed in part 2 includes a brief description and symptoms, plus a list of possible remedies from one or more of the five therapies; self-care tips are also included. Although some of the body system groups have few entries, the range of illnesses covered is comprehensive. The descriptions are terse, and the list of remedies is often specific. Many of the remedies include cautions such as which substances are to be avoided during pregnancy or with certain medical conditions and symptoms requiring medical attention.

Part 3 is divided into sections on plant and animal remedy sources, elements, compounds and minerals, and food and drink. Each substance includes a few paragraphs on its various uses (homeopathic, herbal, etc.) as well as a "data file" on the properties (herbs and foods), symptom pictures (homeopathic remedies), and extraction method (flower essences), information on dosages, and contradictions when applicable. Like the ailments section, appropriate cautions are included.

The publisher is British and the book does have a British and European slant, which may be confusing to some American readers; for example, suggesting an oil is to be applied "neat." Also, some of the substances are not commonly seen in the United States, such as neroli (bitter orange fruit). Chinese herbs are only mentioned in passing, when there is some overlap with the Western herbs; readers searching for information on Chinese herbs and remedies will have to look elsewhere.

The book can be used as a whole—as an overall guide to incorporating traditional remedies into a healthy lifestyle—or as a reference to individual ailments. The remedies are usually cautious, sensible, and simple enough for most people to adopt. The book is beautifully designed; each page is amply illustrated with color photographs, drawings, and shaded boxed text. Anyone looking for detailed and clear information on traditional Western remedies can find it here.—**Stephen Haenel**

227.   Duke, James A. **The Green Pharmacy: New Discoveries in Herbal Remedies for Common Diseases and Conditions from the World's Foremost Authority on Healing Herbs.** Emmaus, Pa., Rodale Press, 1997. 507p. illus. index. $29.95. ISBN 0-87596-316-1.

The Green Pharmacy is a compendium of herbal treatments for more than 120 common medical conditions. Duke, a world-renowned botanist, has written a book that is highly readable, thorough, and up to date. His approach is a mixture of folklore from around the world combined with clinical research and a large dose of personal anecdotes.

The first part of the book is a guide to using medicinal herbs and includes safety considerations and tips on buying, preparing, and using herbal medicines. The second part is an A to Z listing of diseases and conditions, with descriptions of the conditions and a listing of helpful herbs and foods. The range of maladies covered includes allergies, HIV, insect bites and stings, male and female sexual and genitourinary problems, heart disease, viral infections, Parkinson's disease, asthma, and skin conditions. The list is surprisingly complete, with the exception of children's illnesses, which receive scant attention. The text is sprinkled with recipes and stories of herb lore as well as fine line drawings of many herbs. No bibliography or suggested reading list is included, which would make this an even more useful reference work.

All in all, Duke presents a balanced view of both the advantages and disadvantages of herbs and foods as medicines. He quotes a wide variety of experts—herbalists, naturopaths, physicians, researchers, and the German body Commission E—and provides a full account of the advantages and disadvantages of herbs, especially compared to pharmaceuticals. To his credit, Duke is a bit more guarded than some writers on natural products, often hedging his advice with "herbs that might prove helpful" or "if I had . . . I might try . . . ." Conversely, some of his descriptions of ailments and prescriptions lack the depth of some authorities on natural healing. He often gives details on the chemical constituents of herbs, but this work is not overly technical. His writing is lively and approachable. Using this book is like sitting down with a country herbalist, which lends it a certain charm.—**Stephen Haenel**

228.   Elkins, Rita. **The Complete Home Health Advisor.** Pleasant Grove, Utah, Woodland Publishing, 1995. 388p. index. $17.95pa. ISBN 0-913923-96-6.

The author depends on the cover description, "A Guide to Combining Standard Medical Treatments with Wholistic Alternatives," to convey the purpose of the book; there is no preface. Although her credentials are not stated, the text material would seem to indicate careful preparation. More than 100 common health concerns or "ailments" are described, their standard medical treatment discussed, and alternative treatments and other remedies suggested.

Alphabetically listed topics are treated according to the following formula: definition, causes, symptoms, emergency alerts, standard medical treatments (and side effects), home self-care, nutritional approach, herbal remedies, and prevention. Each of these sections is marked by a black symbol in the margin. For example, a stylized plant design indicates herbal remedies and what they are supposed to do. Some topics are actual disease names; most are common descriptions, such as fever. Earache and backache are listed, but strangely, the most common complaint, headache—which is often treated by home remedies—is not. Also, *hantavirus* is hardly a "common" complaint or ailment.

Using regular medical resources is always recommended. The alternatives discussed are presented as auxiliaries rather than substitutes, and medical advice should be sought before using them. The approach is interpretive, explaining how to understand the condition and seek help, not how to self-treat. Dosages or specific directions are not given. This perhaps justifies placing this oversized work in the consumer health collection as well as considering it as a home handbook. It contains much practical and interesting health information.—**Harriette M. Cluxton**

229. Feuerman, Francine, and Marsha J. Handel. **Alternative Medicine Resource Guide.** Chicago, Medical Library Association and Lanham, Md., Scarecrow, 1997. 335p. index. $49.50. ISBN 0-8108-3284-4.

Readers interested in self-regulated health will be pleased with *Alternative Medicine Resources Guide's* extensive coverage of alternative healing methods. The two librarians responsible for this collection of over 30 noninvasive therapies point out that access to health maintenance information is their objective, and with this goal in mind, they have provided definitions and sources ample enough for novices and explicit enough for professionals.

The book is divided into two sections: resources and bibliography. Resources are extracted from U.S. publications, organizations, universities, treatment resorts, and product suppliers. Systems of alternative medicine mentioned here range from 5,000-year-old methods of healing, such as Ayurveda and herbal therapy, to twentieth-century techniques, such as biofeedback and music therapy. The bibliography section, which is one-third of the book, organizes books, journals, and newsletters including manipulative, sensory, and movement therapies. These entries are based on authors' credentials, understandable ideologies, and universality.

The gratifying element of this work is its success in clearing the misconceptions about the numerous ways to maintain good health. There is no preaching, no judgment, no disdain for conventional medicine. This is a primary guide that will benefit and appease those curious and adventurous enough to take on the responsibility of their own health. As the title says, it is alternative medicine.—**Mary Pat Boian**

230. Goldberg, Burton. **Alternative Medicine Guide to Heart Disease, Stroke, & High Blood Pressure.** Tiburon, Calif., Future Medicine Publishing, 1998. 293p. illus. index. $18.95pa. ISBN 1-887299-10-6.

As increasing numbers of people are turning to alternative methods for the prevention and healing of various illnesses, and are seeking information in guides such as this one. As part of a series published in conjunction with the *Alternative Medicine Digest*, this guide is divided into three main sections treating heart disease, stroke, and high blood pressure. In an introductory statement, the author points out that the book is on alternative methods, and many are not understood or endorsed by the traditional medical community. While he urges readers to discuss the treatments prescribed with their doctors and not to use the book as a substitute for the advice and care of a physician, he also points out that the traditional medical community (including pharmaceutical companies, physicians' trade groups, insurance companies, and some government agencies) is somewhat of a monopoly and has an investment in keeping non-patentable, expensive treatments from the public.

In each of the three areas covered in the guide, the causes of the problem are clearly discussed, along with the self-care options available for prevention related to diet, exercise, and lifestyle changes. The main text describes various alternative therapies, citing both individual cases and research studies that are well documented in standard medical and scientific journals. Accompanying the text are excellent illustrations and diagrams, particularly useful for seeing how certain problems appear in the cardiovascular system. An added feature of the guide is the use of icons in the margins to give further information in smaller print. A small caution sign, for example, alerts the reader to certain risks or contraindications. In addition to the list of citations from footnotes in the text, an index and a list of organizations are found in the appendix. This highly informative, very readable guide should be an excellent introduction to alternative treatments for those with heart problems. The fact that most of the material comes from physicians with traditional training who have turned to alternative methods should be a plus for those who are somewhat fearful of trying something new.—**Lucille Whalen**

231.   Lockie, Andrew, and Nicola Geddes. **The Complete Guide to Homeopathy.** New York, Dorling Kindersley, 1995. 240p. illus. index. $29.95. ISBN 0-7894-0148-7.

This book describes 150 homeopathic remedies arranged in 3 sections: key remedies (15), remedies commonly prescribed by homeopaths (30), and minor remedies (105). Descriptions include common names, sources, parts of sources used, and ailments treated. The selection of remedies in the system of homeopathy presented is based on the patient's "constitutional type," which is determined by a 16-page questionnaire assessing the "inherited or acquired physical, emotional and intellectual makeup" of the patient. The constitutional type associated with each remedy is given.

The latter portion of the book is composed of tables describing symptoms, causes, and remedies (including dosages) for specific diseases and conditions. These are arranged by categories of ailments. The book also includes an excellent short history of homeopathy, a brief discussion of homeopathic theory, and chapters on nutrition and special diets. A directory provides addresses of suppliers of homeopathic remedies. There is also a useful index. The guide is profusely, even excessively, illustrated with exceptionally fine color photographs.

This is an attractive book with solid, basic information for the general reader. However, many potential users will find the theory of constitutional types difficult to accept and may find the questionnaire difficult to use. Consequently, the guide may be a better candidate for circulation than for reference. Further, the questionnaire presents the usual risk of loss of pages or defacing of the book in a library setting.—**Gari-Anne Patzwald**

232.   **The Medical Advisor: The Complete Guide to Alternative & Conventional Treatments.** By the Editors of Time-Life Books. Alexandria, Va., Time-Life Books, 1996. 1152p. illus. index. $39.95. ISBN 0-8094-6737-2.

The Medical Advisor covers 300 diagnoses ranging from common mishaps, such as bee stings and sprains, to such serious problems as diabetes or heart disease. For each condition, there is a short description of the complaint, what causes it, the conventional medical treatment, and alternative therapies, plus prevention suggestions. This book is designed to provide a general understanding of specific illnesses to promote discussions between patients and their physicians. This guide is unusual in that it gives both conventional medical treatments and alternative therapies, such as meditation, yoga, acupuncture, homeopathic preparations, and the like. The editors caution that the natural remedies are not intended to replace traditional allopathic medicine but rather to complement it.

Other notable features of the guide are an index with references to 3,000 ailments, treatments, and medicines, as well as a first aid section with procedures for 21 frequent emergencies. There is also an appendix listing 350 commonly used drugs and herbal remedies, with a notation if it is a prescription or over-the-counter drug, a Chinese or Western herb, or a homeopathic remedy, and any precautions to be taken.

Weighing 7 pounds and encompassing 1,152 pages, this tome is intimidating at first glance. However, it is easy to use, with attractive tables and illustrations. The text is well written and avoids overly technical explanations. This book is a good general reference for individuals with no medical training. At $39.95, it is affordable for both the home and the general library. [R: LJ, 1 Oct 96, p. 68; RBB, 1 Sept 96, pp. 167-168]—**Adrienne Antink Bien**

233.   McKenna, Dennis J., Kenneth Jones, and Kerry Hughes, with Sheila Humphrey. **Botanical Medicines: The Desk Reference for Major Herbal Supplements.** Binghamton, N.Y., Haworth Press, 2002. 1138p. index. $169.95; $79.95pa. ISBN 0-7890-1265-0; 0-7890-1266-9pa.

This is an outstanding resource for comprehensive, evidence-based information on the most widely used herbal dietary supplements in North America and Europe. Revised, updated, and expanded from its 1st edition, titled *Natural Dietary Supplements: A Desktop Reference* from the Institute for Natural Products Research (IPRO), this clearly written, exhaustively researched compendium should become a standard reference in botanical medicine. The authors are professionals in the natural products and dietary supplement field and founders of IPRO, a nonprofit educational and scientific organization. The first author is also Senior Lecturer at the Center for Spirituality and Healing, University of Minnesota, and serves on advisory and editorial boards of several botanical medicine organizations.

The book's 34 monographs cover each supplement's botanical data; history and traditional uses; chemistry; therapeutic applications; well-documented reviews of pre-clinical (animal) and clinical (human) studies; recommended dosages; safety profiles (including toxicology); side effects and contraindications; drug interactions and special precautions; safety recommendations during pregnancy and lactation; and full bibliographies.

Chapters range from 16 pages (cordyceps) to 60 (green tea), and their organizational structure —standardized major headings and subheadings used consistently in all chapters—facilitate clarity and easy comparison. A comprehensive name and subject index, and detailed appendixes on criteria for assessing quality of botanical supplements and the key aspects of the Dietary Supplement Health and Education Act of 1994 (DSHEA), complete the volume. This is a necessary resource for all libraries that serve physicians, pharmacists, and other health care providers and students, and can also benefit serious consumers.—**Madeleine Nash**

234.   **Nerys Purchon's Handbook of Natural Healing.** By Nerys Purchon. St. Leonards, Australia, Sue Hines Books; distr., Chicago, Independent Publishers Group, 1998. 412p. $19.95pa. ISBN 1-86448-645-7.

With people in the United States spending more than $1.5 billion a year on herbal products alone, it is no wonder that books on natural healing have become so popular. Many of these books contain much of the same information. The present work, however, brings a somewhat different perspective to the subject because its author grew up in Wales, which has a long tradition of herbal knowledge, and where she and her family found all the remedies needed for health and healing readily available near their home. After migrating to Australia, she started an herb-growing business and has written several books on various types of natural healing.

The handbook focuses mainly on herbal therapies but also includes information on other forms of natural healing, such as massage and meditation. It is arranged alphabetically but not by just herbs and therapies. Interspersed throughout the texts are various conditions for which these natural therapies are recommended, such as emphysema, hepatitis, and shingles. Furthermore, there are entries for the maintenance of good health, including sections on skin care and liver care. Although there are variations in the entries, for the herbal therapies there is generally a brief section on the part of the herb used, how it works, and conditions for which it is used. For most ailments, there is a description of the condition followed by sections on internal treatment, daily supplements, essential oil treatment, and homeopathic treatment.

Although there is a bibliography at the end of the volume, there is no index. The alphabetic arrangement makes an index less necessary, but it would probably simplify the finding of specific information. The work has a great deal of useful material that is made more easily accessible by its attractive page layout and use of different typefaces for headings. Because of the handbook's somewhat different viewpoint, its easily readable information, and its convenient arrangement, it should be a welcome addition to both public libraries and those academic libraries having alternative health collections.—**Lucille Whalen**

235. O'Mathúna, Donal. Larimore, Walt, ed. **Alternative Medicine: The Christian Handbook.** Grand Rapids, Mich., Zondervan Publishing/HarperCollins, 2001. 503p. index. $19.99pa. ISBN 0-310-23584-7.

This book tells the conservative evangelical Christian how to evaluate alternative medicine. It helps them make medical choices in light of the question, "What would Jesus do?" This well-designed and easy-to-use book is part of a series sponsored by the Christian Medical Association whose goal is to help members become like the Great Physician, Jesus Christ. The editors are well credentialed: O'Mathúna has a doctorate in medicinal chemistry from Ohio State University and Larimore is a medical doctor who works in Medical Outreach for Focus on the Family. They decided to put together a single resource that combines the latest and most accurate information on alternative medicine from two important perspectives—science and Christianity. They researched the science well, including ratings of studies with some documentation. They look to the literal interpretation of the Bible (New International Version) for answers on the spiritual side.

The book is divided into four parts: "An Overview of Alternative and Conventional Medicine"; "God, Health, Healing and the Christian"; "Evaluating Alternative Medicine"; and "Popular Alternative Therapies, Herbal Remedies, Vitamins and Dietary Supplements." The first three sections provide well-written discussion, history, and analysis to help readers understand the theological and practical implications of alternative medicine.

Part 4 is a convenient and concise alphabetic explanation and rating of alternative medicines, from acupressure and aloe to yoga and zinc. Included in the descriptions are study findings, claims, cautions, dosages, further readings, and treatment categories—each scored with one to five happy or sad faces. There is a list of diseases and symptoms with happy face scores for alternative therapies that might be applied. For example "dental pain" gets four happy faces for acupuncture and two for willow bark; "eczema" scores two happy faces for evening primrose oil and four unhappy faces for aloe. The book ends with a scripture index and a subject index.

This book will be highly useful and popular with followers of Focus on the Family and other conservative branches of Christianity. It does a very good job of making a complicated subject clear for its believers. It is not recommended for libraries without this patronage since it advises caution against other well-known therapies—ones that are considered "spiritual dangers" because they have origins from other religions such as Buddhism or New Age. For example, the authors find that Deepak Chopra's approach to health contradicts the biblical approach. This is an excellent book for its limited intended audience.—**Georgia Briscoe**

236. Ody, Penelope. **Natural Health Complete Guide to Medicinal Her**bs. New York, DK Publishing, 2000. 240p. illus. index. $29.95. ISBN 0-7894-6785-2.

Dorling Kindersley (DK) has partnered with the periodical *Natural Health* to publish a revised edition of Ody's *Complete Medicinal Herbal* (see ARBA 94, entry 1666). This edition, like the 1st, is a comprehensive guide to medicinal plants and herbal medicine. Herbalists as well as the general reader will find a wealth of information about the history of herbal medicine in various cultures from ancient time to the present. The A-Z directory of medicinal herbs gives information about each plant's appearance, active parts, applications, and preparation. Also included are cautionary notes warning of potential problems, such as interaction with other herbs or drugs and conditions under which the herb should not be used.

The compendium of common ailments and illnesses is organized by body system, with advice on appropriate remedies for each disorder. A case history accompanies each group. There is an extensive section on growing herbs and preparing and administering herbal remedies. Illustrated step-by-step directions are provided for preparing ointments, tinctures, and infusions. Details such as preparation equipment needed, proportions, and safe standard dosages are given.

The final section gives advice on consulting an herbalist. There is a short bibliography, a glossary, and a resource list. The index provides access by subject and by both common and Latin names of herbs. Beautiful color illustrations are an outstanding feature of the guide. There are other nice touches, like herb related literary quotes, accompanying each entry.

Despite the publisher's blurb that claims that text has been completely revised, most of the text and illustrations are taken from the earlier edition. Also, many of the same illustrations were used in Chevallier's *Encyclopedia of Medicinal Plants* (see entry 202). That said, there is new subject matter included in the text and minor reorganization of the information presented. Ayurvedic and Chinese tonics now merit their own section and are covered in more depth. There are also new sections on male reproductive and endocrine disorders. Australian bush herbs and South American herbs are now covered as well as more Native American plants. The revised guide is attractive and authoritative and can certainly hold its own with the many other titles on this popular subject.—**Marlene M. Kuhl**

237.   Russo, Ethan. **Handbook of Psychotropic Herbs: A Scientific Analysis of Herbal Remedies for Psychiatric Conditions.** Binghamton, N.Y., Haworth Press, 2001. 352p. index. $69.95; $29.95pa. ISBN 0-7890-0718-5; 0-7890-1088-7pa.

The stated purpose of this book is to introduce the concepts of herbal treatment for mental or nervous conditions and to serve as a reference of current research on herbal agents. The primary audience is mental health professionals and other interested persons, including students and laypersons. The book is divided into three main parts. Part 1 contains an introductory chapter and chapters on the U.S. history of regulation of botanicals (herbs) and a broad overview of research methodology. Part 2 is comprised of information on specific conditions and the herbs used to treat them. Each condition has its own chapter and a discussion of herbs used for its treatment. Helpful sections on individual herbs include synonyms, botany, phytochemistry, history of use, preparation of extracts, toxicity and side effects, published studies, and cost. A chapter on miscellaneous herbal agents includes research performed on aromatherapy and essential oils; additionally, this chapter contains a historical literature review of research on cannabis. Part 3, "Clinical Case Studies," examines 9 cases the author or others have treated with herbal medicine.

Logically organized, the text contains both a glossary and an index. It is well documented and contains an extensive bibliography of research cited. This book is recommended for professionals and students in mental health, interested laypersons, and academic and medical libraries with collections on alternative or complementary treatments.—**Lynn M. McMain**

238.   Schiller, Carol, and David Schiller. **Aromatherapy Oils: A Complete Guide.** New York, Sterling Publishing, 1996. 160p. illus. index. $14.95pa. ISBN 0-8069-6112-0.

An inexpensive alphabetized guide to types and uses of fragrant and stimulating oils, this compendium offers students, librarians, health workers, merchants, and consumers an overview of the role of aromatic oils in health treatments, relaxation, and stress relief. Containing simple explanations and indistinct line drawings of plants from which oils are extracted, the work opens with a thumbnail history of aromatherapy since the time of the Egyptian pharaohs. A three-page chapter on safe selection and handling of oils warns of the danger to eyes and sensitive skin as well as to pregnant and lactating women. Comments on the dangers of mixing aromatherapy with alcohol are also included. A one-sentence warning about the interference of oils with medication leaves much to the imagination. Remaining chapters discuss vegetable oils and butters, essential and infused oils, methods of use, blending oils, and categories of oil properties. The authors conclude with a cross-reference of botanical names, a list of plant families, a glossary, a bibliography, and an index.

The book presents information on individual oils in brief commentaries. Each entry contains botanical and common names, the family name, and the method of extraction. A history of each oil covers its use from numerous ancient cultures. Practical uses are brief to the point of uselessness, as in the comment that oil of fir balsam needles "lessens pain." Documented properties are also listed in terse, one-word commentary. For example, marjoram heads a laundry list of uses: analgesic, anaphrodisiac, antibacterial, antifungal, antioxidant, antiseptic, antispasmodic, antistress, antitussive, and antiviral, to name a few. The authors are preoccupied with long lists, which give little useful information to readers. The index lacks significant ties to common ailments such as arthritic joints, sleeplessness, and headaches. Overall, the work provides little more than an alphabetic listing of oils and vague applications to human needs.—**Mary Ellen Snodgrass**

239. Stengler, Mark. **The Natural Physician's Healing Therapies.** Paramus, N.J., Prentice Hall, 2001. 562p. index. $30.00. ISBN 0-7352-0250-8.

While this publication has the trappings of a reference book, it is more of a self-help book offering cures for a multitude of illnesses. Its main section gives descriptions of 89 substances and practices designed to cure illness and promote good health. Each entry provides background information, some history, and data on dosage and possible side effects along with a chart telling what the specific therapy is recommended for. These sections typically provide anecdotal support either from Stengler's observations or from the reports of friends, relatives, and patients. There are a few vague references to research findings.

The "References" section provides some, but not much, evidence for the therapies. Some of the references are to scientific journals, some are to Chinese traditional medicine, and some are to naturopathic journals. Many of the references contain the phrases "one study showed . . ." and "a few studies show . . ." Further, an examination of the problems to be cured for specific therapies finds little correspondence with the references. For example, arsenicum album is recommended for seven problems: allergies, anxiety, asthma, arthritis, cancer, ulcers, and the flu. But there only three references: one argues in favor of homeopathic treatments, one describes the use of arsenicum with rats given arsenic, and one describes its use with childhood diarrhea. This lack of correspondence is a common weakness of the reference section. Further, there are cures for which there is not even meager referential support. A major weakness of this book is that it does not provide satisfactory research support for its claims, suggesting that its readers remain cautious.

For those who seek cures, there is a "Quick Cure Finder" with the problems alphabetically arranged. The index is nicely done and should prove useful. Without a research base, this book is not likely to be useful to physicians and others in the medical profession. The general reader who looks for research to support therapeutic claims will be disappointed. Perhaps only those who are indifferent to such concerns will want this book, as well as those who look for easy, quick cures. The latter, using only the treatments offered in this book, might find themselves in difficulty. —**Bertram H. Rothschild**

240. Wardwell, Joyce A. **The Herbal Home Remedy Book: Simple Recipes for Tinctures, Teas, Salves, Tonics, and Syrups.** Pownal, Vt., Storey Communications, 1998. 169p. illus. index. $14.95pa. ISBN 1-58017-016-1.

Wardell is a self-taught herbalist and director of a nonprofit sustainable lifestyle organization. The 1st chapter offers practical advice on plant identification, even for the botanically challenged; gathering plants (with an eye toward conservation); and storage. Other chapters address selection of ingredients and equipment; making teas, tinctures, salves, vinegars, and syrups; drawings and descriptions of 25 useful herbs and their uses; stocking the home medicine cabinet;

blending herbs; an alphabetic arrangement of symptoms and remedies; and finally, a discussion of the spirit of herbalism. Wardell cautions readers that information in the book is not to be construed as medical advice and that anyone should discuss health concerns with their primary health care practitioner. The book is folksy and warm, with careful directions and recipes for making teas, salves, syrups, and tonics, which are interspersed with Native American folktales. Sidebars warn about potential problems, cite proverbs, and provide common sense advice. There is a helpful list of suggested books for a home remedy library, which is organized by topic, a list of suppliers of materials, and educational organizations. There are also a table of metric conversions and a useful index. *The Herbal Home Remedy Book* is recommended for personal or consumer health collections.—**Constance Rinaldo**

DENTISTRY

241. **Oxford Handbook of Clinical Dentistry.** 2d ed. By David A. Mitchell and Laura Mitchell. New York, Oxford University Press, 1995. 799p. illus. index. $36.50pa. ISBN 0-19-262602-7.

The cover of this work touts, "Dental students are going to love this book." This reviewer would agree and would add, "*Dentists* are going to love this book." The handbook is divided into the more or less traditional subspecialties of dentistry, for example, paedodontics and periodontology, but it also has sections on practice management and syndromes of the neck and head. A clever graphic in the table of contents allows one to flip directly to the primary sections without looking at page numbers. The book also contains two bound bookmarks to aid in use, and is in a convenient pocket-sized format.

The work is comprehensive in scope, but necessarily limited in detail and depth. It is presented in a logical, well-written manner, with an index and several useful reference sections. As dentistry continues to specialize and dentists are increasingly finding it necessary to revise and professionalize their practice, this work provides a crucial reference. Specialists can use it for finding information on practice and theory outside their area of expertise, general practitioners can use it for finding information in detail they cannot always be expected to know, and students should find it invaluable for surviving the rigors of an increasingly complex profession. The complications of the treatment of older patients, those living with AIDS or other severe illnesses, and the explosion of new pharmacology have come together to force dentists to become sophisticated diagnosticians, subtle and knowledgeable drug therapists, and adept referral consultants. A good reference work can aid in enhancing professionalism.

The handbook's only drawback for U.S. dentists and students is its political and clinical orientation toward U.K. dentistry. That orientation will prove especially confusing because the book does not use the American tooth numbering system. A suggestion to the authors and publishers would be an appendix or side-by-side comparison of the two systems. The value of the book, however, overcomes these drawbacks. All students, dentists, and dental schools will find this a useful and well-used reference.—**Luiz Alberto Cardoso**

FORENSIC MEDICINE

242. **Forensic Medicine Sourcebook.** Annemarie S. Muth, ed. Detroit, Omnigraphics, 1999. 574p. index. (Health Reference Series). $78.00. ISBN 0-7808-0232-2.

This source is another title from the reputable Health Reference Series by Omnigraphics. Apart from offering the layperson information on forensic medicine, there are several items that make this book attractive to consumers who are seeking certain forensic data. One is the death investigation systems in the United States and Canada that list states and provinces, and the death and injury statistics of the United States that include the top 10 leading causes of death. The other is the timeline of forensic medicine and the employment of biotechnology and multimedia for the advances of crime investigation. Also, the forensic glossary and resources listed are helpful additions.

The book's 55 chapters are arranged into 7 parts, including an overview, crime scene and laboratory investigation, forensic medicine/science subspecialties, emerging forensic subspecialties, advances in crime investigation, the courtroom, and additional helpful information. The section on using computer-aided victim identification and new technology inventions for crime detection is intriguing. The various subspecialties, such as forensic odontology, forensic geology, and forensic engineering, are well defined. Timely topics on DNA testing, drug detection, evidence analysis, accident reconstruction, explosives, statistical data, fingerprinting, product tampering, and autopsies are presented. Burns and rape topics are not thoroughly listed, and the principles on the clinical aspects are not fully analyzed. It is noted that materials from this book were collected from governmental and private agencies, as claimed by the publisher. There are references and notes in some chapters for readers to further locate additional information. On the whole, this is a useful current source for those seeking general forensic medical answers.—**Polin P. Lei**

GERIATRICS

243. **Physical and Mental Issues in Aging Sourcebook.** Jenifer Swanson, ed. Detroit, Omnigraphics, 1999. 660p. index. (Health Reference Series). $78.00. ISBN 0-7808-0233-0.

This new volume in Omnigraphics' Health Reference Series is designed to provide the layperson with a convenient source of information about symptoms, conditions, and diseases commonly encountered by the elderly. The main body of the book is divided into 9 sections covering cardiovascular concerns, pulmonary concerns, oral health and digestive concerns, musculoskeletal and skin concerns, metabolic concerns, sexual and reproductive concerns, concerns about the senses, pain and aging, and mental concerns. Many of the 70 individual chapters provide sources for additional information, and 2 chapters are devoted to identifying resource organizations and agencies, including state agencies on aging. Also included are a feeble glossary and a good index. The book's source material is taken primarily from government publications distributed by the National Institutes of Health, the Federal Drug Administration, and the National Institute on Aging. Most of this material is reasonably current although some of the reprinted and excerpted publications have original publication dates from as early as 1993. A major weakness of the work is the lack of cross-referencing from chapter to chapter. Although the major health problems of aging are covered, this is not a comprehensive sourcebook. The level of writing should be accessible to individuals with a high school reading proficiency. Recommended for public libraries. —**Bruce Stuart**

GYNECOLOGY AND HUMAN REPRODUCTION

244. **Encyclopedia of Birth Control.** Vern L. Bullough, ed., with others. Santa Barbara, Calif., ABC-CLIO, 2001. 349p. illus. index. $75.00. ISBN 1-57607-181-2.

The *Encyclopedia of Birth Control* contains alphabetically organized entries, helpful *see also* notations, and lists of references used. Several of the entries are signed by the authors. Appendix

1, "World Survey of Birth Control Practices," accurate to 1998, contains valuable information including population, birth rate, and total fertility rate (when known) for 184 countries. Appendix 2, "Print and Nonprint Resources," has an excellent list of books, libraries, journals, databases, and organizations. The organizations section in appendix 2 lists both pro-choice and pro-life organizations. Unfortunately, this is one of the only areas to show such impartiality.

Entries such as "Violence against Abortion Providers" and "Christian Hostility to Birth Control" have very little to do with birth control and a lot to do with emotionalism and a vitriolic attack on the pro-life point of view—specifically Christianity. Entries on Muslim and Jewish religious attitudes toward birth control, simply titled "Islam" and "Judaism and the Jewish Tradition," lack the obvious bias evident in the entries dealing with Christianity. The editors of this book intentionally use inflammatory, prejudicial language to convey their personal beliefs. A better selection, with a more balanced perspective and objective manner, is Oryx Press's *Encyclopedia of Birth Control* by Marian Rengel (see entry 251). [R: Choice, Nov 01, p. 485]—**Lynn M. McMain**

245.   **Encyclopedia of Reproduction.** Ernst Knobil and Jimmy D. Neill, eds. San Diego, Calif., Academic Press, 1998. 4v. illus. index. $495.00/set. ISBN 0-12-227020-7.

This encyclopedia is a comprehensive resource encompassing all aspects of reproduction as it relates to the entire animal kingdom. The 4-volume set represents the collaborative effort of 700 authors whose expertise ranges from zoology to animal husbandry, obstetrics, and gynecology. Arranged alphabetically, each entry is written to be a self-contained article. A topical outline provides a brief preview of the article and other important subtopics contained within. A glossary of terms, a summary introduction, cross-references to related articles, and a reading list are also provided in each entry.

Reading a volume straight through is rather interesting given the alphabetical arrangement. The article titled "Artificial Insemination in Humans" is immediately followed by "Asexual Reproduction." Knowing and using the correct terminology to locate information becomes very important. To assist readers in locating specific topics there is an extensive subject index in the fourth volume and article titles are listed under broad subject categories in the first volume. The terms found at the beginning of each article are defined in the context of the article they are used in. If the same term appears in other articles, the details of the definition may vary slightly. A comprehensive glossary of terms is found in the fourth volume.

Readers with extensive subject knowledge may find some of the articles lacking. Also, many of the articles will be outdated in a very short time. However, this is a comprehensive resource for students and the educated public at large. Academic and large public libraries will find it most useful.—**Vicki J. Killion**

246.   **The Encyclopedia of Reproductive Technologies.** Annette Burfoot, ed. Boulder, Colo., Westview Press, 1999. 404p. index. $85.00. ISBN 0-8133-6658-5.

The Encyclopedia of Reproductive Technologies is a rare find, a resource on a technical subject that is both comprehensible and academic. Articles are written in a clear and concise style about a broad variety of medical, technical, legislative, ethical, and historical topics. The credentials of the Canadian sociologist who edited this text and the contributing authors are impressive. The roster of contributors includes medical faculty and researchers, social scientists, ethicists and philosophers, activists, and feminists. The contents are balanced and well researched, with further reading recommendations for each topic.

The text is organized into chapters on the history of reproduction, early reproductive technology, early infertility treatments, advanced infertility technology, and reproductive genetics. Brief articles within chapters discuss the technologies and risks; ethical concerns related to treatments; legislative issues in a variety of developed nations; and genetic topics, such as fetal tissue and embryo research, cloning, and genetic screening. An acronym list provides a quick reference resource for the confusing jumble of shorthand references within this field. The detailed subject index is invaluable because this encyclopedia follows a thematic approach to organization rather than an alphabetical approach. A selective but highly relevant number of illustrations are distributed throughout the text. This overview resource would be an excellent addition to collections serving college students and health consumers researching fertility options.—**Lynne M. Fox**

247.   **Family Planning Sourcebook.** Amy Marcaccio Keyzer, ed. Detroit, Omnigraphics, 2001. 520p. index. (Health Reference Series). $78.00. ISBN 0-7808-0379-5.

Like all the books in Omnigraphics' Health Reference Series, *Family Planning Sourcebook* is a collection of freely available articles from prominent governmental and organizational Websites. According to the preface, it was "designed to provide women and men with objective information on family planning issues and contraceptive choices . . ." (p. xi). The chapter on preconception planning is from the Mayo Clinic's Website, whose URL has changed since the sourcebook's publication. The Website includes more than a half dozen hotlinks (e.g., "What is Fetal Alcohol Syndrome?") not reprinted in this book.

The chapter on infertility is a reprint from a 1997 FDA consumer article, with various methods of treatment discussed briefly but thoroughly. There are also chapters on adoption, abortion, sterilization for men and women, and emergency contraception (popularly known as the "morning after" pill). Information is presented in an unbiased, readable manner, and the sourcebook will certainly be a necessary addition to those public and high school libraries where Internet access is restricted or otherwise problematic. It may be considered an optional purchase for consumer health libraries that have more complete and current information.—**Martha E. Stone**

248.   Kranz, Rachel. **Reproductive Rights and Technology.** New York, Facts on File, 2002. 262p. index. (Library in a Book). $45.00. ISBN 0-8160-4546-1.

The issues surrounding abortion and reproductive technology are some of the most sensitive in today's American society. Facts on File, in its series Library in a Book, offers a reference guide to the history and current status of some of these topics. Regrettably, this volume, written by an author with no professional health care education and limited historical training, has severe weaknesses that negate most of its potential usefulness.

In several of this book's sections the author presents a very biased, feminist, pro-choice perspective that is inappropriate for a reference text. At several places she states her personal fear that the Supreme Court will overturn *Roe v. Wade*, and that President Bush will find a way to further hamper women's access to abortion and birth control. She is also concerned that hospital mergers putting formerly public hospitals under Catholic control will severely limit women's reproductive rights.

Most of the text is an historical presentation of the struggle in the United States over birth control and abortion. Unfortunately the author only provides partial information, leaving out many key individuals and events in this story. She totally ignores the pioneering work of Dr. Robert Dickinson who convinced the American Medical Association to accept birth control as a legitimate medical procedure in 1937 and Margaret Sanger's successful effort to overturn much of the Comstock Law in the 1936 court case *U.S. v. One Package*. In the section listing major individuals in abortion's history the author not only leaves out Dickinson but also ignores the pro-birth control activities of such leaders as Mary Ware Dennett and Clarence James Gamble. The most useful section in this volume is the coverage of significant court decisions on abortion (e.g., *Roe v. Wade*, *Webster v. Reproductive Health Services*). One chapter includes helpful charts listing the current legal status of abortion rights issues in every state: mandatory waiting period, restrictions on minors, public funding for abortions. The author does not claim that her annotated bibliography of books and journal articles on the history of reproductive rights and techniques is comprehensive. Still any such list should provide the major works in this area, including *From Private Vice to Public Virtue* (1978) by James Reed, *On the Pill* (1998) by Elizabeth Watkins, *Contraception and Abortion in 19th-Century America* (1997) by Janet Brodie, and *Abortion in America: The Origins and Evolution of National Policy, 1800-1900* (1979) by James Mohr. These and other serious flaws make this volume unacceptable as a reference work for any library.—**Jonathon Erlen**

249.   Melloni, J. L. **Melloni's Illustrated Dictionary of Obstetrics and Gynecology.** Edited by I. G. Dox and H. H. Sheld. Pearl River, N.Y., Parthenon, 2000. 401p. illus. $39.95pa. ISBN 1-85070-710-3.

This dictionary defines more than 15,000 terms related to obstetrics and gynecology in simple everyday language. The 300 clear illustrations help the reader understand a word's meaning and expand on its definition. This feature is especially helpful in defining anatomical terms. Pronunciations are given and there is also a list of abbreviations used in obstetrics and gynecology. Although the book is a paperback, the binding is sturdy, the layout is excellent, and the type is large enough to read. The work would be even more useful if it included the more common drugs used in obstetrics and gynecology.

Large medical libraries may want a copy in both reference and circulation. All medical libraries should add a copy to their circulating collections since this dictionary will be useful for physicians, nurses, nursing and medical students, and others in allied health areas. It is recommended. [R: Choice, Feb 01, p. 1059]—**Natalie Kupferberg**

250.   **Pregnancy and Birth Sourcebook.** Heather E. Aldred, ed. Detroit, Omnigraphics, 1997. 737p. index. (Health Reference Series, vol.31). $75.00. ISBN 0-7808-0216-0.

This reference book is one of the many sourcebooks from Omnigraphics that health sciences libraries are acquiring for their reference collections. The format is similar to the rest of the Health Reference Series. Some expectant mothers can use this book to identify differences between the normal discomforts of pregnancy and the symptoms that may signal medical problems. The source materials are collected from individual publications and excerpted documents produced by the National Institutes of Health (NIH), its sister agencies and subagencies, and other reliable medical associations. Thus, the contents presented are authoritative and can be used to help women understand, prevent, detect, treat, and cope with the miscellaneous health concerns of pregnancy and childbirth. Most of the basic information is about all aspects of pregnancy and birth. There are 40 chapters in this book, which are arranged in 8 parts: planning for pregnancy, maternal care during pregnancy, fetal development during gestation, labor and delivery, postpartum and prenatal care, pregnancy in mothers with special concerns, disorders of pregnancy, and a glossary. Some chapters discuss common topics that are worth noting, including immunization and pregnancy, genetic counseling, drugs and pregnancy, over-the-counter drugs, amniocentesis, nutrition, weight gain, breast cancer and pregnancy, breast-feeding, mental health, and multiple births. There are historical and statistical data inserted in several chapters. In addition, the detailed index makes it easier to locate information within the book. This resource is recommended for public libraries to have on hand.—**Polin P. Lei**

251.   Rengel, Marian. **Encyclopedia of Birth Control.** Phoenix, Ariz., Oryx Press, 2000. 285p. illus. index. $55.00. ISBN 1-57356-255-6.

Birth control is an area of interest both to those concerned with social or legal policy and those who want information on their own options. This work could be useful in both areas. Articles in dictionary format cover methods of birth control and abortion, information on the human reproductive system, attitudes of particular religions, history and status of birth control in specific countries, issues and controversies, articles on individual influences in the field, and areas of ongoing research.

A guide in the front lists articles by area of interest. Each article lists sources for further information, and there is also an extensive bibliography. Rengel is a writer rather than a health professional—she draws on her medical information primarily from recent physiology texts, which she cites. Information included is very current, covering after-the-fact methods of birth control only recently or not yet available in the United States, such as RU-486 and PREVEN. Information on countries is selective rather than comprehensive, and the medical information may be too technical for some readers. Nevertheless, this book contains a great deal of up-to-date, useful information and is recommended for all types of libraries. [R: LJ, Jan 01, p. 92]—**Marit S. Taylor**

252.   Turkington, Carol, and Michael M. Alper. **The Encyclopedia of Fertility and Infertility.** New York, Facts on File, 2001. 308p. index. (Facts on File Library of Health and Living). $71.50. ISBN 0-8160-4154-7.

More than 15 percent of American women have received some form of fertility treatment. When confronted with difficulty in conceiving or carrying a baby to term, a couple is introduced to a new, seemingly impenetrable, language of laboratory terms, diagnoses, and fertility techniques. There are numerous decisions to be made and economic, lifestyle, and ethical factors to be considered. This encyclopedia is a simple yet comprehensive layperson's guide to the modern fertility field.

The authors of the encyclopedia are the head of the largest fertility center in the United States and an experienced science journalist. Their combined efforts have created an effective tool for educating the patient, with Alper contributing the expertise and Turkington ensuring the work will be accessible to the layperson. The first 245 pages of the book are an alphabetic listing of terms associated with human reproduction, conditions that can interfere with fertility, fertility treatments, and names of fertility-related organizations. Entries range from just a few sentences to several pages, and for major conditions, drugs, and techniques include statistics, contraindications, possible side effects, and discussions of ethical considerations where appropriate. In many cases, the authors work to dispel the myths and misunderstandings that are so prevalent in anything dealing with human reproduction.

There are six appendixes, including a list of fertility-related organizations with their telephone numbers, addresses, and Websites; a short bibliography; advice on selecting and interviewing a specialist; and a state-by-state list of fertility centers. All of these features, as well as the text itself, will be valuable resources to patients and health care workers and educators. [R: Choice, April 02, p. 1398]—**Carol L. Noll**

OPHTHALMOLOGY

253.   Cassin, Barbara. Rubin, Melvin L., ed. **Dictionary of Eye Terminology.** 4th ed. Gainesville, Fla., Triad, 2001. 286p. illus. $26.50 spiralbound. ISBN 0-937404-63-2.

The 4th edition of the *Dictionary of Eye Terminology* differs in two ways from the 3d edition (see entry 254). First, many entries have been rewritten to ensure that the definitions are as clear as possible for the intended audience of laypeople, students, and medical support staff working in eye-related fields. Second, in order to meet the objective of keeping the book the same size as the previous edition, types of diseases, surgeries, conditions, and so on have been grouped together in one place and the reader is directed to that point with many cross-references. For instance, definitions of the many types of *scotoma* (blind spot)—such as absolute, central, eclipse, relative, ring, and scintillating—are grouped together under scotoma, instead of separately in the alphabetic body of the book. Because of this strategy, space has been freed up to allow for additional new terminology to be added with only a modest increase in pages. The additional terms are largely in the area of new technology and drugs.

This dictionary continues to occupy a unique niche in the ophthalmology field for its focus on concise and clear definitions geared toward students and others working in the eye care field. Because of the considerable number of new entries, libraries that own the 3d edition will want to purchase this latest edition. Eye care support staff and students will want their own copy to slip into their lab coat pocket.—**Elaine F. Jurries**

254. **Dictionary of Eye Terminology.** 3d ed. By Barbara Cassin and Sheila A. B. Solomon. Melvin L. Rubin, ed. Gainesville, Fla., Triad, 1997. 283p. $24.95 spiralbound. ISBN 0-937404-44-6.

This is the 3d edition of a dictionary of ophthalmic terminology geared toward laypeople, students of optometry and ophthalmology, and medical support staff working in eye-related fields. The 1st edition (see ARBA 85, entry 1592) was published in 1984 and the 2d edition in 1990 (see ARBA 92, entry 1672). Written in plain English, each entry is identified by a category (drug, surgical procedure, symptom, function, and the like) and contains a pronunciation key if needed, synonyms, and a concise definition. Comparison to the 2d edition finds them nearly identical in page length, but because of a slightly larger page size, the more current edition contains approximately 1,000 more entries. Terms new to the 3d edition cover new laser procedures, drugs, surgical techniques, medications, and general medical conditions that affect the eye.

This dictionary occupies a unique niche, because *Stedman's Ophthalmology Words* (Williams & Wilkins, 1992) serves as a source to validate the spelling and accuracy of eye terms (no definitions), and *Dictionary of Visual Science* (4th ed.; see ARBA 90, entry 1691) is intended primarily for professionals. The dictionary under review is a definite acquisition for medical libraries and institutions supporting eye-related health programs. —**Elaine F. Jurries**

255. **Physicians' Desk Reference for Ophthalmic Medicine 2002.** 30th ed. Montvale, N.J., Medical Economics Data, 2001. 344p. $61.95. ISBN 1-56363-410-4.

The *Physicians' Desk Reference for Ophthalmic Medicines 2002* is a completely revised and updated edition of an annual reference work that provides eye-care professionals with current, comprehensive FDA-approved guidelines on ophthalmic pharmaceuticals and equipment as well as critical updates on new and revised drugs and adverse reactions. The work is composed of the following sections: "Pharmaceuticals in Ophthalmology" (which includes mydriatics and cycloplegics, anesthetic agents, diagnostic agents, and off-label drugs); "Suture Materials"; "Ophthalmic Lenses"; "Vision Standards and Low Vision"; a full-color "Product Identification Guide"; "Pharmaceutical and Equipment Product Information"; and "Intraocular Product Information" (which includes drug information and poison control centers listed in alphabetic order by state). The first section consists of four indexes to locate product information: a manufacturer's index; a product name index; a product category index; and an active ingredients index.

The well-organized format of the *Physicians' Desk Reference for Ophthalmic Medicines 2002* facilitates ease and rapid accessibility of information. It is recommended for the libraries of those medical centers and medical schools that offer specialized ophthalmology or optometry services, as well as for medium to large general medical centers and schools. Public libraries with substantial consumer health collections may also find this work a useful addition to their reference collections.—**Rita Neri**

256. **Quick Reference Glossary of Eyecare Terminology.** 3d ed. Joseph Hoffman and Janice K. Ledford, eds. Thorofare, N.J., Slack, 2002. 327p. $24.00pa. ISBN 1-55642-472-8.

This compact volume provides both technical and general medical terms used in ophthalmic practices throughout the United States. This edition has been updated to include new concepts and terms, with an emphasis on refractive surgery, laser surgery, and opticianry. Terms are listed in alphabetical order and provide easy-to-understand definitions. *See* references are provided when necessary. New to this edition are 20 appendixes, which make this edition much more valuable than the 2d edition. These appendixes include lists of acronyms and abbreviations, systemic disorders and their effects on the eye, ophthalmic drugs, a list of the types of lasers used in eye surgery, Websites related to eye care, and a list of suggested readings, just to name a few. This compact dictionary will be handy for medical libraries as well as those working in an office or lab.—**Shannon Graff Hysell**

257.   Rubin, Melvin L., and Lawrence A. Winograd. **Taking Care of Your Eyes: A Collection of the Patient Education Handouts Used by America's Leading Eye Doctors.** Gainesville, Fla., Triad, 2003. 270p. $24.95pa. ISBN 0-937404-61-6.

For most of us, there will come a time when we or a family member will need our first pair of glasses or bifocals, contemplate contact lenses or LASIK surgery, or have some kind of eye problem. When that day comes, this book is an excellent starting point to begin the education.

As the title indicates, this is a collection of brief informative summaries gleaned from handouts originally used by eye doctors to help their patients understand an eye condition or procedure. The handouts have been brought together and grouped into eight sections: eye injuries, refractive errors and their corrections, eye muscle problems and other conditions affecting children, cataracts, glaucoma, common eye conditions, less common eye conditions, and helpful information. Among the topics discussed within these sections are types of glaucoma, allergies to makeup, sports eye injuries, getting used to bifocals, amblyopia (lazy eye), LASIK, how to put in eyedrops, and retinal detachment. The authors' writing style is geared toward the layperson, and medical jargon is kept to a minimum. Public libraries will find this book a useful reference to recommend to users searching for information on eye topics.—**Elaine F. Jurries**

PEDIATRICS

Dictionaries and Encyclopedias

258. **The Cambridge Encyclopedia of Human Growth and Development.** Stanley J. Ulijaszek, Francis E. Johnston, and Michael A. Preece, eds. New York, Cambridge University Press, 1998. 497p. illus. index. $95.00. ISBN 0-521-56046-2.

This book has an introduction and a history of human growth and development. The contents of this publication include information on measurement and assessment, patterns of human growth, genetics of growth, fetal growth, postnatal growth and maturation, behavioral and cognitive development, clinical growth abnormalities, the human lifespan, and the future. A favorite feature is the excellent biographies of people important in the field of human development. There are many excellent charts and graphs for help in understanding the complex subject matter. Although the encyclopedia includes many technical terms, there is a glossary in the back as well as a good index and bibliographies. *The Cambridge Encyclopedia of Human Growth and Development* is best suited for reference collections in larger public libraries and in academic libraries. [R: BL, 15 Oct 98, p. 437]—**Theresa Maggio**

259.   **Children's Health.** Dawn P. Dawson, ed. Englewood Cliffs, N.J., Salem Press, 1999. 2v. illus. index. $185.00/set. ISBN 0-89356-944-5.

The vast subject of children's health presents daunting challenges for both parents and health providers. This 2-volume reference tool, although not claiming to be definitive or to be used in place of professional medical advice, does provide excellent overview guidance for those overseeing the health of youngsters, from newborns through age 18.

This encyclopedia is written by 142 authors, mostly M.D.s and Ph.D.s, and contains 324 alphabetically arranged entries, 90 of which have been republished from *Magill's Medical Guide* (see entry 165). Entries vary in length from 100 to 3,500 words and are accompanied by 173 useful photographs, graphs, and charts. The entries range in coverage from broad health concerns (bleeding, discipline) to specific diseases (bulimia, scabies). Some essays deal with basic childhood developmental issues (growth, senses), whereas others describe the responsibilities of pediatric health specialties (dentistry, urology). Entries' contents vary depending on their length. The majority contain the basic description of the disease or topic, key terms, causes and symptoms, treatment and therapy, and possible outcomes. The longer essays also include a list of suggested readings. A separate resources section contains names, addresses, telephone numbers, and URLs for organizations to consult for further information and assistance. Thorough indexing and cross-referencing make these volumes easy to use.

This clearly written reference guide is an important addition to the reference collections of both medical and public libraries and will prove very useful for health professionals and the general public. [R: LJ, 15 Sept 99, p. 68; BL, 1 Dec 99, p. 733]—**Jonathon Erlen**

260.   Coleman, Jeanine G. **The Early Intervention Dictionary: A Multidisciplinary Guide to Terminology.** 2d ed. Bethesda, Md., Woodbine House, 1999. 410p. $17.95pa. ISBN 1-890627-05-4.

The 2d edition of this revised and updated dictionary reflects the ever-changing and expanding role of the early intervention field in identifying and treating infant and early childhood special needs. Hundreds of medical, therapeutic, and educational terms are defined that have been commonly used in current literature, reports, and discussions. The aim has been to foster understanding and collaboration among families of young children with developmental delays and disabilities, and those professionals providing services for them. This collaboration could then enhance the development of effective and comprehensive programs for children with special needs.

Entries, ranging in length from one line to one paragraph, are prefaced by a pronunciation guide, and define terms as they apply to early intervention or child care and development. Cross-references add to the volume's usefulness. Appendixes have charts and tables providing health and nutritional information.

Early intervention is the best recourse in helping children with specific problems, and the dictionary part of the publisher's "Special-Needs Collection" supplies a common foundation for these efforts. Future editions could include other terms used in describing age-appropriate behavior, such as "separation anxiety" and "permanence," and would be welcome references. [R: Choice, Jan 2000, p. 908]—**Anita Zutis**

261.   Darragh, Frances, and Louise Darragh Law. **Healing Your Child: An A-Z Guide to Using Natural Remedies.** New York, Marlowe & Company/Avalon Publishing Group; distr., Emeryville, Calif., Publishers Group West, 2000. 273p. index. $13.95pa. ISBN 1-56924-614-9.

The authors, both registered natural health practitioners, have written this handbook as a guide for parents and caregivers seeking alternative remedies to heal their child's illnesses, disorders, and injuries. The most up-to-date advice is provided for long-term solutions, emergency procedures, resistance and immunity, and combining remedies. Throughout the handbook, the authors advise readers of when they should seek professional medical attention for various ailments. Also, many of the alternative treatments included in the handbook are intended to complement other treatments that a child is going through.

Entries are organized under individual illnesses as opposed to specific symptoms. In each entry the authors discuss the course the illness takes and its possible cause, what symptoms to expect, and what immediate action to follow. They then describe how to make use of herbs, homeopathic remedies, and cell salts. Descriptions of side effects, aftereffects, and possible complications are also included. A bibliography, an index, and a list of natural suppliers conclude the work.

This guide is recommended for parents and caregivers who prefer alternative and natural treatments for ailments. But, as the authors state, not all ailments can be treated successfully by herbs, homeopathic remedies, and cell salts. Professional medical doctors should always treat serious illnesses and emergencies. In this handbook, however, parents and caregivers may find some helpful remedies for less serious ailments such as acne, bites and stings, chicken pox, and much more.—**Cari Ringelheim**

262. Markel, Howard, and Frank A. Oski. **The Practical Pediatrician: The A to Z Guide to Your Child's Health, Behavior, and Safety.** New York, W. H. Freeman, 1996. 364p. index. $16.95pa. ISBN 0-7167-2897-4.

Books on child care are among the most popular and useful items in public library collections. *The Practical Pediatrician*, a new source written by two professors of pediatrics, is a fine addition to the literature. Arranged alphabetically by subject and written in lay language, it is reassuring and easy to use. The authors emphasize the positive aspects of parenthood and encourage mothers and fathers to trust their instincts, ask questions, and love their children.

Entries range in length from one paragraph to several pages. They cover both medical (ear infections, abdominal pain) and behavioral subjects (aggression, toilet training). They also offer practical advice on shopping with young children and choosing health care providers. The major strengths of the book include an emphasis on safety, with detailed first aid information and a fold-out chart on child-proofing the home, and discussions of important contemporary issues, such as computers/the Internet, television, latchkey children, divorce, and firearms in the home. Black-and-white illustrations supplement the text. There are also detailed growth charts and tables of what should be included in well-child examinations from birth to eight years of age.

Although this book lacks the depth of the American Academy of Pediatrics's *Caring for Your Baby and Young Child: Birth to Age 5* (Bantam Books, 1993), it is an excellent ready-reference source. *The Practical Pediatrician* is a good choice for circulating parenting collections as well. [R: LJ, 1 Nov 96, p. 62; RBB, 1 Sept 96, p. 170]—**Barbara M. Bibel**

263. Weaver, David D., and Ira K. Brandt. **Catalog of Prenatally Diagnosed Conditions.** 3d ed. Baltimore, Md., Johns Hopkins University Press, 1999. 682p. index. $110.00. ISBN 0-8018-6044-X.

This Johns Hopkins University Press publication was originally published in 1989 listing 445 prenatal diagnosed conditions. The 2d edition arrived in 1992 with 601 conditions. The 3d edition presents 940 conditions, a 56 percent increase over the previous edition. As the identification of new genes is rapidly growing, this book serves as a reference to provide "more diagnostic information to a larger number of women who carry fetuses with a wider array of problems."

Using this reference source is not as difficult as it seems. The book is divided into 3 parts. The 1st is the text, then comes the massive references alphabetically sorted by author, and the last part is the exhaustive index with the numerical index at the end. The text is divided into chapters discussing chromosomal anomalies; congenital malformations, deformations, disruptions, and related disorders; dermatologic disorders; fetal infections; hematologic disorders and hemaglobinopathies; inborn errors of metabolism; other prenatal conditions, tumors, and cysts; and multiple congenital anomalies of unknown etiology. Each condition has been assigned a reference number that is modeled after the one used by Victor A. McKusick in the book *Mendelian Inheritance in Man* (repr. ed.; Books Demand). The change in reference numbers and names since the 2d edition is explained in a short table. When the information on Short Rib-Polydactyly Syndrome, Majewski Type, was compared between the 1st edition and the 3d edition, it was found that not only does the current edition give differential diagnosis and syndrome notes, it also conveys specific information about the conditions or findings by using a list of superscripts attached to the references listed at the end of the condition. This helps in identifying the particularly useful references for readers. Some conditions have extra information, such as treatment modality, methods and findings, prenatal treatment, and prenatal diagnosis. Abbreviations used in this book are also carefully grouped for easy reading.

Prenatal care is important to women and prenatal diagnosis is essential to determine the health of fetuses before birth. With the help of molecular genetic technology, the practice of prenatal care will become more accurate and simple. This book serves as a guide for such information needs.—**Polin P. Lei**

Directories

264.   **The Complete Directory for Pediatric Disorders, 2002/03.** 2d ed. Lakeville, Conn., Grey House Publishing, 2002. 1120p. index. $190.00; $165.00pa. ISBN 1-930956-62-2; 1-930956-61-4pa.

265.   **The Complete Directory for Pediatric Disorders. http://www.greyhouse.com.** [Website]. Millerton, N.Y., Grey House Publishing. $215.00/year subscription; $300.00/year subscription (w/print directory). Date reviewed: May 02.

Caring for a child who has a serious illness or a genetic or congenital disorder can be a challenge. *The Complete Directory for Pediatric Disorders*, first published in 2000 (see ARBA 2001, entry 1458), provides information and resources to help healthcare practitioners and parents get the support that they need. The 2d edition has 7 new chapters: "Eating Disorders," "Lead Poisoning," "Sleep Apnea," "Post-Traumatic Stress Disorder," "Physical and Sexual Abuse," "Hypertrophic Cardiomyopathy," and "Syncope." It also has several chapters covering broad subject areas, such as dental conditions and preventable childhood infections. Medical editor Alan Friedman, of Yale University, and a team of associates reviewed all of the material in the book.

The *Directory* has three major sections. The first covers specific disorders. The alphabetic entries include the name of the disorder and synonyms; a description; and information on symptoms, physical findings, related disorders, cause, treatment, and resources. The latter may include associations, support groups, government and nonprofit agencies, libraries and research centers, media sources, and Websites. Section 2 covers general resources: government agencies, national associations, research centers, libraries, media resources, and camps. Section 3 explains the human body systems. A glossary, guidelines for obtaining information, and three indexes (alphabetic, subject, and geographic) complete the work.

The Complete Directory for Pediatric Disorders is a valuable resource for medical, consumer health, and large public libraries. Although the reading level is high, it provides concise, thorough descriptions of disorders in lay language and offers help with extensive resource lists. The new edition is also available as an online subscription with continuous updates. The online edition gives the user access to more than 5,500 disorder-specific and general resources. Librarians that cannot afford it will find much of the same information available on MedlinePlus at *http://www.medlineplus.gov.*—**Barbara M. Bibel**

Handbooks and Yearbooks

266. **American Academy of Pediatrics Guide to Your Child's Nutrition: Making Peace at the Table and Building Healthy Eating Habits for Life.** William H. Dietz and Loraine Stern, eds. New York, Villard/Random House, 1999. 234p. index. $23.00. ISBN 0-375-50187-8.

This helpful guide for parents and other caretakers gives advice on working with the picky eater and myriad other issues involving the nutrition of children from infancy through adolescence. Written in a narrative style with many case studies of common problems, this book is entertaining reading as well as full of authoritative advice from the doctors of the American Academy of Pediatrics. The first five chapters are an overview of nutrition for children through all the stages of their early life. Many of the questions that parents ask their doctors are discussed. For example, breast-feeding and what to order a child when eating out are both discussed here. Chapters on nutrition basics; outside influences (e.g., television, grandparents, childcare providers); eating disorders; alternative diets and supplements; and allergies round out this useful book.

There are a number of other books that address the topic of children's nutrition. An equally authoritative work, *The Yale Guide to Children's Nutrition* (see entry 276), contains essentially the same information, with the addition of 100 pages of recipes designed to entice children to eat better. *Mom's Guide to Your Kid's Nutrition* (Alpha Books, 1997) is a popular rendition of advice on children's nutrition.

This guide is a worthy addition to the nutrition collection of all public libraries. Academic libraries that have an education, nutrition, nursing, or medical program will also find it useful. —**Elaine F. Jurries**

267. **American Academy of Pediatrics Guide to Your Child's Symptoms: The Official, Complete Home Reference, Birth Through Adolescence.** Donald Schiff and Steven P. Shelov, eds. New York, Villard/Random House, 1997. 256p. index. $18.95pa. ISBN 0-375-75257-9.

As we approach the millennium, the American Academy of Pediatrics is now giving parents a reference guide to a child's symptoms. This is a no-nonsense book written and reviewed by members of the American Academy of Pediatrics. This guide is one of a series of guides for parents developed by this Academy. The included information is derived from the consensus of accepted pediatric practice. However, this book does not provide the ultimate solution to caring for children in need of medical care. It is a means to provide the needed and ever-changing information. This reference guide is divided into 2 sections. One section is a list of more than 100 most common childhood symptoms, and the other section is an illustrated first aid manual and safety guide.

The 1st section is presented in 3 parts according to age: early infancy (first three months), later infancy and childhood, and adolescence. In each area, the symptoms are listed alphabetically according to their common names. If the user looks up fever, a general and clear description is given. It even mentions normal temperature variations according to time of day. The chart following is easy to follow. Each symptom is described in general, then proceeds with advice on when to call your pediatrician, questions to consider, possible causes, action to take, or illustrated boxes.

The 2d section is an illustrated first aid manual and safety guide, which is a reference tool for parents dealing with unexpected emergencies or minor mishaps. This information is valuable for parents to administer first aid before seeing the pediatrician in case of emergency. Again, there are 2 sections with this segment and the 1st section is divided into 2 parts: how to administer first aid and frequently used first aid measures. The 2d section is a guide to safety and prevention and a guide to food safety.

The index at the end is well put together and thorough. Every parent with small children should keep one of these guides by the Academy at home. Public or school libraries might consider adding this item for reference.—**Polin P. Lei**

268. **American Medical Association Complete Guide to Your Children's Health.** Edward S. Traisman, Karen Judy, and Mary Jane Staba, eds. Chicago, American Medical Association, 1999. 710p. illus. index. $39.95. ISBN 0-679-45776-3.

This volume is the latest entry in the American Medical Association's (AMA) health library that includes the similar *American Medical Association Family Medical Guide* (see ARBA 83, entry 1462). This book, however, is designed specifically for parents of children, newborn to age 21, to help them take control of their children's health in this age of mutating insurance plans and impersonal, clinic-based managed care.

The guide is divided into three sections. The first, on the healthy child from birth to adolescence, is six chapters on normal development and growth. It discusses normal changes and growth patterns, developmental milestones, and problems to look for. It has very good discussions and guidelines for nutrition, exercise, sleep, and discipline for each age group. The second section, on caring for a child's health, gives advice on selection of pediatricians and other health professionals, discusses day-care options, and gives timetables for routine tests, immunizations, and dental care. It even goes into such overlooked but important topics as how to childproof a home and other methods of accident prevention.

The third section of the book is a very complete medical encyclopedia. It opens with 50 pages of symptom flowcharts to help parents diagnose problems and decide whether a doctor's visit is warranted. What follows is over 300 entries on childhood diseases and conditions, all clear, concise, and illustrated when necessary.

The *Columbia University Department of Pediatrics Children's Medical Guide* (see entry 270) is a somewhat similar home health reference published just a few years ago. This new AMA offering is less graphics based and colorful, but more comprehensive. Either work is a good choice for home use, but this comprehensive and detailed AMA volume is a better selection for library reference.—**Carol L. Noll**

269. **Breastfeeding Sourcebook.** Jenni Lynn Colson, ed. Detroit, Omnigraphics, 2002. 388p. index. (Health Reference Series). $78.00. ISBN 0-7808-0332-9.

Breastfeeding Sourcebook, like all the titles in Omnigraphics' Health Reference Series, is a collection of freely available articles and Websites. In 8 parts and 64 chapters it covers all major areas, including rationale for breastfeeding versus bottle feeding, preparation, breastfeeding during early weeks and later in infancy, the issues of working mothers, and a variety of difficult and special situations including teenage mothers and illnesses of the mother or the infant. "Breastfeeding the Baby with Special Needs" is reprinted from http://www. lalecheleague.org. "Is it Safe to Lose Weight While Breastfeeding?" is a news release from the National Institute of Child Health and Human Development located at http://www.nichd.nih.gov. "Breastfeeding the Adopted Baby" is also freely available, although its URL (http://users.erols.com/cindyrn/24.htm) is not given.

Particularly useful is the information about professional lactation services and chapters on breastfeeding when returning to work, which includes a sample letter to an employer requesting accommodations for nursing mothers.

There is a glossary, a list of medications to avoid when breastfeeding, legal rights of nursing mothers, annotated breastfeeding resources (e.g., books, magazines, associations), and an index. *Breastfeeding Sourcebook* will be useful for public libraries, consumer health libraries, and technical schools offering nurse assistant training, especially in areas where Internet access is problematic.
—**Martha E. Stone**

270.   **Columbia University Department of Pediatrics Children's Medical Guide.** By Steve Z. Miller and Bernard Valman. New York, DK Publishing, 1997. 216p. illus. index. $29.95. ISBN 0-7894-1443-0.

It is the sad truth that the growth of managed care, health maintenance organizations, and insurance plans that can force families to switch doctors almost annually has meant that parents must be more knowledgeable than ever about their children's health problems. This quick-reference guide can help parents with that ever-important question, "Should I call the doctor, or can I treat this problem myself?" Along the way, the book also educates readers on normal growth patterns, self-help strategies for numerous conditions, and the meaning of the diagnosis and treatment options they may receive when they do visit a medical clinic.

The book is divided into 4 sections. The 1st describes normal childhood anatomy and development and gives advice on nutrition, home safety, and advice on living with an infant. Here, as elsewhere in the book, much of the information is displayed in easy-to-use charts and illustrations, which emphasize the wide range of growth patterns and behavior that can be considered normal. The 2d section, which comprises the majority of the book, is made up of 41 symptom charts, which are flow charts to help parents assess a child's condition and make an initial diagnosis. As in other guides of this type, such as the *AMA Family Medical Guide* (see ARBA 83, entry 1462), the goal is not to replace the doctor but to help parents decide whether a trip to the doctor is necessary, and if so, how urgent. The flow charts take initial symptoms, such as "painful joints," and by posing a series of questions lead the reader to a possible diagnosis. Most charts also include self-help advice on relieving the problem. A 3d section discusses the diseases and disorders to which children are prone. It is essentially a brief medical encyclopedia, arranged by body systems, such as skeletal, digestive, and so forth, profusely illustrated and written in an easy-to-understand, question-and-answer format. Finally, there is a first aid guide section, which includes illustrated how-tos on choking, rescue-breathing, and cardiopulmonary resuscitation. All place the emphasis on treatment of children, which may be different from similar techniques for adults.

This is an outstanding resource, produced by two doctors from one of the finest pediatric departments in the country. It is authoritative, comprehensive, and easy to use.—**Carol L. Noll**

271.   **Infant and Toddler Health Sourcebook.** Jenifer Swanson, ed. Detroit, Omnigraphics, 2000. 585p. index. (Health Reference Series). $78.00. ISBN 0-7808-0246-2.

This book is a welcome updated information source for parents with infants and toddlers up to the age of three. At times, raising infants and toddlers might cause confusion. There are answers in this book to cover questions about health issues, nutrition, immunizations, and common illnesses. This is one of the many sourcebooks from the popular Health Reference Series. Its contents are well researched—collected from a wide range of government agencies, nonprofit organizations, and journals—and are useful for parents who wish to know more about the care, hygiene, and growth of their young children.

The 7 major parts are comprised of 80 chapters. The newborn section introduces the normal newborn, statistics, and certain illnesses and concerns such as SIDS (Sudden Infant Death

Syndrome). The nutrition section talks about breast milk, formula, solid foods, food labeling, and vegetable nutrition. The well-baby care section describes routine health check-ups, developmental milestones, recommended vaccinations, vision and hearing screening, and so on. The tips for parents section provides advice for parents on a wide range of common concerns, such as how to choose a health care provider, bathing, communication, dental care, diaper rash, teething, thumb-sucking, and much more. The section covering common medical concerns during early childhood presents the most common health problems in infants and toddlers, such as allergies, asthma, birthmarks, colds, ear infections, fevers, and others. The safety and first aid section provides advice on keeping children safe at home and with caretakers. The additional help and information section includes a list of important terms and a directory of resources. Websites and e-mail addresses are also provided.

The 34-page index at the end of the book is a plus. However, readers must not treat this book as an encyclopedic work for infant and toddler care. There are areas of care not included in this sourcebook and there are no illustrations. Nevertheless, this is a good source for general use.
—**Polin P. Lei**

272. **Pediatric Cancer Sourcebook.** Edward J. Prucha, ed. Detroit, Omnigraphics, 1999. 587p. index. (Health Reference Series). $78.00. ISBN 0-7808-0245-4.

Although people often think of cancer as being terminal, the fact is that many cancers, especially those often found in children, are treatable and often curable. This sourcebook looks specifically at those cancers that frequently are diagnosed in infants, children, and adolescents. These include leukemias, brain tumors, sarcomas, and lymphomas, among others. The book is divided into 5 parts: "Common Childhood Cancers," "Treatments and Therapies," "Coping Strategies and Other Information for Parents," "Financial Information for Families of Children with Cancer," and "Additional Help and Information." The 1st section takes each of the cancers mentioned above and explains their signs and symptoms and how they can be treated. "Treatments and Therapies" discusses chemotherapy, radiation, and transplants as well as discusses what the side effects of these treatment often are. "Coping Strategies and Other Information for Parents" give parents practical information, everything from discussing cancer with children to getting one's health care to cover treatments. "Financial Information for Families of Children with Cancer" gives basic advice on dealing with insurance providers and obtaining financial assistance for treatments. "Additional Help and Information" provides everything from defining terms related to cancer to giving names, addresses, and Websites for foundations that support cancer patients. An index concludes the work. Because of this volume's emphasis on pediatric cancer it will be a valuable addition to all libraries specializing in health services and many public libraries.—**Shannon Graff Hysell**

273. **Policy Reference Guide of the American Academy of Pediatrics: A Comprehensive Guide to AAP Policies Issued Through January 2000.** 13th ed. Elk Grove Village, Ill., American Academy of Pediatrics, 2000. 1349p. index. $79.95pa. ISBN 1-58110-040-X. ISSN 1522-4716.

According to the introduction of this volume, this guide is "designed as a quick reference tool for Academy members, staff, and other interested parties" (p. xi). It notes that policies are reviewed every three years. Until a revision is approved or retired, the current policy remains in effect. Beginning with the 3d edition in 1990, this book has been published on an annual basis. The approximately 375 policy statements are arranged alphabetically. The full text of the statement is included as well as its authors and, if appropriate, bibliographic references and tables. The statements' lengths range from 1 page (e.g., "Generic Prescribing, Generic Substitution, and Therapeutic Substitution") to 18 pages ("Newborn Screening Fact Sheets") . The latter includes a table listing all states and the types of hospital screening programs available for newborns. A wide range of topics are covered, from triathlon participation to car seats for premature infants, issues related to HIV, vaccination, cancer, and health supervision issues for children with a variety of syndromes. There is an index by committee of authorship and a subject index. This guide is an appropriate purchase for academic medical libraries and libraries serving inpatient or outpatient pediatric practices.—**Martha E. Stone**

274. Rozario, Diane. **The Immunization Resource Guide: Where to Find Answers to All Your Questions About Childhood Vaccinations.** 4th ed. Burlington, Iowa, Patter, 2000. 245p. index. $13.95pa. ISBN 0-9643366-5-0.

This text provides the reader with a valuable resource that pertains to childhood immunizations. The beginning of the book discusses vaccinations and includes definitions, modern vaccinations, and religious and social issues surrounding vaccinations.

Within the body there are book reviews and resources. The book review section contains books for parents and health care providers and books that discuss vaccination safety and effectiveness, philosophical objections, current research, legal exemptions, government programs, the history of vaccination, homeopathy and vaccines, international travel, and vaccination programs around the world. Within each summary, the author included information such as the author and publisher, date of publication, and where the publication can be located.

The resources section contains topics such as vaccination organizations, health organizations, vaccine injuries, pediatric vaccines, and publishers. This section is well presented and is easy to use. A section of acronyms and an index are included at the end of the book.

A valuable resource, this book would be appropriate for an adult reader, with or without medical training. Parents, educators, and health care providers may find this to be an invaluable resource.—**Paul M. Murphy III**

275. **The 3 a.m. Handbook: The Most Commonly Asked Questions About Your Child's Health.** William Feldman, ed. New York, Facts on File, 1998. 224p. illus. index. $17.95pa. ISBN 0-8160-3802-3.

This book comprises 18 chapters on a variety of topics of interest to parents of children of all ages. The editor and the authors, all pediatricians, are associated with Toronto Hospital for Sick Children; some work in pediatric subspecialties. The authors write from the point of view of problems as parents experience them. The chapters address such issues as fever, feeding, crying, rashes, vomiting and diarrhea, behavior and learning, pain, and emergencies. Areas of anticipatory guidance, such as toilet training, safety, and immunizations, are also discussed. One chapter addresses specific common conditions, such as roseola, asthma, bronchiolitis, and chickenpox. In a unique chapter the authors explain clinical research and offer ideas about deciding to have a child participate in a research study.

The book is nicely laid out. The print is pleasant to read, with simple illustrations. Each chapter has a highlighted sidebar illuminating a specific point, such as preventing night awakenings (sleep chapter) and hints on breast-feeding (feeding chapter). Important problems that must be distinguished from normal are pointed out, such as persistent snoring and risks of dehydration (diarrhea and vomiting chapter). Confusing things, like some medical tests, are clearly explained. The emergency chapter is located at the end and easy to find.

Although this book is from a Canadian point of view, nearly everything pertains to U.S. medicine as well. Some terms are not usual American parlance, but that will not confuse the average parent. Most parents will find this a helpful and sensible book. The small list of support telephone numbers is very eclectic. No Websites are listed.—**Margretta Reed Seashore**

276.   **The Yale Guide to Children's Nutrition.** William V. Tamborlane and others, eds. New Haven, Conn., Yale University Press, 1997. 415p. illus. index. $18.00pa. ISBN 0-300-07159-8.

In searching the national online catalog, one finds more than 8,000 books published on the subject of nutrition for children and infants. At least 80 books are published with a similar title, including such words as "children's nutrition." However, the guide under review is broad based and has arrived in a timely fashion to enlighten modern parents who have concerns for their children's diet and to provide dietary recommendations.

The Yale Guide is a compilation from more than 50 contributors—physicians, dietitians, nurses, and social workers—writing on a wide spectrum of nutrition-related topics, such as physiology, psychology, health and diseases, social problems, concerns and myths, dietary intake and recommendations, grocery shopping and eating out, and sensible recipes provided by chefs throughout the United States. The editors attempt to be comprehensive in order to address many popular questions adults and children may have about childhood nutrition (e.g., acne and diet). Even though this book is devoted to the nutritional needs of normal children, there are tips on how to deal with special feeding problems, such as cleft palate.

This resource is presented in six parts, from infancy to adolescence: "Developmental Nutrition"; "Common Concerns"; "Beyond the Basics: Special Challenges in Nutrition"; "Building Blocks for Good Nutrition"; "Eating In, Eating Out"; and "Recipes." Appendixes include growth charts, recommended dietary allowances, and a recipe conversion table. The editors' mission in publishing this book was to bring to parents awareness of the importance of good nutrition for the future health of their children. *The Yale Guide* is recommended as a general reference guide for parents who wish to promote healthy eating habits for their children. Also, this is a good reference book for public or health sciences libraries. [R: LJ, 15 Feb 97, p. 129]—**Polin P. Lei**

277.   Entry omitted.

278.   Zand, Janet, Rachel Walton, and Bob Rountree. **A Parent's Guide to Medical Emergencies: First Aid for Your Child.** Garden City Park, N.Y., Avery Publishing, 1997. 186p. illus. index. $11.95pa. ISBN 0-89529-736-1.

No parent likes to think about the possibility of accidents, but the fact is that with children involved, the next medical emergency is just around the corner. This simple paperback is a testament to the Boy Scout's motto—be prepared. The volume has two purposes. First, it shows parents what steps to take before an accident occurs—phone numbers to have ready, supplies to have on hand, measures to take to prevent accidents, even what type of attitude will best reassure a frightened child. There is vital advice on the often overlooked topic of designating legal surrogates to make medical decisions in the parents' absence. Second, the book contains a quick, easy-to-use guide describing what to do in a number of emergencies. Included is advice on treating specific types of poisoning, animal bites, seizures, and just about all the other types of injuries to which children are prone.

In most cases, the information included in this guide is easy to find, easy to read, and the best possible advice in the situation. One idiosyncrasy of this particular volume is that one of the authors is an herbalist and specialist in Oriental medicine, so many of the standard treatments are followed by advice on herbal and homeopathic regimens, which many readers may find puzzling.

Although this guide will have some use as a reference book, it is not designed to sit on a library shelf. Rather, it should be in an accessible place in the home, with all the emergency numbers on the inside cover filled out, the home safety checklist gone over, and the home emergency medical kit already assembled.—**Carol L. Noll**

PODIATRY

279. **Podiatry Sourcebook.** M. Lisa Weatherford, ed. Detroit, Omnigraphics, 2001. 380p. index. (Health Reference Series). $78.00. ISBN 0-7808-0215-2.

Information on podiatry, the field of medicine that specializes in foot care, is essential to a variety of people, from those suffering accident injuries to those with long-term illnesses such as diabetes and AIDS. This new volume in Omnigraphics' Health Reference Series provides reprinted articles from medical sources such as the National Institute of Aging, The National Institute of Arthritis and Musculoskeletal and Skin Diseases, *Podiatry Today*, and the Mayo Foundation for Medical Education and Research, among many others. The full citation of each source is printed at the first page of each chapter.

This book has four parts, which are then broken down into several related chapters. Part 1 is an overview of the foot and provides chapters with information on topics such as the importance of finding the right fit in shoes, foot pain prevention, and pregnancy and the foot. Part 2, titled "Foot Conditions," discusses common foot problems, including bunions, tarsal tunnel syndrome, and structural deformities. Part 3 discusses diseases that commonly effect foot health (e.g., diabetes, arthritis, AIDS). Part 4 discusses injuries to the foot due to accidents and sports. The final section provides a glossary and a list of medical resources and foot safety resources for more information (with address, telephone and fax numbers, and e-mail and Website addresses).

There is a lot of information presented here on a topic that is usually only covered sparingly in most larger comprehensive medical encyclopedias. Consumer health libraries may want to consider this book for purchase as well as some larger public libraries.—**Shannon Graff Hysell**

280. Tremaine, M. David, and Elias M. Awad. **The Foot & Ankle Sourcebook: Everything You Need to Know.** Los Angeles, Calif., Lowell House, 1995. 324p. illus. index. $26.00. ISBN 1-56565-150-2.

In today's world, with people living longer and more active lives, the phrase "oh, my aching feet" can be heard more and more often. The authors (an orthopedic surgeon and an information specialist) set out to write a user's guide to the human foot, as much to prevent foot problems as to help sufferers treat them. The 18 chapters in this book discuss normal feet and the mechanics of walking and running, describe a variety of congenital problems that can appear in infants and children, and cover in detail the numerous ailments that can beset the feet of adults as they age. There is particular emphasis on sports injuries, occupational foot problems, and especially diabetic foot problems, which are the third leading cause of hospital admissions in the United States.

Throughout the text, the authors give excellent, practical advice in lay terms. They cover both self-help suggestions and advice on when it is best to consult a professional. For most injuries and problems, possible courses of treatment are discussed, and typical recovery times are given. Also included are a glossary of terms and an extensive list of agencies and support groups concerned with foot and ankle problems.—**Carol L. Noll**

SPECIFIC DISEASES AND CONDITIONS

AIDS

281.   **AIDS.** 1996 ed. Suzanne B. Squyres, Mark A. Siegel, and Nancy R. Jacobs, eds. Wylie, Tex., Information Plus, 1996. 124p. index. $12.95pa. ISBN 1-57302-025-7.

Information Plus is a for-profit group of former teachers who got together in 1990 to publish current information for middle and high school students doing library research. Students will learn that information if they call the toll-free telephone number on the back cover of *AIDS*. The book itself omits a statement of purpose, the background or credentials of the various in-house writers, a glossary, and a title page. Students writing a term paper or giving an oration on AIDS who find this book in the school library may overlook these points, however, and think only that they have found a gold mine. The 1996 edition of *AIDS* is filled with charts, graphs, quotations, and information in 11 well-organized chapters. Students will write and speak with authority after only a few sessions with *AIDS*. Although the book is scheduled for revision in 1998, one problem may pervade the way Information Plus creates their books. The chapters appear to be written by different people with little coordination between them. Information is both repetitive and inconsistent. With a sparse and incomplete index—one page—students would have a hard time relocating any inconsistencies they discover in their notes. For example, there is no index entry for "women," so it would be difficult to cross-check and question a statement on page 30 ("The actual number of AIDS cases in women is declining . . .") with one on page 101 ("Women now account for roughly 40% . . . of all HIV infections . . ."). Completeness is another issue. The role of the protease inhibitors is slighted in a number of places: how these drugs have increased the cost of care and decreased settlements and how some persons with AIDS cannot tolerate the inhibitors. Reverse transcriptase inhibitors and viral load need to be defined and explained, the role of monkeys and the origin of AIDS clearly resolved, and the opportunistic infections described more fully. Students may find that a trip to their local AIDS service organization will provide current information and firsthand experience to supplement the Information Plus book.—**Pete Prunkl**

282.   **The AIDS Crisis: A Documentary History.** Douglas A. Feldman and Julia Wang Miller, eds. Westport, Conn., Greenwood Press, 1998. 266p. index. (Primary Documents in American History and Contemporary Issues Series). $49.95. ISBN 0-313-28715-5.

This text, geared toward high school and college students, is the latest in a series on controversial contemporary issues from Greenwood Press. The focus is not on medicine and science, but rather the "social, political, psychological, public health and cultural" aspects of the history of AIDS. The book provides short excerpts from accepted professional or governmental publications and is organized under 9 comprehensive topical chapters ranging from the history of the epidemic to ethics, developing countries, special populations, and the future. A full range of viewpoints are represented. The editors provide an introductory chapter, an additional introduction to each topical chapter, and a brief comment on each entry. The full citation for each excerpt is given, and each chapter ends with a suggested reference list, which allows the user to pursue the topic in more depth. The book is well indexed for ease of use, and is written at a level appropriate to the target audience. A glossary of terms is included for those unfamiliar with the complex language of AIDS.

One concern about his work is that some students might see this reference as an ending point. This reviewer would hope that students are encouraged by this text to read the entire primary source rather than relying on the excerpts. The book then becomes much like an encyclopedia, a starting point for their learning. *The AIDS Crisis* is highly recommended for college and high school libraries.—**Mary Ann Thompson**

283. **AIDS Sourcebook.** 2d ed. Karen Bellenir, ed. Detroit, Omnigraphics, 1999. 751p. index. (Health Reference Series, v.48). $78.00. ISBN 0-7808-0225-X.

The 63 chapters in *AIDS Sourcebook* are complete or excerpted documents from 16 U.S. government agencies, 3 nonprofit organizations, and 1 United Nations program. Omnigraphics found, compiled, and edited the documents, which were originally published between 1993 and 1998. As one might expect from government publications, the writing style is terse, factual, and advice-based. Quotations and case studies, which might personalize the topics, are almost totally absent. Content is authoritative, scientific, and as complete as one will find. With the exception of the 90-page glossary, articles are quite short, averaging 8 pages, an ideal length for high school and college students. Areas covered include general AIDS information, statistics and trends, information for people living with AIDS, prevention, and research. This work is highly recommended. —**Pete Prunkl**

284. **The Body: An AIDS and HIV Information Resource. http://www.thebody.com/index.shtml**. [Website]. New York, N.Y., Body Health Resources Corporation. Free. Date reviewed: Oct 02.

This Web resource, sponsored by The Body Health Resources Corporation, is designed to help both HIV/AIDS patients and those researching AIDS find the most up-to-date and authoritative articles and information on the most current research in the field. The site provides links to 20,000 documents on such topics as prevention of the spread of AIDS, HIV testing, treatment strategies, antiviral medications, HIV/AIDS in newborns and children, and side effects of drugs and co-infections. The sponsors of the site provides information from experts and organizations within the field of AIDS and states that, while some information may be contradictory, it is presented here with the idea that "airing such differences will lead to the advancement of social, political, and medical thought." The site also provides a forum board where users can ask experts AIDS-related questions on such topics as treatment, safe sex, and pain management. This site is updated daily, which contributes to its usefulness and accuracy. This site is highly recommended for use in research in university libraries.—**Shannon Graff Hysell**

285. **Encyclopedia of AIDS: A Social, Political, Cultural, and Scientific Record of the HIV Epidemic.** rev. ed. Raymond A. Smith, ed. New York, Penguin Books, 2001. 782p. index. $25.00pa. ISBN 0-14-051486-4.

Contributors to this encyclopedia were asked to write with a "mainstream consensus" perspective, thereby providing coverage for a wide range of topics that might otherwise remain unintelligible to the average reader. For the most part, this editorial goal has been accomplished. The result is a series of brief (2-5 pages) signed articles, arranged alphabetically, and accompanied by cross-references and selected resources for further reading. Topics range from abstinence to writers, economics to transplantation, African Americans to Protestant churches—in short, a tapestry of sociopolitical, scientific, cultural, and subcultural perspectives and concepts.

The time frame for topics covered is from 1981 through 1996. As such, this volume is to be used as a historical encyclopedia of AIDS, rather than as an up-to-the-minute resource. A disclaimer placed on the contents page signals the reader that this work is not to be used for medical advice; nor should it be construed as a definitive guide to related law and legal issues. And in the introduction to this edition, it is indicated that this paperback edition is really to be considered an update to the 1998 hardback edition of the same title, and published by Fitzroy Dearborn. A full index supplements the main text.

As an overview with historical perspectives, the work can easily be used by many researchers as a starting point. However, it is likely to need replacing every three to five years, since even AIDS suffers from revisionist historical methodologies. Many libraries might want to opt for an even more general introduction to the topic, and consider purchase of this volume to appease the information needs of those who are already somewhat versed in the topic.—**Edmund F. SantaVicca**

286.   **HIV and AIDS: A Global View.** Karen McElrath, ed. Westport, Conn., Greenwood Press, 2002. 290p. index. (A World View of Social Issues). $49.95. ISBN 0-313-31403-9.
The spread of HIV/AIDS worldwide during the past two decades has had a major impact on world health. Every nation and region (Sub-Saharan Africa) has faced its own unique series of challenges created by this disease—economic, social, cultural, and medical. This edited work presents the historical and current efforts of 16 countries/regions to handle these demanding health-related issues. This volume is part of A World View of Social Issues series, which attempts to compare and contrast how different societies in the first and third worlds confront significant social problems such as drug addiction, poverty, and women's rights.
Each chapter follows a similar pattern, describing the country or region, presenting a very brief history of HIV/AIDS in that area, discussing current policies and legislation to handle this crisis, and projecting possible future activities to combat the spread of this illness. The authors of these chapters vary greatly in their AIDS experience, coming from such diverse backgrounds as sociology, criminal justice, anthropology, and policy-making. While most authors have AIDS-related publications listed in AIDSLINE a few have no publications listed in this database. The chapter on HIV/AIDS in the United States presents an overly brief, superficial history of this disease in America. A clearly written section discussing the numbers and demographics of PWAs, 1981-1999, and the problems of AIDS-based discrimination follow this historical account. The amount and types of AIDS research being conducted in the late 1990s and the importance of AIDS-related work of nongovernmental organizations are discussed. A short conclusion challenges the United States to confront its AIDS future. The bibliography, while listing some primary documentation, fails to include many potentially useful publications one would expect to find.
Overall, this work may be of limited use for academic and public libraries but this volume lacks the depth required for medical and health care libraries. Individuals interested in obtaining in-depth information about HIV/AIDS in specific countries or regions should be encouraged to do an AIDSLINE search that easily provides more current and complete material on this subject. —**Jonathon Erlen**

287.   **HIV/AIDS Internet Information Sources and Resources.** Jeffrey T. Huber, ed. Binghamton, N.Y., Harrington Park Press/Haworth Press, 1998. 165p. index. $34.95; $19.95pa. ISBN 0-7890-0544-1; 1-56023-117-3pa.
This volume is both a collection of essays dealing with the state of information regarding HIV and AIDS as well as a valuable reference tool that analyzes and profiles information that is accessible via the Internet and World Wide Web. It was also simultaneously published under the same title as a special issue of *Health Care on the Internet* (1998). Among the topics and perspectives covered are strategies for creation of Websites by AIDS community-based organizations, a profile of AIDS service organizations on the Internet, strategies for networking of organizations, the use of Websites as educational tools aimed at at-risk populations, resources available for HIV-positive children and adolescents, Websites that provide information relevant to HIV and women, HIV-related news and discussion groups and their use as support tools, resources and services available through the National Institutes of Health, relevant resources from the Centers for Disease Control, Internet resources pertaining to complementary and alternative medicine and

HIV/AIDS, Internet resources that can be used for clinical management of HIV disease, and Internet resources regarding the development of antiretroviral drugs. A full index complements the essays.

Each of the essays is written by an individual with expertise in the area presented. As appropriate, full bibliographic references and URLs are given. All essays are well organized and quite readable. All in all, the work is a valuable addition to any reference collection, given the abundance of information presented—to be updated in time.—**Edmund F. SantaVicca**

288.   Huber, Jeffery T., and Mary L. Gillaspy. **Encyclopedic Dictionary of AIDS-related Terminology.** Binghamton, N.Y., Haworth Press, 2000. 246p. $59.95; $24.95pa. ISBN 0-7890-0714-2; 0-7890-1207-3pa.

Clear and concise definitions aimed at the general reader are the highlight of this reference tool. Arranged alphabetically, the volume presents a variety of terms related to AIDS and to disciplines or areas that have some relevance to the topic. Here the user can find legal, social, psychological, and religious terms, as well as those that pertain to medicine, care giving, insurance, pharmacology, and other areas. Whether reading an article or book, using the Internet, or writing a research paper, users can avail themselves of this dictionary as a handy thesaurus for synonyms, usage for standard abbreviations, and understanding the interrelationships of various concepts. Discipline-specific and popular terms are interfiled and cross-referenced for ease of use and understanding. Slang and colloquial idioms are also included.

A separate appendix provides directory and contact information to more than 70 governmental agencies and entities in the United States. In addition to name, address, and telephone number, listings include URLs, fax numbers, and contact information for specialized services. Although the price may keep this title from being in every academic or public library, it should receive strong consideration for purchase for those collections where interest and research in AIDS is significant.—**Edmund F. SantaVicca**

289.   Lerner, Eric K., and Mary Ellen Hombs. **AIDS Crisis in America: A Reference Handbook.** 2d ed. Santa Barbara, Calif., ABC-CLIO, 1998. 323p. index. (Contemporary World Issues). $45.00. ISBN 1-57607-070-0.

A welcome revision and update of information contained in the original edition, this valuable reference tool serves as a basic introduction to the subject of AIDS, as well as a resource for various facets and issues related to the topic. The work opens with a general overview including history, scientific perspectives, government response, and predictions for the future. This is followed by a quite detailed chapter treating the chronology (through 1997) of significant events related to AIDS. Short biographies of key people who have played some role in the AIDS crisis are also included. The remaining chapters focus in turn on facts and statistics, official government reports, and legal aspects and issues surrounding AIDS. Coverage throughout these chapters is somewhat uneven, generally encompassing 1997, and sometimes 1998.

Of great value to the individual seeking further information are the two final chapters of the work. The first functions as a directory of agencies, organizations, hotlines, and other assistance programs throughout Canada and the United States. Directory information as well as descriptions of purpose and scope are included. The last chapter focuses on reference materials, and includes both print (books, newsletters, pamphlets, anthologies, personal accounts, photographic works) and nonprint (films, videos, CD-ROMs, Websites). The whole is supplemented by a glossary, index, and biographical profile of the authors.

Although the work suffers, by necessity, of not being as up-to-date as possible, it does present a solid overview and introduction to its topic. Recommended for high school, public, and college libraries, with the understanding that it must be complemented by electronic and periodical literature.—**Edmund F. SantaVicca**

290.   Walter, Virginia A., and Melissa Gross. **HIV/AIDS Information for Children: A Guide to Issues and Resources.** Bronx, N.Y., H. W. Wilson, 1996. 261p. index. $35.00. ISBN 0-8242-0902-8.

A remarkable handbook and resource guide aimed at improving information services for children and adolescents, this book is arranged in 5 major sections. The initial 4 provide discussions, overviews, and profiles of issues surrounding children and AIDS. Among the many topics covered are children with AIDS, family issues, concepts of information needs, information-seeking behaviors, information gaps, availability of materials, what libraries can do, readers' advisory and reference services, booktalks, curriculum development, bibliographies, and so on. Each of these 4 sections provides a list of references.

It is the 5th section of this work that provides the reader with an impressive annotated bibliography of resources—both fiction and nonfiction—appropriate for children. Separate sections are provided for annotation of resources pertinent to adoption and foster care, compassion, death and dying, emotions, ethics and values, family, friendship, health and nutrition, homelessness and poverty, homosexuality, illness and disease, medical care, safety and survival, self-esteem, sex education, sexual abuse, social action, and substance abuse. Resources for adults are also included, as well as an appendix that provides evaluation criteria and a checklist for the selection of relevant titles. Four indexes—by grade level, recommendation level, author, and title—conclude the work.

This work should be in every school and public library, as well as in any environment where people address or counsel on issues of AIDS and children. The book is an impressive addition to the literature of AIDS and of children.—**Edmund F. SantaVicca**

291.   Watstein, Sarah Barbara, with Karen Chandler. **The AIDS Dictionary.** New York, Facts on File, 1998. 340p. index. $45.00; $24.95pa. ISBN 0-8160-3149-5; 0-8160-3754-Xpa.

This work will find its greatest audience among students, social service and health care organizations, and health care workers and administrators. With more than 3,000 entries, this dictionary includes terms pertinent not only to the basic biological and medical aspects of the disease but also to the financial, legal, psychological, emotional, political, and social aspects of HIV and AIDS. Most of the entries are short (5 to 10 lines), whereas others are quite lengthy. Cross-references to related entries are given throughout. A valuable quality is the inclusion of terms that may not be currently used but that are found in the early literature of the disease.

Appendixes include a list of frequently used abbreviations; a statistical profile of the epidemic through 1996; and a select list of resources that includes associations and organizations, education and training centers, journals and newsletters, and a comprehensive list of Internet and World Wide Web sites available on a variety of topics. A separate three-page bibliography completes the volume.

The authors are careful to indicate that this work is not exhaustive and that the fields of HIV and AIDS are constantly changing. Keeping this in mind, it is still hard to imagine an academic, public, or high school library that would not benefit from adding this tool to its reference collection. [R: BL, 15 Sept 98, p. 256; Choice, Nov 98, pp. 498-499]—**Edmund F. SantaVicca**

Allergies

292. Allergies Sourcebook. 2d ed. Annemarie S. Muth, ed. Detroit, Omnigraphics, 2002. 580p. index. (Health Reference Series). $78.00. ISBN 0-7808-0376-0.

First published in 1997, the *Allergies Sourcebook* has been completely revised and updated to include the latest information about common allergies. With an advisory board of librarians and a physician as medical consultant, the editor has selected relevant material from publications produced by the National Institutes of Health, the Environmental Protection Agency, nonprofit organizations, magazines, journals, and Websites. Full citations appear for all sources.

The book has six sections. Part 1 is a general overview, with an explanation of the allergic response, statistics, a summary of recent research, and information about the impact of allergies on daily life. Part 2 covers specific allergies and their effects on health. There is information about the symptoms, diagnosis, and treatment of respiratory, skin, and eye allergies as well as anaphylaxis. There are also chapters about multiple chemical sensitivity and a brief but interesting article about the potential link between Meniere's Disease and allergies. Part 3 discusses food allergies and intolerances, explaining the difference between these conditions and dispelling the myths about them. The next two sections describe the common allergy triggers (e.g., pet dander, molds, pollens, latex, venoms) and the diagnostic tests, treatment options, alternative therapies, and wellness aids that allergy patients may use. The last section of the book contains a glossary and lists of organizations that offer information and other resources for those living with allergies.

Since one out of five Americans is allergic to something, the *Allergies Sourcebook* is a welcome resource. The information is up-to-date and written at the high school level. Although most medical encyclopedias cover allergies at a basic level, this book brings a great deal of useful material together. The information about air cleaning systems and the objective evaluation of alternative therapies is especially useful. This is an excellent addition to public and consumer health library collections.—**Barbara M. Bibel**

293.   Lipkowitz, Myron A., and Tova Navarra. **The Encyclopedia of Allergies.** 2d ed. New York, Facts on File, 2001. 340p. index. (Facts on File Library of Health and Living). $66.00. ISBN 0-8160-4404-X.

Millions of individuals suffer from allergies and their symptoms vary widely, ranging from sneezing to life-threatening anaphylaxis. *The Encyclopedia of Allergies* was written by an allergist and a nurse for both allergy sufferers and nonsufferers to better understand the nature of allergies. The work contains new and updated information on allergies, allergens, symptoms, tests, medications, treatments (both traditional and nontraditional), and much more, and is written in an easy-to-understand style. The entries are arranged in alphabetic order and include such topics as allergy shots, asthma, immune system, and myths about allergies and asthma. Also included are more than 40 tables that cover subjects such as occupational allergens and weeds that cause hay fever in the United States and Canada.

The *Encyclopedia* has an informative timeline of allergy and immunology that begins with the death of Egyptian pharaoh Menes from anaphylaxis after a wasp sting in 2640 B.C.E. and continues up through 2001 with the publication of Dr. Jean Ford's report on the devastating impact of asthma. Appendixes provide information on the following topics: major pollen areas of the United States and Canada, available Radioallergosorbent Tests (RAST) for allergies, allergy organizations, and guidelines for the operation of camps for asthmatic children by the Consortium on Children's Asthma Camps. A bibliography (with most of the references being published in 1992 or earlier) and an index are included. *The Encyclopedia of Allergies* is a highly informative resource and is recommended for all consumer health collections.—**Rita Neri**

Alzheimer's Disease

294. **Alzheimer's Disease Sourcebook.** 2d ed. Karen Bellenir, ed. Detroit, Omnigraphics, 1999. 524p. index. (Health Reference Series, v.26). $78.00. ISBN 0-7808-0223-3.

This new edition of the *Alzheimer's, Stroke, and 29 Other Neurological Disorders Sourcebook* (see ARBA 94, entry 1862) is actually a very different book. The 1st edition provided mainly descriptive information about a wide range of neurological diseases; this 2d edition narrows its focus to diseases producing dementia. It is not only more current but also provides more practical assistance to those who fear these diseases or who must deal with an afflicted loved one. The wide-ranging information included is reprinted, like that in its predecessor, but is drawn not only from U.S. government agencies but also from medical journals and organizations, such as the Alzheimer's Association. The initial section summarizes what is known about Alzheimer's and its occurrence. What used to be called senility is far from universal; only 5 to 6 percent of elderly people suffer from Alzheimer's or related dementias. An overview of warning signs and diagnostic information help the consumer understand what are and what are not signs of a serious problem. Another section covers other diseases of the aged causing dementia, such as Huntington's Disease and Multi-Infarct Dementia, which is the result of a series of strokes causing brain damage. Parts 3, 4, and 5 of this work cover recent developments in prevention and treatment research, information on long-term care of patients, and guides to where those caring for an Alzheimer's patient can find assistance (including directories of federal, state, community, and other assistance programs), and a bibliography. Compilations of reprinted articles can be uneven in style and possibly in currency. Nonetheless, this book provides a wealth of useful information not otherwise available in one place. This resource is recommended for all types of libraries.—**Marit S. Taylor**

295.   Moore, Elaine A., with Lisa Moore. **Encyclopedia of Alzheimer's Disease: With Directories of Research, Treatment and Care Facilities.** Jefferson, N.C., McFarland, 2003. 401p. illus. index. $55.00. ISBN 0-7864-1438-3.

The *Encyclopedia of Alzheimer's Disease* is co-authored by a mother-daughter team who have written on medical subjects before. Elaine A. Moore has worked in a hospital laboratory for more than 30 years and her daughter, Lisa Moore, is a policy analyst for the federal government. This guide is arranged in four sections. The first section, "The Encyclopedia," provides hundreds of definitions related to Alzheimer's disease and its symptoms. Topics discussed include brain anatomy, disease pathology, the process of the disease, current research and treatment, and caregivers and government programs. The second section is a directory of long term and day care facilities for Alzheimer's patients. It is organized alphabetically first by state and then by city. Each center listed includes the name of the center, the address and telephone number, type of facility, number of nurses or caretakers, and whether the facility is privately or government owned. Section 3 lists research facilities alphabetically by state, with contact information. The final section lists resources for families and caretakers of Alzheimer's patients, including books, pamphlets, clinical trials, legal assistance, and Internet resources, just to name a few. The volume concludes with an index.

This resource will be valuable to those just diagnosed with Alzheimer's disease and their family members. It should be made available in health care libraries and larger public libraries. —**Shannon Graff Hysell**

296.   Powell, Lenore, with Katie Courtice. **Alzheimer's Disease: A Guide for Families and Caregivers.** 3d ed. Cambridge, Mass., Perseus, 2002. 396p. index. $18.00pa. ISBN 0-7382-0598-2.

Powell has designed this work to aid the families and caregivers of Alzheimer's sufferers and to help them deal with the multitude of difficult issues they face on a day-to-day basis. Following an introduction, Powell provides information on what exactly Alzheimer's Disease is, how it is diagnosed, and how it is treated. Next, Powell discusses some of the emotions that many patients, family members, and caregivers experience, including denial, anger, depression, guilt, and fear. The middle portion of the book leads readers through the process of the disease and the issues they will face, such as whether or not the patient needs to be placed in a nursing home and dealing with the patients eventual death.

While much of the book is geared for patients as well as relatives and caregivers, the last part of the book is specifically directed to relatives and caregivers and how they need to take care of themselves. Topics such as psychotherapy and adopting a healthy lifestyle to not only maintain better overall health but to also prevent Alzheimer's are covered. A list of organizations, a sample of a resident's bill of rights, a living will, and two memory tests conclude the book, along with chapter notes, a select list of references, and an index.—**Cari Ringelheim**

Arthritis

297.   Lorig, Kate, and James F. Fries. **The Arthritis Helpbook: A Tested Self-Management Program for Coping with Arthritis and Fibromyalgia.** 5th ed. Cambridge, Mass., Perseus Books, 2000. 367p. illus. index. $18.00pa. ISBN 0-7382-0224-X.

Arranged in six parts, this self-help/reference work is devoted entirely to persons afflicted with arthritis. In this latest edition, new information on arthritis medicines and pain reduction techniques, as well as new exercises and instructive illustrations, are included.

The first of the parts provides general information, prognosis, and treatment on arthritis, rheumatoid arthritis, osteoarthritis, osteoporosis, fibromyalgia, and other nagging pains. The second part considers how a patient can manage arthritis. Information such as goals, action plans, and an action plan calendar is provided. Part 3 considers how best to deal with daily activities, such as sitting, standing, lifting, and other types of activities. Black-and-white photographs are included to enhance the text. Part 4 provides the patient with a series of exercises useful for arthritic problems. Flexibility, strengthening, and aerobic exercises are included, along with cartoon illustrations of how best to carry out these exercises. A section on healthy eating is also included, along with food guide charts. Part 5 discusses with the patient how to solve particular problems, such as pain management, a good night's sleep, depression, fatigue, feelings, and communication. Part 6 lays out the medical resources that are available. Such areas as working with a physician, taking drugs (including painkillers), and surgery are considered.

An appendix listing the addresses and telephone numbers of the Arthritis Foundation in each state of the union as well as Great Britain, Canada, Australia, New Zealand are provided, along with fibromyalgia Websites. A subject index concludes the work.

This work is highly recommended for all people suffering from arthritis and arthritic-type conditions. It is also highly recommended for public libraries. *The Arthritis Helpbook* is recommended for college and universities that include self-help books as part of their collection development policy.—**George H. Bell**

Blood and Circulatory Disorders

298. **Blood and Circulatory Disorders Sourcebook.** Linda M. Shin and Karen Bellenir, eds. Detroit, Omnigraphics, 1999. 554p. index. (Health Reference Series, v.39). $78.00. ISBN 0-7808-0203-9.

This volume is a recent publication in a series of books that bring together and index reprints of articles originally published by government health agencies and private disease-related organizations. Omnigraphics has produced more than 45 of these volumes, on topics ranging from AIDS to learning disabilities. The target audience is patients and their families as well as health professionals who are involved with patient education. In all cases articles are clear and easy to understand, written in lay terminology and often providing illustrations. Some are in question and answer form, which is particularly handy for patient education purposes. The 51 chapters include material on specific blood problems, such as anemia, leukemia and bleeding disorders, and articles on diseases of the circulatory system, such as aneurysms, hypertension, and atherosclerosis. A final section discusses blood transfusions and their risks, autologous transfusion, and progress toward safety of the blood supply. There are a glossary of blood-related terms and a list of private and government agency resources for patients that gives addresses, telephone numbers, e-mail addresses, and Websites. Most articles are fairly recent, with copyright dates of 1995 or later. —**Carol L. Noll**

Brain Disorders

299. **Brain Disorders Sourcebook.** Karen Bellenir, ed. Detroit, Omnigraphics, 1999. 481p. index. (Health Reference Series). $78.00. ISBN 0-7808-0229-2.

This is a new addition to the Health Reference Series and is a basic consumer guide of health information about functions of the human brain as well as strokes, seizures, Lou Gehrig's disease, Parkinson's disease, cancer, and other brain disorders. The easy reading style provides readers with information on the complex issues surrounding the brain and its disorders. The text explains the causes and treatments of these diseases, and the book further provides symptoms, diagnostic tests, and coping strategies. There are a few black-and-white illustrations. The 46 chapters are arranged in 7 parts: the human brain including anatomy, EEG, MRI, CT, PET, and brain donation; strokes, including age groups, prevention, Warfarin, carotid endarterectomy, asymptomatic carotid atherosclerosis, and emergency; seizure disorders, including epilepsy and pregnancy, drugs, Felbamate, surgery, traumatic brain injury, febrile seizures, and genetics; Amyotrophic Lateral Sclerosis, including drugs and coping with this disease; Parkinson's disease, including drug therapies and coping mechanisms; other brain disorders, such as tumors, cerebral palsy, headache, narcolepsy, neurotrauma, Tourette's syndrome, and Tuberous Sclerosis; and additional help and information including brain terms, organizational resources for patients with brain disorders, and further reading on brain disorders. In addition to a good index, there are copyrighted articles.

Materials are collected from different government agencies, such as the National Cancer Institute, Agency for Health Care Policy and Research, National Center for Research Resources, National Institutes of Health, and from private organizations such as the American Parkinson Disease Association and the American Academy of Neurology. If readers are familiar with the style Health Reference Series offers, they will also find this source useful. However, these series do not replace professional health advice from health care providers.—**Polin P. Lei**

300.   Turkington, Carol. **The Brain Encyclopedia.** New York, Facts on File, 1996. 316p. index. $40.00. ISBN 0-8160-3169-X.

Research in the neurological sciences has accelerated greatly in recent years. This book aims to summarize for the layperson the status of knowledge about the brain, the body's most important organ. The introduction claims the encyclopedia "provides a guided tour through the brain"—but provision of a map would greatly assist most readers: There are no diagrams or illustrations of any kind. The encyclopedic arrangement of articles of varying length makes browsing intriguing; the book is not a neurological text specifically about the brain.

Small topics alphabetically arranged cover aspects of the brain, its structure and function, disorders, their diagnosis and treatment, and its relationship with other parts of the neurological and endocrinologic systems. There are many terms from psychology and psychiatry, and discussions of drugs affecting the brain—in good or bad ways. Paragraphs under "the brain in history" provide interesting sidelights, as do those under important physiologists and philosophers. There is no entry for "mind," but it is mentioned under "thought," "emotions," "consciousness," and the like.

An appendix list supports organizations, many of which are also described under the entries. There is a glossary of neurological terms and an adequate index. The bibliography is a reading list of recent articles related to the general subject, often readily available in such magazines as *Science News.*

This book succeeds admirably in helping readers to understand what is now known about the brain, and some of what yet needs to be learned about its mysteries. The encyclopedia is highly recommended for school and public libraries and health care workers. [R: LJ, July 96, p. 106; RBB, 15 Sept 96, p. 280]—**Harriette M. Cluxton**

301.   Turkington, Carol. **Encyclopedia of the Brain and Brain Disorders.** 2d ed. New York, Facts on File, 2002. 369p. index. (Facts on File Library of Health and Living). $65.00. ISBN 0-8160-4774-X.

The *Encyclopedia of the Brain and Brain Disorders*, now in its 2d edition, is a thoroughly revised and expanded version of the previous edition. It contains more than 800 clearly and concisely written alphabetically arranged entries on topics associated with the brain and neurology, brain diseases and disorders, brain structure and function, key persons associated with brain research, and associations and societies. The brain diseases and disorders entries include description, cause, symptoms, and treatment.

The work includes topics on alcohol and the brain, Alzheimer's disease, epilepsy, headaches, lead poisoning and the brain, learning disabilities, memory, meningitis, and Parkinson's disease. New topics include Mad Cow disease, new Alzheimer's drugs, human prion diseases, movement disorders, shaken baby syndrome, and vitamin deficiency and the brain. Many of the entries are cross-referenced.

The *Encyclopedia* has extensive additional resources. The appendixes contain a list of self-help organizations arranged by subject, a list of professional organizations, and a list of governmental organizations, all with contact information. There is also a glossary, a bibliography, and an index.

This reference work covers a wide range of topics on the functioning (or malfunctioning) of the brain and provides easy-to-understand information to the lay reader. It is recommended for school and public libraries as well as for organizations that are concerned with these subjects. —**Rita Neri**

302.   Turkington, Carol, and Joseph R. Harris. **The Encyclopedia of Memory and Memory Disorders.** 2d ed. New York, Facts on File, 2001. 296p. index. (Facts on File Library of Health and Living). $66.00. ISBN 0-8160-4141-5.

Memory links our past and future, providing a smooth transition. Its disruption is frightening, upsetting our lives and those of others. This revision and updating of the 1994 edition of *The Encyclopedia of Memory and Memory Disorders* (see ARBA 96, entry 780) presents new findings in the diagnosis and treatment of this crucial health issue. More than 700 entries to terms related to memory and its disorders and diseases are included. The reference is intended to serve a wide audience—detailed coverage for professionals, broad coverage for students, and readable information for general readers.

Entries reflect a wide range of terms relating to memory and range in length from several lines to several pages, as in the case of "Alzheimer's disease" and "Aging and Memory." Clinical terms, key researchers, memory tests, possible causes of disorders, major theories, symptoms, and treatments are included. Suggestions for memory improvement and slowing memory loss are also offered. Numerous cross-references enhance access.

Four appendixes provide lists of additional associations and Websites to contact, as well as monographs and periodicals that offer further information. A glossary of useful terms, an extensive list of references, and an index complete the volume. Whereas rapid advances have been made in scanning and mapping the brain, those involving memory, an integral aspect of human existence, have yet to keep pace. They will undoubtedly be reflected in the new revisions promised of this informative encyclopedia. [R: Choice, Mar 02, p. 1221]—**Anita Zutis**

Cancer

303.   Altman, Roberta, and Michael J. Sarg. **The Cancer Dictionary.** rev. ed. New York, Facts on File, 2000. 387p. illus. index. $40.00. ISBN 0-8160-3953-4.

Co-authored by a former cancer patient and an oncologist, this dictionary provides concise and understandable information for the layperson on more than 2,500 types of cancers. Entries note causes, incidence, symptoms, diagnosis, states, and treatment. Diagnostic tests, surgical procedures, anticancer drugs, radiation and biological therapies, side effects, risk factors, carcinogens, prevention, and support services and organizations are also covered. Extensive cross-referencing is used to lead the reader to the word that is most common and most well known.

Although arranged alphabetically, an index is also included to aid the reader. An additional subject index groups dictionary entries under broad general headings. National associations, support organizations, and cancer research and treatment centers are listed in the appendixes.

While many people use the Internet to search for the very latest information and treatment options, this dictionary can still provide assistance in sorting through the many intimidating terms and procedures associated with cancer. Public libraries will find it a useful addition to their consumer health sections. [R: LJ, Jan 2000, p. 78; BR, Sept/Oct 2000, p. 66]—**Vicki J. Killion**

304.   **Breast Cancer.** [CD-ROM]. By Eileen Kenny. Jacksonville, Fla., Steel Beach Productions, 2001. (Women's Health Series). Minimum system requirements: IBM or compatible Pentium processor. Four-speed CD-ROM. 32MB RAM. 16-bit color. 16-bit sound card. $19.95.

This CD-ROM effectively conveys information on breast cancer facts, risks, screening, prevention, and signs and symptoms in a visually easy-to-understand format. Navigation is clear and simple, and the program starts on its own once the CD-ROM is put into the computer. A mixture of virtual reality, still photographs, and live action video is used to communicate information on procedures such as mammograms and breast self-examination. Information on how often a woman should have these procedures performed is also included. [R: LJ, 1 Oct 01, p. 156]—**Denise A. Garofalo**

305. **Breast Cancer Sourcebook.** Edward J. Prucha and Karen Bellenir, eds. Detroit, Omnigraphics, 2001. 580p. index. (Health Reference Series). $78.00. ISBN 0-7808-0244-6.

In the United States, more than 180,000 women and 1,400 men receive a diagnosis of breast cancer every year. They need information to understand their condition and make decisions about treatment options. The *Breast Cancer Sourcebook*, part of Omnigraphics' Health Reference Series, provides an overview of the diagnosis and treatment of this disease.

The book's 65 chapters are organized into 8 sections. "Assessing Breast Health" discusses breast anatomy and its changes, risk factors, prevention, and self-examination. "Breast Cancer Fundamentals" explains the biology and epidemiology of the disease in males and females. "Evaluating Breast Cancer Risk Factors" covers the influence of genetics, hormones, diet, lifestyle, and environmental pollution. "Mammograms and Other Screening Tools" explains how physicians look for and diagnose breast cancer. "Treatment Options" discusses surgery; radiation; and drug, hormone, and alternative/complementary therapies. "Clinical Trials and Other Research" discusses current studies and explains what clinical trials are and what participants may expect. "Coping with Breast Cancer" deals with the psychosocial, family, and legal issues of cancer. "Additional Help and Information" offers a glossary, a directory of organizations for support, a list of Websites, and a bibliography.

The information in this book comes from government agencies, such as the National Cancer Institute and the Center for Disease Control and Prevention, and from nonprofit organizations. Full citations appear on the first page of each chapter. The broad range of topics covered in lay language make the *Breast Cancer Sourcebook* an excellent addition to public and consumer health library collections.—**Barbara M. Bibel**

306. **Cancer and the Environment: A Bibliography.** Joan Nordquist, comp. Santa Cruz, Calif., Reference and Research Services, 1999. 71p. (Contemporary Social Issues: A Bibliographic Series, no.53). $20.00pa. ISBN 1-892068-04-4.

The Contemporary Social Issues series is unfamiliar to many health sciences librarians, but is a staple in many libraries where students need to gather recent, relevant, and important articles and books for argumentative essays on topics of current interest. The series endeavors to locate and list materials in one resource that would require hours of searching to compile. The 53d volume in the Contemporary Social Issues series offers a bibliography on cancer and the environment. It provides a thorough record of popular, professional, and research articles, books, dissertations, conference proceedings, professional society reports, government publications, organizations, and Websites on various aspects of the theme. Citations are dated from 1990 onward.

As with other volumes in the series, the bibliography is especially strong in offering viewpoints from activist organizations, radical political writers, small presses, and other alternative sources. The slim bibliography is not annotated, but is organized by subjects such as water pollution and cancer, smoking and cancer, breast cancer and environmental pollution, and magnetic fields and cancer. Libraries may purchase individual issues from the series or subscribe to the series from Reference and Research Services in Santa Cruz, California. —**Lynne M. Fox**

307. **The Cancer Handbook.** Malcolm R. Alison, ed. New York, Nature Publishing Group/Grove Reference, 2002. 2v. illus. index. $525.00/set. ISBN 0-333-77659-3.

Research and publications in the field of cancer studies, are rapidly expanding. Journal articles and top quality Websites provide a constant flow of new information on this topic required by both professional health providers and their patients. These two volumes produced by the Nature

Publishing Group are an attempt to combine the recent discoveries about cancer from the basic research sciences and the clinical medicine community.

These volumes are divided into 102 chapters organized by 6 broad categories. Special attention is focused on the causes/prevention of cancers, cancer models, the use of imaging technology for the diagnosis and treatment of these diseases, and a variety of potential therapies for specific types of cancer. A major strength of this text is the use of numerous photographs, medical illustrations, charts, and graphs. Regrettably, the highly technical language used throughout this work seriously interferes with its usefulness for librarians and their nonmedical patrons, despite the inclusion of an extensive glossary.

With the availability of accepted major cancer reference tools such as *Cancer: Principles & Practice of Oncology* by DeVita, *Cancer Medicine* produced under the auspices of the American Cancer Society, and the nearly 6,000 URLs related to the National Cancer Institute whose main Website is http://www.nci.nih.gov/, it is questionable whether it is worthwhile to purchase this book when the information will quickly become dated.—**Jonathon Erlen**

308.   **Cancer Sourcebook.** 3d ed. Edward J. Prucha, ed. Detroit, Omnigraphics, 2000. 1069p. index. (Health Reference Series). $78.00. ISBN 0-7808-0227-6.

Periodicals and publications of government and nonprofit agencies make up the content of the 3d edition of this valuable health information source. Over 80 chapters are organized into 5 major parts. The introductory chapter covers general cancer information and contains an FAQ section. Other sections cover the major types of cancers with the exception of cancers of the female reproductive system and pediatric cancers. These are covered in separate volumes in the series.

The section dealing with the types of cancers is divided into eight subsections covering the major forms of cancer affecting specific body organs and systems. The nature of the cancer, its symptoms, risk factors, and treatment methods are explained. Treatment by stage of the cancer is described as well. Suggestions for further reading appear at the end of each section.

Cancer patients and their families are encouraged to be proactive in the management of their disease. A list of questions to be asked of surgeons and oncologists is provided and participation in clinical trials is encouraged. Also covered are genetic testing, tumor marking, and prevention recommendations for African Americans and people over 65. Suggestions for pain management, diet, and fatigue are covered as well. A glossary and a directory of organizations complete the book.

There have been some changes in this edition. The types of cancers have been reorganized. Endocrine cancers, formerly included with head and neck cancers, now have a separate section. The treatment and therapy section has been expanded to include a list of older and newer chemotherapy drugs, their uses, and side effects. Newer treatment methods such as lasers and stem cell infusion are also covered. Alternative therapies are discussed and include the medical use of marijuana. Missing from this edition are the statistical chapter and illustrations. The useful boldface highlighting of words that are defined in the glossary has also been dropped.

The Health Reference Series continues to be a comprehensive and reliable source of consumer health information. This volume is no exception. It can be effectively used by cancer patients and their families who are looking for answers in a language they can understand. Public and hospital patient libraries should have it on their shelves.—**Marlene M. Kuhl**

309.   **Cancer Sourcebook for Women.** 2d ed. Karen Bellenir, ed. Detroit, Omnigraphics, 2002. 604p. index. (Health Reference Series). $225.00. ISBN 0-7808-0226-8.

First published in 1996, the *Cancer Sourcebook for Women* has been updated to include the latest information about gynecologic cancers, cancer during pregnancy, fertility after cancer treatment, and conditions that may be mistaken for cancer. The material comes from the publications of government agencies, professional associations, and nonprofit organizations. Full citations are provided.

There are sections on breast, cervical, endometrial, and ovarian cancers, as well as chapters about conditions such as fibroid tumors that exhibit symptoms easily confused with cancer. The book also covers cancer screening and prevention, treatment options, recent research developments, and clinical trials. Information about the link between Human Papillomavirus (HPV) and cervical cancer, cancer treatment during pregnancy, and the effects of chemotherapy and radiation on fertility and sexuality will be useful for patients. The coverage of strategies for coping with treatment side effects and helping children understand their mother's illness are helpful too. A glossary, resource list, and information about the Family and Medical Leave Act complete the book. This volume from Omnigraphics' Health Reference Series is an excellent addition to collections in public, consumer health, and women's health libraries.—**Barbara M. Bibel**

310. **Encyclopedia of Cancer.** 2d ed. Joseph R. Bertino, ed. San Diego, Calif., Academic Press, 2002. 4v. illus. index. $800.00/set. ISBN 0-12-227555-1.

It is hard to imagine that anyone, outside of a specialist, would be able to remain current with the vast knowledge and new research in the field of cancer. The updated edition of this encyclopedia does offer a quick reference for the scientist or health care professional "desiring information [on cancer] outside their area of expertise." More than 220 entries on the topics of epidemiology, causation, science, and treatment have been contributed by cancer specialists from around the world. Individual entries average 5 to 10 pages in length. The entries are presented alphabetically in a standard format, starting with a topical outline and glossary and ending with a short bibliography and cross-references. Each volume begins with a table of contents for all four volumes in the series. The encyclopedia is written in a highly technical language appropriate to the scientist, physician, or medical student. Therefore, the reference is not appropriate for the layperson. The *Encyclopedia of Cancer* is recommended for medical libraries or specialty libraries serving health care professionals or scientists.—**Mary Ann Thompson**

311. **The Gale Encyclopedia of Cancer: A Guide to Cancer and Its Treatments.** Ellen Thackery, ed. Farmington Hills, Mich., Gale, 2002. 2v. illus. index. $275.00/set. ISBN 0-7876-5609-7.

One expects the best from the Gale Group and *The Gale Encyclopedia of Cancer: A Guide to Cancer and Its Treatments* does not disappoint. This 2-volume set contains more than 450 entries alphabetically arranged and signed, with excellent photographs and illustrations, a comprehensive index, and outstanding appendixes. There are entries for cancer types and cancer drugs. Entries regarding cancer types have the additional "Questions to ask the Doctor" and "Key Terms," and end with a "References" category, which is helpfully subdivided into books, organizations, and other resources. The level of language used is appropriate for laypersons as well as undergraduate and graduate students in the health sciences.

The appendixes contain superb contact information, such as the National Cancer Institute's designated Comprehensive Cancer Centers, National Support Groups, and Government Agencies and Research Groups. This outstanding resource will be a treasure in any public, high school, community college, or undergraduate library. [R: LJ, 1 May 02, p. 90; Choice, April 02, p. 1397]—**Lynn M. McMain**

312. **Prostate Cancer Sourcebook.** Dawn D. Matthews, ed. Detroit, Omnigraphics, 2001. 340p. index. (Health Reference Series). $78.00. ISBN 0-7808-0324-8.

The *Prostate Cancer Sourcebook* is another entry in the expanding series of Omnigraphics' Health Reference Series. As with other titles in the series, this addition is a valuable resource for health care consumers seeking information on the subject. Recent statistics indicate that 16 percent of American men will experience prostate cancer and that this number will probably grow as men's life spans increase. The demand for reliable, readable information will continue to grow.

Once again Omnigraphics presents a difficult subject with sensitivity, and even appropriate humor, to reassure and inform the reader. The sourcebook contains statistics; definitions; diagrams; explanations of physiology, diagnosis, and treatment; lists of support and advocacy organizations; and information for caregivers, family, and cancer survivors. The source of information is compiled and reprinted from a variety of sources: government documents, news sources, Websites, and original material written by health professionals specifically for the sourcebook. A small section addresses concerns about insurance and financial matters. The sourcebook also includes information on alternative and complementary treatment issues.

The topics addressed in the sourcebook anticipate many of the questions health consumers ask when facing decisions about prostate cancer. A detailed index allows convenient access to specific information, while the table of contents outlines the parts of the book for the casual browser. All text is written in a clear, easy-to-understand language that avoids technical jargon. Any library that collects consumer health resources would strengthen their collection with the addition of the *Prostate Cancer Sourcebook.*—**Lynne M. Fox**

Chronic Fatigue Syndrome

313. Patarca-Montero, Roberto. **Concise Encyclopedia of Chronic Fatigue Syndrome.** Binghamton, N.Y., Haworth Press, 2000. 160p. index. $24.95. ISBN 0-7890-0922-6.

There is so much to be learned about chronic fatigue syndrome. Montero has collated research publications from the past three years and presented readers with his own summation in this text. As noted in the references section, the cited materials are over 64 pages versus the 87 pages of content. There are *see* references to lead readers to the appropriate terms, and many concepts are written in medical convictions. In short, this is a concise book for researchers as well as sophisticated patients who seek advanced information for their own benefits.

The book includes a list of abbreviations used, A to Z contents, notes, and an index. The A to Z contents list a high caliber of topics relating to cardiovascular medicine, endocrinology, epidemiology, immunology, infectious diseases, neurology, psychiatry, and psychology. As medical sciences are changing, this book might need updating as the author suggested including evidence-based medicine and other new therapeutic findings. There is so much consumer information on chronic fatigue syndrome; this book serves as a backbone for scientific reading. [R: RUSQ, Winter 2000, p. 183]—**Polin P. Lei**

Diabetes

314. **American Diabetes Association Complete Guide to Diabetes.** Alexandria, Va., American Diabetes Association, 1996. 446p. index. $29.95. ISBN 0-945448-64-3.

Diabetes is a disorder that affects more than 16 million Americans—approximately 1 of every 17 people. With a statistic this staggering, the demand for accurate written information about the disease is obviously high. Indeed, there are innumerable texts written on various aspects of diabetes, including a number of popular guides. The highly respected American Diabetes Association has responded with yet another resource book that is a compilation of the best self-care techniques for the diabetic.

Written in a positive, easily understood style, this guide covers all the practical matters that the diabetic must know in order to enjoy a long, healthy life. The different types of diabetes (Type I, Type II, and gestational) are described and a general management plan given for each. A chapter on the health care team that may be especially needed by the person with diabetes (e.g., physician, dietitian, exercise physiologist, podiatrist, eye doctor, mental health counselor) is extensive. Detailed information is given on insulin and how to use it. Techniques for monitoring blood glucose levels are clearly described. A chapter on diabetes tools provides a description of such items as blood glucose meters, test strips, and lancets that are currently available for the diabetic. Other key pieces of the diabetes management plan, proper diet, and exercise are outlined.

Although diabetes can be controlled, there can be complications, such as cardiovascular disease, eye problems, nerve damage, and infections. These complications are discussed and preventive advice given. Because diabetes affects not only the person with the disorder but also family, friends, and coworkers, a chapter is devoted to discussing emotional, psychological, and discrimination issues that may result. A glossary, various appendixes, and a resource list round out this useful guide.

The *Joslin Guide to Diabetes* (Simon & Schuster Trade, 1995), written by doctors at the world-renowned Joslin Diabetes Center (affiliated with Harvard University) is similar in content. The two resource books differ mostly in organization and physical layout. For example, the American Diabetes Association guide contains large margins on each page that may be used by the individual to add personal notes. This is a guide for everyone who is touched by diabetes: the individual with a long history of the disease, the person newly diagnosed with diabetes, and others who desire to be supportive and better informed. The work is highly recommended for personal purchase and for all types of libraries.—**Elaine F. Jurries**

315.   **Diabetes A to Z: What You Need to Know About Diabetes—Simply Put.** 3d ed. Peter Banks and Sherrye Landrum, eds. Alexandria, Va., American Diabetes Association, 1997. 195p. illus. index. $11.95pa. ISBN 0-945448-96-1.

Diabetes A to Z is described in the preface as an encyclopedia of diabetes. This book is supposed to tell one everything one needs to know about diabetes in clear and simple terms. It is interesting to note the disclaimer of the American Diabetes Association on the verso of the title page about the accuracy of the information in this book. According to the preface, "the information in each entry will help you understand how to balance your diabetes care with a full and active lifestyle." Helpful tips for coping with the social and emotional challenges are presented for the person with diabetes. Much of the information in this book is not supported by the newest writings and research on diabetes care. Some of the newer writings suggest high protein, low fat, low carbohydrate diets for treating diabetes patients. There is no mention in the book that diet can reverse its damaging effects. After reading all the possibilities of complications from the disease, a newly diagnosed diabetic could find the information in this book terrifying.

The encyclopedic style of the book makes it easy to use. The charts and tables are easy to read and serve as a helpful guide through the topics. The alphabetic listings provide quick, easy access to the subjects. The fact that the American Diabetes Association does not support the content in this book, although it is their own publication, is reason enough not to purchase it.—**Betty J. Morris**

316.   **Diabetes Sourcebook.** 2d ed. Karen Bellenir, ed. Detroit, Omnigraphics, 1999. 688p. illus. index. (Health Reference Series, v.3). $78.00. ISBN 0-7808-0224-1.

This giant comprehensive volume is designed as an overview for laypersons to help them recognize the risk factors associated with diabetes, to identify symptoms, and to acquire the proper medical care. Of the 16 million Americans who suffer the illness, there are still 8 million people who remain undiagnosed. Medical professionals recommend that all adults age 45 and older should be tested for diabetes, and high-risk people under 45 should be tested as well. Based on these sheer numbers alone, this book serves a unique purpose for those people who are diabetic or for those who are high-risk candidates.

The new edition takes into account the changes in diabetic care since the first edition in 1994. According to the preface, the new volume contains 95 percent revised or new material. The 67 chapters of the book are divided into 8 parts. The parts of the book focus on broad areas of interest whereas the chapters relate to single topics. Part 1, "Diabetes Prevalence," offers statistical information about diabetes in the United States. Part 2, "Types of Diabetes and Related Disorders," describes the risk factors and symptoms for the major types of diabetes and related disorders. Part 3, "Diabetes Management," provides practical suggestions for managing the disease and reducing complications. Part 4, "The Role of Diet and Exercise in Diabetes Management," examines the relationship between diabetes management and the lifestyle factors of diet and exercise. Part 5, "Insulin and Other Diabetes Medicines," provides information about the different types of insulin, other medications, and drug interactions of special concern to diabetics. Part 6, "Complications of Diabetes," explains the major complications of diabetes, describes how they develop and provides treatment information. Part 7, "Research Initiatives," reports on diabetes research and the path toward further investigation. Part 8, "Additional Help and Information," provides a diabetes dictionary, sources for cookbooks and recipes, a bibliography of diabetes information, financial help sources, and a directory of diabetes organizations.

A comprehensive index provides easy access to information in the book. Material for this volume was collected from a wide array of government and private agencies. Copyrighted articles from a variety of sources have been reprinted throughout the book. In the commitment to provide ongoing coverage of important medical developments in the field of diabetes, the editors ask the readers to share their medical concerns for the next volume. This comprehensive book is an excellent addition for high school, academic, medical, and public libraries serving clientele with a broad range of medical concerns about diabetes. This volume is highly recommended. —**Betty J. Morris**

317.   Petit, William A., Jr., and Christine Adamec. **The Encyclopedia of Diabetes.** New York, Facts on File, 2002. 374p. index. (Facts on File Library of Health and Living). $71.50. ISBN 0-8160-4498-8.

This encyclopedia is an outstanding example of what can happen when a highly knowledgeable medical specialist is teamed with a talented medical writer—informative, accurate information is presented in a clear, intelligible style. It begins with an overview of the history of diabetes and key historical events in the development of treatments for this disease. Entries follow that examine key issues: the variant types, medications and other therapies, associated illnesses and complications, and demographics of diagnosed populations. The volume continues with appendixes that give contact information for diabetes-related organizations, research centers, and programs; Websites for further information; medications used in diabetic care; and tables of calculated body mass indexes. It concludes with a bibliography and a very thorough index.

Written for both consumers and professionals, the goal of the authors is to educate people who have diabetes about the disease, how to control its effects, and how to avoid serious complications. The goal is to prevent its development in people not diagnosed, encourage them to help those affected, and advocate for further research. This book admirably succeeds in its goals.—**Susan K. Setterlund**

Digestive Disorders

318. **Digestive Diseases and Disorders Sourcebook.** Karen Bellenir, ed. Detroit, Omnigraphics, 2000. 335p. illus. index. (Health Reference Series). $48.00. ISBN 0-7808-0327-2.

Part of Omnigraphics' Health Reference series, this excellent handbook provides a layperson's overview of both common and uncommon digestive ailments. The digestive system is explained, along with the common diagnostic tests that are performed on the upper and lower digestive tracts. Some common myths are refuted (such as spicy foods causing ulcers), and the digestion-related side effects of common medicines are summarized.

The diseases covered range from common indigestion, heartburn, constipation, and diarrhea to Zollinger-Ellison Syndrome. Each ailment is described and alternative names are given. Each entry lists symptoms, treatments, risk factors, and so on. A separate table provides the statistics on incidence, prevalence, mortality, hospitalizations, physician office visits, prescriptions, and procedures as of 1987. Each entry is written by a recognized expert in the field. Often the entries are copied from patient handbooks provided by associations or organizations that deal directly with patients. An appendix lists digestive disease organizations. This title would be an excellent addition to all public or patient-research libraries.—**Susan B. Hagloch**

Eating Disorders

319. Cassell, Dana, and David H. Gleaves. **The Encyclopedia of Obesity and Eating Disorders.** 2d ed. New York, Facts on File, 2000. 290p. index. $55.00. ISBN 0-8160-4042-7.

It is not surprising in a society preoccupied with being thin that the health industry is finding that more and more people are suffering from eating disorders and obesity. This book, first published in 1994 (see ARBA 95, entry 1678), aims to define the terms most often used by the health professionals treating these illnesses as well as those terms used by the diet industry and the pharmaceutical companies. The introduction is a six-page historical overview of obesity and eating disorders. It covers a lot of ground in a few pages by discussing different cultural ideas about body weight, the psychological ties to eating disorders that have been found, and the current struggle that exists between societal ideals and reality. Following the introduction are the A to Z definitions of terms. These include many psychology terms, medical terms, and definitions of drugs in the weight loss industry. Terms also included famous diets (e.g., Weight Watchers, Jenny Craig) and fraudulent products found in the weight loss industry. Seven appendixes follow the list of terms, which include a chronology, sources of information, eating disorder centers, and Websites of interest. A bibliography and an index conclude the volume.

Considering how prevalent obesity and eating disorders are in our society, all libraries should have one if not several volumes on the subject. This would be a good choice because it covers a wide array of topics and is written in a way that anyone, from high school students to adults, will understand. This volume is recommended for any public library's reference collection. [R: BL, 1 Dec 2000, pp. 748-750]—**Shannon Graff Hysell**

320. **Eating Disorders: A Reference Sourcebook.** 2d ed. Raymond Lemberg and Leigh Cohn, eds. Phoenix, Ariz., Oryx Press, 1999. 253p. index. $49.50. ISBN 1-57356-156-8.

Eating disorders, such as anorexia nervosa and bulimia, pose a grave danger to the health of thousands of Americans each year. This volume dispels the myths surrounding these disorders and is well grounded in research on the topic. Essays covers such topics as the causes and symptoms of eating disorders, body-size acceptance, eating disorders in males, eating disorders in athletes, feminist perspectives on eating disorders, and the treatment that is available.

Eating Disorders: A Reference Sourcebook is the 2d edition of *Controlling Eating Disorders with Facts, Advice, and Resources* (Oryx, 1992). New to this edition is an updated state-by-state list of facilities and programs for treating eating disorders, and the section on selected resources has been substantially expanded, listing books, articles, audiovisual materials, electronic resources, and Websites. An annotated list of Internet addresses for sites with information on eating disorders is a valuable resource. Also included is a new section on organizations, associations, hotline counseling services, and support groups. Bibliographic references and an index are included.

A personal account by Meredy Humphreys entitled "Death of a Scalesman" depicts the suffering of an anorexic and her struggle day in and day out to overcome it. This poignant account is accompanied by a case study by the editor. This single volume is uplifting and offers hope to anyone seeking assistance with coping with an eating disorder. [R: BR, Sept/Oct 99, pp. 70-71]—**Marilynn Green Hopman**

321.   **Eating Disorders Sourcebook.** Dawn D. Matthews, ed. Detroit, Omnigraphics, 2001. 304p. index. (Health Reference Series). $78.00. ISBN 0-7808-0335-3.

The *Eating Disorders Sourcebook*, edited by Matthews, is part of Omnigraphic's Health Reference Series. Its coverage includes anorexia nervosa, bulimia nervosa, binge eating, body dysmorphic disorder, pica, laxative abuse, and night eating syndrome. The publication is divided into the following sections: "Introduction to Eating Disorders"; "Types of Eating Disorders"; "Causes and Adverse Affects"; "Treatment and Prevention"; "Specific Concerns Related to Children and Adolescents"; and "Additional Help and Information." The information on frequently asked questions about eating disorders is excellent. There are also helpful bibliographies and links to eating disorder Websites. It compares favorably with Oryx Press's *Eating Disorders: A Reference Sourcebook* (2d ed.; see entry 320), but this publication's information is more current and accurate, particularly in regards to Website addresses. It is recommended for the reference collection of large public libraries.—**Theresa Maggio**

Endocrine and Metabolic Disorders

322.   **Endocrine and Metabolic Disorders Sourcebook.** Linda M. Shin, ed. Detroit, Omnigraphics, 1999. 574p. index. (Health Reference Series, v.36). $78.00. ISBN 0-7808-0207-1.

Presently there are 44 titles on various medical topics in Omnigraphics' Health Reference Series. Because of the success of this series, Omnigraphics intends to expand the series to 58 volumes in 1999. *Endocrine and Metabolic Disorders Sourcebook* follows a similar format of the other sourcebooks. Generally the sourcebooks are written in easy-to-read text and are designed for consumers seeking health-related information on certain medical disorders. These sourcebooks intend to be comprehensive in scope, but supplementary sources will still need to be acquired for any in-depth clinical information on disorder.

There are a total of 58 chapters in the volume at hand. Part 1 begins with an introduction to the endocrine system and human metabolism. The other 5 parts contain information on the glands and their disorders. Part 2 lists pancreatic and diabetic disorders, with nutritional recommendations and exercise control. Part 3 is on adrenal gland disorders and has only 4 chapters. Part 4 is on pituitary and growth disorders and includes a chapter on acromegaly. Part 5 is on thyroid and parathyroid disorders, which is extremely useful for a percentage of the general public. Part 6 provides information on other disorders of endocrine and metabolic functioning, such as hypercalcemia, PKU, FMEN1, galactosemia, and more. There are a few illustrations and charts to illustrate growth rate and locations of glands. Although some Websites are included for certain organizations and associations, it would be useful if more appropriate links were inserted, such as PDQ, NCI, or NIDDM for the electronic-savvy readers. Some chapters give suggested readings, other resources, or references. The index at the end is thorough, and readers will have no problem in locating "the information on the glands of the endocrine system, its components, the hormones it regulates, and the metabolic consequences of various disorders." Omnigraphics has produced another needed resource for health information consumers.—**Polin P. Lei**

323. Martin, Constance R. **Dictionary of Endocrinology and Related Biomedical Sciences.** New York, Oxford University Press, 1995. 785p. $75.00. ISBN 0-19-50633-4.

Noting that it is impossible for many professionals to keep up with the changing concepts and terminology of the many facets of endocrinology and related sciences, the author conceived this dictionary as a reference tool fostering mutual understanding, no matter which subspecialty or scientific discipline is being practiced. Much of the same information is of value to both.

Among the areas covered are endocrine physiology; hormones, neurotransmitters, and other regulatory factors; and terms relating to endocrinology drawn from other biomedical sciences. Although human physiology is emphasized, considerable attention is given to other species. Acronyms are numerous. The definitions are designed to be readily understood by readers who may be unfamiliar with specific terms, but are composed in highly technical language. Frequently, entries are accompanied by diagrams of chemical structure. These were produced by an ISIS/Draw program from Molecular Design Limited.

Considerable scientific acumen is needed for effective use of this scholarly, highly detailed, and extensive dictionary on endocrinology and aspects of biology, biochemistry, immunology, genetics, and the like, interrelated with this complicated subject. The book should be a valuable resource for many medical and research institutions, but it is not for general libraries. [R: Choice, Feb 96, p. 930]—**Harriette M. Cluxton**

Genetic Disorders

324. **Genetic Disorders Sourcebook.** 2d ed. Kathy Massimini, ed. Detroit, Omnigraphics, 2000. 768p. index. (Health Reference Series). $78.00. ISBN 0-7808-0241-1.

Since the 1st edition of the *Genetic Disorders Sourcebook* (1996) there have been advances in the study of gene detection. Researchers are already able to identify most genes associated with cystic fibrosis, Down syndrome, hemophilia, Huntington's disease, and sickle cell anemia, although no cures have been found. This handbook is divided into eight parts. Part 1 discusses the nature of genes, genetic disorders, and genetic screening, discussing gene make-up and how genes are inherited from one generation to the next. Part 2 focuses on disorders involving extra, absent, broken, or rearranged chromosomes, which results in Down syndrome and fragile X syndrome (which causes mental retardation). Parts 3 through 6 discuss blood clotting disorders (e.g., hemophilia), disorders of blood cells (e.g., sickle cell anemia), inborn errors of metabolism, and lysosomal storage diseases (e.g., Gaucher's disease, Tay-Sachs disease). Each of these parts discusses the diseases associated with these genetic disorders and what the symptoms and current research in the field is. The work ends with a section titled "Additional Help and Information," which provides a glossary, tips to help parents cope with their child's illness, and a list of organizations that can provide further information on specific topics surrounding genetic disorders.

This volume is written mainly with the layperson in mind and will be most beneficial in public libraries needing materials to supplement their popular medicine collection.—**Shannon Graff Hysell**

325. **Handbook of Genetic Communicative Disorders.** Sanford E. Gerber, ed. San Diego, Calif., Academic Press, 2001. 270p. illus. index. $84.95. ISBN 0-12-280605-0.

This work, edited by Sanford Gerber, a former professor of communication disorders and long-time author, has put together this work on the role of genetics in communicative disorders specifically with the practicing health clinician in mind. Gerber himself admits that he is not an expert on genetics but, instead, represents clinicians that need easy-to-understand and reliable information on genetics and how they relate to communicative disorders. The introduction provides the background on communicative disorders and defines the language that is used in the volume. Chapter 2 addresses what is known about genetics involvement in communicative disorders and how it has been researched so far (e.g., twin studies, sibling studies, the use of animals as models). The next several chapters use case studies to explain the role of genetics in hearing disorders, speech disorders, and autism and dyslexia. The last two chapters bring up the issue of ethics in genetics and how much science should do to alter or change the genetic make up of people. All of the contributors of this work are listed at the beginning of the volume along with their professional affiliation and address.

This work will be useful in health libraries and the health collections of academic libraries. This information is readable and current and all essays include extensive lists of references along with the work's concluding bibliography.—**Shannon Graff Hysell**

Hearing Disorders

326. **Singular's Illustrated Dictionary of Audiology.** By Lisa Lucks Mendel, Jeffrey L. Danhauer, and Sadanand Singh. San Diego, Calif., Singular; distr., Albany, N.Y., Thomson Learning, 1999. 357p. illus. $71.50. ISBN 1-56593-950-6.

This dictionary on audiology terms is intended for use by clinicians, teachers, researchers, equipment manufacturers, speech-language pathologists, and general physicians who deal with the hearing impaired or audiology in general. There are 4,500 terms listed here, each about one to two sentences in length. The work is extensively cross-referenced. There are words in bold typeface in many definitions, which indicates that the word has a separate entry of its own. Words that require a more detailed description than can be provided here refer readers to the *Audiologists' Desk Reference, Volume 1 and 2*. The appendixes at the end of the volume will be useful to professionals and students in the field of audiology. They provide a list of acronyms in the field, a list of illustrations and their credits used in the volume, and measurements used in the field. The most useful appendix provides 23 topical categories with words related to that category listed beneath. This will be especially useful to students trying to find related topics to the subject they are researching. This volume will be useful in medical libraries that serve those in the field of audiology as well as larger public libraries.—**Shannon Graff Hysell**

327. Turkington, Carol, and Allen E. Sussman. **The Encyclopedia of Deafness and Hearing Disorders.** 2d ed. New York, Facts on File, 2000. 294p. index. (Facts on File Library of Health and Healing). $55.00. ISBN 0-8160-4046-X.

This volume is part of the Facts on File Library of Health and Living series, which aims to provide both general and professional readers with up-to-date, comprehensive information on health-related issues. The 2d edition of this title (see ARBA 93, entry 1656, for a review of the 1st edition) has some 800 entries on topics ranging from parts of the ear and diseases to clinical terms, specialists, devices and equipment, and organizations for the deaf or hearing impaired. The entries make up the bulk of the volume. New to this edition are expanded entries on autoimmune inner ear disease, cochlear implants, the American Academy of Audiology, Pendred's Syndrome, and the relationship between smoking and hearing loss. The 14 appendixes in this volume contain a lot of information that library patrons will most likely be interested in, such as statewide services for the hearing impaired, directory information of organizations, periodicals of interest to deaf people, summer camps for hearing impaired children, and bibliographic information on sign language dictionaries, to name a few. A nine-page bibliography and an index conclude the volume.

Although certainly not the only reference work on deafness, this volume is an easy-to-use source for the general reader. It will be most valuable in large public libraries.—**Shannon Graff Hysell**

Heart Disorders

328.   **Healthy Heart Sourcebook for Women.** Dawn D. Matthews, ed. Detroit, Omnigraphics, 2000. 336p. index. (Health Reference Series). $48.00. ISBN 0-7808-0329-9.

Healthy Heart Sourcebook for Women is divided into 6 parts with 39 chapters and covers such topics as risk factors for stroke with chapters on depression, cholesterol and age at menopause. Other topics discussed are treatment and control strategies including the outlook for women after bypass surgery, hormone replacement therapy (pros and cons of estrogen replacement therapy and postmenopausal hormones), and dietary issues (fiber, coffee, meal plans, and recipes). Like all the titles in the Omnigraphics series, it is a collection of articles from a variety of sources. The chapter on women and heart attacks comes from a 1996 article in *The Nurse Practitioner*. The chapter on passive smoking comes from a 1996 article in the *Harvard Health Letter* and the quiz on women's heart disease and stroke comes from the Canadian women's magazine *Chatelaine*. The 1996 Website (www.nhlbi.nih.gov/health/public/heart/other/homocyst.txt) from the National Heart, Lung, and Blood Institute (NHLBI) is the source of the chapter on homocysteine and heart disease. Other chapters, such as the one covering risk factors like smoking and high blood pressure, is excerpted from the NHLBI's *Heart Healthy Handbook for Women*. As with all Omnigraphics titles, there are useful tables (e.g., leading causes of death for American women, interpretation of blood cholesterol levels, and a sample walking program). There is an index and a brief glossary as well as an annotated list of resources with complete contact information and URLs when available. Because of the lack of information specific to women on this topic, this book is recommended for public libraries and consumer libraries, especially those where Web access is problematic.—**Martha E. Stone**

329.   **Heart Diseases and Disorders Sourcebook.** 2d ed. Karen Bellenir, ed. Detroit, Omnigraphics, 2000. 612p. illus. index. (Health Reference Series). $78.00. ISBN 0-7808-0238-1.

Heart disease continues to be the leading cause of death in the United States, with an estimated 57 million Americans living with some type of cardiovascular disease. This reference book, another in the Health Reference series, updates the previous edition entitled *Cardiovascular Diseases and Disorders Sourcebook* published in 1995.

Many advances have occurred in the arena of heart disease research since 1995 and this new edition updates research findings, treatment options, and statistics. As in the previous edition, this book is a compilation of documents and excerpts from government agencies such as the National Institutes of Health, Centers for Disease Control, National Heart, Lung and Blood Institute, and the U.S. Food and Drug Administration. The volume also contains copyrighted articles produced by organizations like the American Heart Association and Johns Hopkins Intelihealth, and articles from respected periodicals such as Harvard Heart Letter, Mayo Clinic Health Letter, and Tufts University Diet and Nutrition Letter. Given the source of the information, all of the chapters are quite readable, accurate, and geared toward the average consumer.

The 2d edition has been extensively reworked and consists of 6 major parts and 66 separate chapters. The major divisions are: the introduction; understanding your heart; preventing heart disease; common types of heart problems; medications, interventions, and other treatment options; cardiac rehabilitation; and additional help and information. The section on additional help and information contains a glossary of heart terms; a bibliography of heart-healthy cookbooks; a listing of Spanish-language publications available from the National Heart, Lung, and Blood Institute; and a directory of resources for heart patients.

There are innumerable books written about heart disease, but this work stands out as an imminently accessible resource for the general public. *Heart Diseases and Disorders Sourcebook* is recommended for the reference and circulating shelves of school, public and academic libraries. —**Elaine F. Jurries**

Liver Disorders

330. **Liver Disorders Sourcebook.** Joyce Brennfleck Shannon, ed. Detroit, Omnigraphics, 2000. 591p. illus. index. (Health Reference Series). $78.00. ISBN 0-7808-0383-3.

This work, which is part of Omnigraphics' Health Reference Series, provides a thorough overview of liver complications. It has been designed and written in a manner that makes referencing specific liver disorders easy.

The work is divided into 10 parts, each containing several chapters. Topics discussed include liver mechanics and maintenance, medical tests, liver distress, the effects of drugs on the liver, liver cancer, hepatitis, genetically based liver disease, other diseases of the liver, and liver transportation, among other information. Throughout the text are several illustrations. Although they are not in color, they are still effective. In addition, the text that accompanies the illustrations provides sufficient explanations. The end of the work has useful resources, including additional contacts for information, a glossary of terms, and a reference section on the remaining Health Reference Series.

This volume will be a valuable resource for adult readers and will complement home libraries. Medical professionals may also find this text to be useful as a tool for obtaining general medical information on the liver.—**Paul M. Murphy III**

Lung Disorders

331. **Asthma Sourcebook.** Annemarie S. Muth, ed. Detroit, Omnigraphics, 2000. 627p. index. (Health Reference Series). $78.00. ISBN 0-7808-1381-7.

Asthma Sourcebook is the most recent offering in the Health Reference Series from Omnigraphics. As with all books in the Health Reference Series, *Asthma Sourcebook* consists of documents and articles from various sources, such as federal government departments and agencies, private organizations, and professional journals.

Presented as basic consumer health information, the book covers a wide variety of topics about asthma, including diagnosis and treatment, management, medications, theories of causes, and alternative prevention ideas. Interestingly, part 2, "Asthma Statistics," contains over 100

pages on asthma statistical data, a more useful resource for secondary and lower division undergraduate students than consumers. Part 8, "Additional Help and Information," contains a small but helpful glossary, a chapter on resources, an index, and the obligatory catalog of other Health Reference Series titles. The chapter of resources has valuable contact information, including Web and e-mail addresses, for traditional organizations such as the Allergy and Asthma Network-Mothers of Asthmatics and Asthma and Allergy Foundation of America, as well as nontraditional sources such as the Center for Complementary and Alternative Medicine Research in Asthma. This informative text is recommended for consumer health collections in public, secondary school, and community college libraries and the libraries of universities with a large undergraduate population.
—**Lynn M. McMain**

332.   **Lung Disorders Sourcebook.** Dawn D. Matthews, ed. Detroit, Omnigraphics, 2002. 678p. index. (Health Reference Series). $78.00. ISBN 0-7808-0339-6.

This book discusses "basic consumer health information about emphysema, pneumonia, tuberculosis, asthma, cystic fibrosis, and other lung disorders . . . ." This title is a great addition for public and school libraries because it provides concise health information on the lungs. Readers can start with this reference source and get satisfactory answers before proceeding to other medical reference tools for more in-depth information.

There are six parts to this reference tool: an introduction, "Types of Lung Disorders," "Diagnosis," "Treatment," "Risks and Prevention," and "Additional Help and Information." The introduction presents the history, anatomical functions, environment, and disorders of the lung. A few black-and-white illustrations are inserted. It would be great if there was a CD-ROM included on the animated lungs. The types of lung diseases are listed in question-and-answer format with short and concise answers. At the end of each chapter there is information for where readers can get more information from support groups. "Diagnosis" explains how the various tests are done, such as body plethysmography, bronchoscopy, and chest MRI. The section on "Treatment" provides explanations on inhalation, ventilation, nebulizer, and other treatments. "Risks and Prevention" discusses the dangers of smoking, asbestos, radon, formaldehyde, air pollution, and ozone generators. "Additional Help and Information" provides a glossary as well as contact information for national organizations for lung cancers, asthma resources, and sleep disorder clinics. Most of the general research documentations are from Centers for Disease Control and Prevention (CDC) and Department of Health and Human Services (DHHS) as well as many other governmental entities—generally authoritative sources. However, readers should not treat this book as a replacement for medical professional care but use it as a good guide for health education on lung disorders.—**Polin P. Lei**

333.   Navarra, Tova. **The Encyclopedia of Asthma and Respiratory Disorders.** New York, Facts on File, 2003. 410p. index. $71.50. ISBN 0-8160-4467-8.

Respiratory problems are associated with at least 4 of the 10 leading causes of death in the United States. In addition, many people, across all age groups, suffer from chronic respiratory diseases. This book, compiled by a registered nurse, brings together a wealth of information on the topic of respiratory diseases, with a particular emphasis on asthma. The contents would be of help to health care professionals as well as the lay public. The major section of the reference includes more than 1,000 alphabetized entries, with definitions or explanations in language that will be accessible to the average adult. Of particular value in this section are the inclusion of medications, listed by generic and brand name, and two extensive tables of plants that lead to hay fever, including the period of pollination during the calendar year. A second section of appendixes includes a variety of statistical and diagnostic and management information. Entries include such things as morbidity and mortality data on the major respiratory diseases, common medications (with dosages and side effects), treatment flow charts, and the use of complementary and alternative therapies. The book concludes with a directory listing of professional and lay organizations related to the diseases. The information contained in the book is accurate and current to 2002. This resource is recommended for public and college libraries, as well as the personal libraries of families coping with respiratory diseases.—**Mary Ann Thompson**

Osteoporosis

334.   **Osteoporosis.** 2d ed. Robert Marcus, David Feldman, and Jennifer Kelsey, eds. San Diego, Calif., Academic Press, 2001. 2v. illus. index. $399.95/set. ISBN 0-12-470862-5.

Perhaps the best thing that can be said about a medical text book is that a person with little interest in the subject or much of a medical background can read, understand, and actually find chapters of the book very interesting. This is such a book. If a medical library only collects one book on osteoporosis this should be it. All aspects of the disease are covered with eight new chapters added since the last edition published in 1996. The topics include basic anatomy and physiology of bone, pathophysiology, risk factors for the disease, the role of nutrition and physical exercise in the development of osteoporosis, as well as treatment. All chapters contain lists of up-to-date references with many photographs, illustrations, graphs, and tables. What makes this book accessible to the nonspecialist is that most chapters clearly explain introductory concepts. For example, the chapter entitled "Design Considerations for Clinical Investigations of Osteoporosis" explains the various types of research studies and their strengths and limitations.

Of course, no book on any medical subject can be completely up to date, but in light of the current controversy on hormone replacement therapy, the chapter "Estrogens and Osteoporosis" is quite timely. The chapter discusses the FDA's recent decision "to rescind estrogen's osteoporosis treatment indication" (p. 577) and points out that taking estrogen may cause an increased risk of cardiovascular events. The chapter's authors do suggest waiting for the results of the Women's Health Initiative to shed further light on the controversy.

Other nice features of this book are that the type and layout are easy to read and its wide margins make photocopying possible. This sourcebook is highly recommended for all medical libraries.—**Natalie Kupferberg**

335.   **Osteoporosis Sourcebook.** Allan R. Cook, ed. Detroit, Omnigraphics, 2001. 584p. index. (Health Reference Series). $78.00. ISBN 0-7808-0239-X.

The Health Reference Series has long been a champion to deliver consumer type of health information to the general public. These resources are comprehensive in scope and easy reading for all. Abundant research and expert opinions are included in all of these publications, and the *Osteoporosis Sourcebook* is of no exception. This is a timely resource for those baby boomers that may one day suffer from osteoporosis. The unusual inclusions in this book are the sections on "How to Find a Doctor" and "Taking Supplements for Osteoporosis," which might prove to provide answers to common questions asked by many of the sufferers of this disease.

This book is in seven sections: "Introduction: A Quick Review"; "The Nature of Osteoporosis"; "Facts and Figures for Osteoporosis"; "Related Conditions"; "Osteoporosis Risk Factors and Prevention"; "Diagnosis, Treatment, and Coping Strategies"; and "Additional Help and Information." For those who are interested in data on African, Asian, and Latino women suffering from this ailment, chapters 12 and 14 provide some venue for this information. This book is thorough to include osteoporosis for men as well. Apart from that, this book is also strong on the treatment aspects providing not one but several alternatives for consideration.

A glossary and a directory of resources add an additional outlet for readers to seek assistance from the right source. As usual the thorough index provides a bonus to readers. This 1st edition includes the complete catalog of books in the Health Reference Series, with clips of reviews. This is a good reflection of how solid the Health Reference Series publications are. Once again, this resource is recommended as a great reference source for public, health, and academic libraries, and is another triumph for the editors of Omnigraphics.—**Polin P. Lei**

Poisoning

336.   Morelli, Jim. **Poison! How to Handle the Hazardous Substances in Your Home.** Kansas City, Mo., Andrews and McMeel, 1997. 258p. illus. index. $9.95pa. ISBN 0-8362-2721-2.

There is no doubt about it, Morelli has cornered the market on toxicological information for consumers. Although this book is not a replacement for expert assistance, especially during a toxicological emergency, it may decrease the possibility of having such an emergency by providing a necessary element for increased consumer awareness. Readers will learn what to do about the various poisons that lurk in their homes, gardens, and medicine cabinets. According to the author, we live in a toxic dump. However, this book will "add a note of rationality to the mysterious world of poisons . . . by tearing down some enduring myths." Creative and humorous, this conversational volume takes the "science" out of "scientific" jargon. It puts the information at the reader's fingertips in a user-friendly format, and it makes learning fun.—**Sue Lyon Mertl**

337.   True, Bev-Lorraine, and Robert H. **Dreisbach. Dreisbach's Handbook of Poisoning: Prevention, Diagnosis, and Treatment.** 13th ed. Pearl River, N.Y., Parthenon, 2002. 696p. index. $49.95pa. ISBN 1-85070-038-9.

The introduction to this updated edition notes the high yearly incidence of exposures, illnesses, and fatalities from poisons. Speed is vital to survival and recovery from poisoning, and this book sets out to provide "a concise summary and quick reference" for diagnosis and treatment. The introductory chapters give general information about prevention, diagnosis and treatment, and medical and legal issues surrounding poisons and poisoning. The 31 chapters follow, covering all types of poisons, from the more obvious occupational and household products to self-ingested chemicals and snakebites. The chapters are organized under the general categories of agricultural, industrial, household, medicinal, and animals and plants. Each individual entry is no more than two pages long. Each poison is presented in a structured format: introduction, clinical and laboratory findings, acute and chronic treatments, prevention, and prognosis. Medical references cited are timely, generally from the late 1990s. The language and content of the book is appropriate to health care professionals, poison control centers, and scientists. The actual size of the book (a pocket-sized reference) makes it portable. This is an absolute essential reference for emergency rooms, poison centers, and emergency response personnel.—**Mary Ann Thompson**

338.   Turkington, Carol. **The Poisons and Antidotes Sourcebook.** New York, Checkmark Books/Facts on File, 1999. 408p. index. $35.00. ISBN 0-8160-3959-3.

The Poisons and Antidotes Sourcebook is designed to inform readers about dangerous materials that may be within their own home without their knowledge of their dangers or of how to treat them in case of deadly contact. The book includes information on such common items as household poisons; insecticides and fertilizers; poisonous spiders and snakes; drugs; and poison ivy and other toxic plants. Part 1 of the work contains tips on what to do in a poison emergency, how to make one's home safe, food poisoning, and what poisons are associated with what symptoms. The book then is arranged into A to Z entries. These entries explain what the poison is, the symptoms

that will occur, and treatment. The book is extensively cross-referenced. At the end of the work are several appendixes that provide hotline telephone numbers in case of emergency, newsletters, organizations, regional poison control centers, and Websites for more information. A glossary, reference section, and index conclude the work. The information provided in this guide is both in-depth and valuable. The work will be useful in both personal libraries and public reference collections.
—**Shannon Graff Hysell**

Parkinson's Disease

339.   Weiner, William J., Lisa M. Shulman, and Anthony E. Lang. **Parkinson's Disease: A Complete Guide for Patients and Families.** Baltimore, Md., Johns Hopkins University Press, 2001. 256p. index. (A Johns Hopkins Press Health Book). $19.95pa. ISBN 0-8018-6556-5.

The authors state that this book is for the patients and their families to better understand Parkinson's disease and to give them information on new treatments and how the disease will impact their lives. The text starts with a diagnosis since the disease can mimic six other diseases and explains what happens to the brain to cause the disease. It also makes it quite clear there is no cure for the disease. The first six chapters chart the disease from the beginning stages—from diagnosis to moderate levels and on to advanced levels of the disease. Each chapter describes the different changes in the body the disease causes and how the patient's day-to-day life will change also. Later chapters go into more detail on how doctors diagnosis the disease and distinguish it from other neurological diseases, the drug therapies used to treat the symptoms and how they interact in the body, alternative treatments that work in combination with the drugs to maintain the patient's quality of life, and surgical treatments. Another chapter covers information on current research and the last chapter lists frequently asked questions with answers. The book has a list of resources for more information from groups or foundations, which includes the name, address, telephone number, Website, and a brief description. There is also an extensive index.

The book is written for the average nonmedical person in clear, concise language. The definitions and descriptions are easy to understand. The book does not talk down to the reader even though it approaches the subject from the viewpoint that the reader knows nothing about the subject except its name and that it involves tremors. This guide is highly recommended for all public libraries and medical or health libraries that serve as patient educators. The book is well worth the cost.—**Betsy J. Kraus**

Sexually Transmitted Diseases

340.   Marr, Lisa. **Sexually Transmitted Diseases: A Physician Tells You What You Need to Know.** Baltimore, Md., Johns Hopkins University Press, 1998. 341p. index. $39.95; $16.95pa. ISBN 0-8018-6042-3; 0-8018-6043-1pa.

This text addresses a topic that is of increasing importance and yet is still considered by many to be taboo. The book has two primary components. Part 1 discusses what readers need to know about sexually transmitted diseases (STDs) and part 2 is called the "Encyclopedia of STDs." This approach is beneficial because part 1 provides readers with an overview of what they should know regarding anatomy, symptoms, STD examinations, communication skills, and safe sex. Part 2 is a natural transition as it explains the STDs, including STD signs and symptoms, treatment options, and statistics.

The medical terminology and statistics will not be overly complex for the adult reader to understand. The illustrations are easy to interpret and they correspond directly to the contents of the book. The resources, a glossary of terms, and references are provided in the latter portion of the text. Contact information, including telephone numbers, mailing address, and Website, has been included when possible.

This text provides valuable information that has been presented in a professional and concise manner. Although it could be included in any medical library, it could easily complement a number of libraries (i.e., public, home, health care clinic) as a source of valuable information. It may also be useful as a reference resource for individuals involved in teaching courses that discuss sexually transmitted diseases.—**Paul M. Murphy III**

341. **Sexually Transmitted Diseases Sourcebook.** 2d ed. Dawn D. Matthews, ed. Detroit, Omnigraphics, 2001. 538p. index. (Health Reference Series). $78.00. ISBN 0-7808-0249-7.

Omnigraphics' Health Reference Series produces books with basic consumer health information on various topics, in this case on sexually transmitted diseases (STDs). The books in the Health Reference Series are compilations of documents and articles previously published by private or government sources.

Sexually Transmitted Diseases Sourcebook is divided into seven main parts: an introduction, types of STDs, risk and prevention issues, diagnosis and treatment, issues related to youth, other issues, and additional information. The additional information includes a useful glossary and a comprehensive index. The parts are divided into 50 chapters. Most of the chapters end with useful references or suggested readings.

The interesting chapter on nonsexual transmission of STDs addresses the disease risks of tattooing and piercing. The chapters on adolescents and STDs provide beneficial information for both parents and teens. This 2d edition differs from the previous edition in organizational structure, increased emphasis on a larger variety of STDs, and is updated with more recent material.

This book would be useful for persons who require a review or overview of material on STDs. This text is recommended for consumer health collections in public libraries, and secondary school and community college libraries. [R: BL, 15 April 01, p. 1582]—**Lynn M. McMain**

Skin Disorders

342. Boyd, Alan S. **The Skin Sourcebook.** Los Angeles, Calif., Lowell House, 1998. 404p. illus. index. $22.95pa. ISBN 0-7373-0003-5.

The Skin Sourcebook should not be confused with the plethora of beauty and skin care books. This text transcends the beauty book genre, offering instead a clear and easy-to-understand consumer health dermatology resource. *The Skin Sourcebook* would be a valuable addition to any library fielding consumer health inquiries in the area of dermatology. Prior to the publication of this work, consumer health questions on dermatology were referred to more technical dermatology textbooks, or to consumer health magazines with less authoritative sources of information. The author of this work, Alan S. Boyd, is an experienced Vanderbilt University dermatologist with specialties in dermatology and psoriasis care.

The health of the skin is the focus of well-indexed chapters on skin care and therapy, dermatitis, skin cancer, and diseases and conditions affecting the skin. The chapters include short descriptions of conditions; discussions of commonly prescribed topical, ingested, or injectable preparations and medications; and suggestions for self-diagnosis. The color illustrations of skin conditions at the center of this book provide a visual reference guide usually reserved for more expensive and technical atlases of dermatology. Unfortunately, neither the index nor the chapter text refers the reader to the illustrations. Readers must find topics of interest in the index, identify the chapter that includes the topic, then find the group of illustrations under that chapter heading.

Three appendixes provide additional resources, including a list of commonly prescribed medications along with dosage and drug interaction notes. Another appendix suggests possible conditions indicated by major symptoms. The third appendix includes organizations that provide information and support to patients. An extensive bibliography lists resources used in the preparation of the book. This work will be a useful resource for multiple types of libraries serving patrons with health care concerns.—**Lynne M. Fox**

343. **Burns Sourcebook.** Allan R. Cook, ed. Detroit, Omnigraphics, 1999. 604p. illus. index. (Health Reference Series). $78.00. ISBN 0-7808-0204-7.

Annually, some 1.25 million burns are reported to medical personnel in the United States, including 5,500 burn fatalities, making burn injuries one of the nation's leading causes of accidental death. This latest volume in the Health Reference Series from Omnigraphics is an important resource for both health professionals and the general public in dealing with the problems created by burn injuries. Drawing from governmental, medical, and scientific literature, the editors provide a lot of knowledge pertaining to the prevention and the appropriate handling of a wide variety of burns.

This book is divided into 7 easy-to-use sections. Beginning with burn statistics, the following segments discuss the types and degrees of burns, the variety of treatment protocols, issues of rehabilitation and living with the long-term effects of burns, preventive measures to safeguard homes and businesses from burn hazards, and emergency and first-aid procedures for burn victims. A final brief section lists some of the major additional societal and institutional burn resources that are available. Illustrations and bibliographies provide additional useful information throughout this volume, which also includes a comprehensive index.

Burns are a serious public health problem in the United States. This key reference guide is an invaluable addition to all health care and public libraries in confronting this ongoing health issue.—**Jonathon Erlen**

344. Turkington, Carol A., and Jeffrey S. Dover. **The Encyclopedia of Skin and Skin Disorders.** 2d ed. Illustrated by Birck Cox. New York, Facts on File, 2002. 436p. illus. index. (Facts on File Library of Health and Living). $71.50. ISBN 0-8160-4776-6.

First published in 1996 as *Skin Deep: An A-Z of Skin Disorders* (see ARBA 97, entry 1333), the authors have completely revised and updated this encyclopedia. Turkington is a medical writer and Dover is a clinical professor of dermatology at the Yale University School of Medicine and the Dartmouth Medical School. The new edition has over 1,100 alphabetic entries covering a wide variety of topics related to the skin.

The entries range from one sentence to one page in length. They include specific skin disorders (e.g., alopecias, various skin cancers), other diseases that affect the skin (e.g., Addison's Disease, Kawasaki Disease), drugs (e.g., isotretinoin, neomycin), cosmetic procedures (e.g., Botox, chemical face peel), associations (e.g., Interplast, Lupus Foundation of America), cosmetics (e.g., nail hardeners, permanent makeup), and related topics (e.g., sunscreens, cosmetic labeling). Black-and-white line drawings illustrate some entries. A series of appendixes cover cosmetic ingredients, types of skin lesions, support organizations for diseases and conditions, and professional associations. The information about cosmetics is very useful because it includes color additive terms and ingredients to avoid, such as allergens, irritants, and carcinogens. A glossary, bibliography of professional and lay sources, and an index complete the work. Most sources listed in the bibliography are from the 1990s. *The Encyclopedia of Skin and Skin Disorders* will be very useful in public and consumer health libraries since questions about skin care and disease are common.—**Barbara M. Bibel**

345.   Wood, Corinne Shear. **An Annotated Bibliography on Leprosy.** Lewiston, N.Y., Edwin Mellen Press, 1997. 176p. (Studies in Health and Human Services, v.30). $89.95. ISBN 0-7734-8441-8.

A carefully prepared work published by Edwin Mellen Press, this reference source presents an up-to-date bibliography and a "panoramic view" on Hansen's disease. It appears that each reference is reviewed and selected for medical professionals, social scientists, and for those who wish to know more about this disease. The author admits that this book is not intended to be comprehensive in scope, but includes collective contributions on international publications and journal articles from different global sites such as India, Australia, Germany, Switzerland, and Africa.

The work features 14 chapters. The first few chapters are on leprosy related to historical, social, and biblical concerns. A few references in these chapters were published in the eighteenth century and are worth exploring. For the clinical aspects, there are chapters on research and fieldwork, treatment, diagnosis and rehabilitation, epidemiology, compliance studies, control and prevention, and immunology. Women and children with leprosy are separately listed. In addition, publications on biographies, literature, and texts on leprosy are listed to enlighten the curious mind. However, the health education chapter could be enriched a little. Overall, the concise annotations help to define the scope of the items and to identify the source country of work performed. The author clarifies whether the annotations are the original author's summary or an abstract. The index of authors is alphabetic and thorough. However, it would have been useful if a list of keywords had been included. In general, this is a great resource and a good compilation of publications on this disease. Academic libraries should consider acquiring this title to add to the reference collection. [R: Choice, July/Aug 98, p. 1834]—**Polin P. Lei**

Sleep Disorders

346.   **Sleep Disorders Sourcebook.** Jenifer Swanson, ed. Detroit, Omnigraphics, 1999. 439p. index. (Health Reference Series). $78.00. ISBN 0-7808-0234-9.

This text, which is part of Omnigraphics' Health Reference Series, contains more than 400 pages of useful information relating to sleep. The book is divided into 6 parts and contains 53 chapters.

Part 1, "Understanding Sleep Requirements and the Cost of Sleep Deprivation," discusses topics such as why we need sleep and power napping. Part 2 contains 11 chapters that explore "Sleep Through the Lifespan." Topics include "What Is Sudden Infant Death Syndrome" (SIDS), "Common Bedtime Trauma," and "Sleep in Older Persons." Part 3 discusses major sleep disorders. The 15 chapters cover topics such as sleep apnea, snoring, narcolepsy, insomnia, and sleepwalking. Part 4, "Sleep Medications," focuses on medications that may be used to either enhance or facilitate sleep. Four chapters are dedicated to medications such as Melatonin, benzodiazepines, and over-the-counter options. Part 5 has 9 chapters that focus on "Sleep and Other Disorders." This section of the book explores the effects and relation between sleep and coexisting illnesses. Part 6, the last 4 chapters of the book, provides the reader with a glossary of terms and an extensive list of references. The inside of the front and back covers of this book lists a complete catalog of the Health Reference Series. This text will complement any home or medical library. It is user-friendly and ideal for the adult reader.—**Paul M. Murphy III**

347.   Thorpy, Michael J., and Jan Yager. **Encyclopedia of Sleep and Sleep Disorders.** 2d ed. New York, Facts on File, 2001. 314p. index. (Facts on File Library of Health and Living). $66.00. ISBN 0-8160-4089-3.

This revised and updated 2d edition contains recent research and breakthroughs and reflects current science and understanding of sleep and sleep disorders. Important terms and significant facts are cross-referenced and indexed. Terms covered include those for syndromes, medications, disorders, individuals, organizations, treatments, symptoms, and conditions. The readable and informative material is useful to the layperson as well as the professional. Extensive appendixes include a state-by-state listing of sleep centers and laboratory members of the AASM, Websites, and international and diagnostic classifications of sleep disorders. A bibliography is also included.
—**Denise A. Garofalo**

SPEECH PATHOLOGY

348.   Singh, Sadanand, and Raymond D. Kent. **Illustrated Dictionary of Speech-Language Pathology.** San Diego, Calif., Singular; distr., Albany, N.Y., Thomson Learning, 2000. 287p. illus. $45.00. ISBN 1-56593-988-3.

This specialized dictionary was developed to meet the needs of the broad range of disciplines now contributing to, and working in, the field of communication science and communication disorders. The goal of the compilers is to aggregate the terms and concepts that have "migrated" to this field, and to define them in light of speech and language norms and pathology. They have succeeded in their goal. The entries include terms, phrases, and concepts specific to the discipline, but also terms associated with anatomy and physiology, pathology, and various psychological and health-related theories. Main entries are printed in bold, larger-than-average font to facilitate use. Black-and-white photographs, diagrams, graphs, and tables are interspersed. Particularly helpful are the simple anatomical illustrations. Four appendixes are included: commonly used abbreviations, the international phonetics alphabet, an alphabetized listing of illustrations, and a short chapter on physical quantities and units. This reference would be invaluable to students and practitioners in the field of communication science and disorders. In addition, it would be appropriate for health science libraries and institutions, such as chronic and rehabilitation hospitals, long-term care facilities, or special schools serving persons with communication disorders.
—**Mary Ann Thompson**

SPORTS MEDICINE

349.   Potparic, O., and J. Gibson. **A Dictionary of Sports Injuries and Disorders.** Pearl River, N.Y., Parthenon, 1996. 155p. $35.00. ISBN 1-85070-686-7.

This text is presented in traditional dictionary form. Overall, the print is easy to read. Topics defined/discussed range from "abstinence syndrome" to the "glasgow coma scale" and "zygoma fractures." Some of the definitions will require the reader to have a medical terminology background in order to understand them.

Unfortunately, there are no pictures or illustrations in the text. Having them would have enhanced some of the definitions or conditions mentioned in the text. In addition, there is no table of contents and no index, either of which would probably make this text easier to use.

The work is designed to be used primarily by individuals with a medical background or by athletes themselves. However, adult readers who are involved or interested in sports will probably find this text to be of benefit as a reference source in conjunction with other texts. It is a good reference for general sports injuries.—**Paul M. Murphy III**

350. **Sports Injuries Sourcebook.** 2d ed. Joyce Brennfleck Shannon, ed. Detroit, Omnigraphics, 2002. 592p. index. (Health Reference Series). $78.00. ISBN 0-7808-0604-2.

This new edition is completely reorganized, with 8 main parts subdivided into 58 chapters compared to the 1st edition's 5 parts and 46 chapters (see ARBA 2000, entry 1441). There are newly discussed sports and activities such as home trampolines, BB guns, motor scooters, horse-related activities, mountain biking, sledding, ice hockey, and water-related activities. Additionally, there is expanded information on sports and athletic injuries in mid-life and elderly persons.

As with all sourcebooks in the Health Reference Series by Omnigraphics, this book provides general information regarding sports and athletic injuries specifically geared to consumers. The articles are usually reprints from other sources, primarily professional organizations and the federal government. The only caveat is while most of the articles are one to two years old, there are some articles up to four years old and a few that are undated. Despite that, this is an excellent reference for consumers and it is recommended for public, community college, and undergraduate libraries.—**Lynn M. McMain**

SURGERY

351. Haeger, Knut. Roy Calne. **The Illustrated History of Surgery.** 2d ed. London, Harold Starke Publishers and Chicago, Fitzroy Dearborn, 2000. 295p. illus. index. $50.00. ISBN 1-57958-319-9.

In recent years scholars have published numerous major histories of surgical specialties, including neurosurgery, cardiac surgery, and orthopedics. Still many readers prefer an overview survey text on surgery's origins and development. Haeger's revised volume is a competent work to meet this request. This book is intended for both physicians and the general reader, although the latter probably will find it most useful. The revised edition of the original 1988 study adds material on recent advances in transplantation and minimal invasive surgical procedures.

In less than 300 pages the author surveys the evolution of surgery as a medical specialty, from trepanation in the earliest of times through modern transplant procedures. There is very limited discussion of Chinese and Indian surgical concepts, with the vast majority of the text focusing on European and American surgical advances. The greatest strength in this volume is the wonderful collection of color and black-and-white illustrations, depicting various surgical procedures and the pioneers who developed them. Although there are some factual errors that demonstrate that the author has failed to keep up with some of the recent historical scholarship, such as the incorrect date for Galen of Pergamon's death, taken as a whole this text presents the traditional stories in a sound, scholarly fashion.

This book is an adequate, general survey of many of the major surgical innovations throughout history. Readers interested in a more in-depth treatment of the history of this medical specialty should consult Owen Wangensteen's massive work, *The Rise of Surgery* (Midewiwin, 1978), or Zimmerman's and Veith's *Great Ideas in the History of Surgery* (repr., 1993). For most casual reader's, however, Haeger's volume will prove more than sufficient to answer their questions about surgery's past.—**Jonathon Erlen**

352. **Reconstructive and Cosmetic Surgery Sourcebook.** M. Lisa Weatherford, ed. Detroit, Omnigraphics, 2001. 374p. illus. index. (Health Reference Series). $48.00. ISBN 0-7808-0214-4.

Many guides to cosmetic surgery have been published in the past few years as the demand for appearance enhancing cosmetic surgery has increased. These guides have lacked information on medically necessary reconstructive surgeries. The *Reconstructive and Cosmetic Surgery Sourcebook* from Omnigraphics is an excellent reference that addresses cosmetic and medically necessary reconstructive surgeries. Omnigraphics has established itself as a publisher of quality consumer health information with the Health Reference Series sourcebooks. The sourcebooks compile information from the World Wide Web, medical texts, journal articles, and other sources into a valuable reference work. An advisory board reviews the sourcebooks to ensure accuracy and quality of information.

The topics addressed in the sourcebook anticipate many of the questions health consumers ask when facing decisions about reconstructive or cosmetic surgery. The reference is divided into short chapters that address common types of surgeries and their alternatives. Many articles also address emotional and social concerns related to plastic surgery. One section is devoted to statistics on reconstructive and plastic surgeries. Chapters also address practical matters, such as choosing a surgeon or dealing with insurance issues. Black-and-white photographs and drawings illustrate stages of surgery and recovery. A helpful glossary defines common surgical, anatomical, material, and equipment terms. A detailed index allows convenient access to specific information, while the table of contents outlines the parts of the book for the more casual browser. All of the text is written in a clear, easy-to-understand language that avoids technical jargon. The style of the prose is calm and reassuring, discussing the many positive outcomes now available due to advances in surgical techniques. Any library that collects consumer health resources would strengthen their collection with the addition of this fine sourcebook.—**Lynne M. Fox**

353. **Transplantation Sourcebook.** Joyce Brennfleck Shannon, ed. Detroit, Omnigraphics, 2002. 610p. index. (Health Reference Series). $78.00. ISBN 0-7808-0322-1.

The last quarter century has seen tremendous advances in transplantation technology. Currently, transplants are available for a number of organs (e.g., kidney, liver, heart) and tissues (e.g., skin, corneas, bone marrow). Along with these advances have come a number of daunting questions for potential transplant patients, their families, and their health care providers. This reference text is the best single tool to address many of these questions.

Nine broad sections, divided into 50 chapters, present important, clearly written information discussing a wide variety of transplantation issues. Who are potential transplant recipients? Where should they go to be evaluated and placed on the transplant waiting list? What are the financial aspects of receiving a transplant? How will receiving a transplant change the rest of the patient's life? Specific material is provided on organ and tissue transplantation topics, pediatric transplantation concerns, organ donation centers, and the future of transplantation. A final section presents a useful glossary of transplantation terms and lists of transplant organizations, donor centers, and major transplant hospitals nationwide.

This volume is a new addition to the outstanding Health Reference Series, which features standard medical and health care reference works. It will be a much-needed addition to the reference collections in health care, academic, and large public libraries.—**Jonathon Erlen**

4 Men's and Women's Health

354. **American Medical Association Complete Guide to Men's Health.** Angela Perry and Mark Schacht, eds. New York, John Wiley, 2001. 502p. illus. index. $34.95. ISBN 0-471-41411-5.

Health guides for the lay public have traditionally been directed at women's health, children's health, or family health. By focusing solely on men's health and illness, this book helps to fill a major gap in the health information and advice literature. Edited by a reliable source, the American Medical Association, the book is a comprehensive guide to health and disease issues for men across the lifespan. The reference begins with a thorough discussion of "The Healthy Man" and holistic advice on how to stay healthy. Chapters on diet and nutrition, exercise, mental health, routine health screenings, and major health risks are included. Reproductive health is covered in a separate section. The book concludes with 14 chapters discussing common medical concerns for individual bodily systems. A unique but timely addition is a chapter on cosmetic surgery. The book is written in simple language that will be accessible to a majority of lay readers. The content is accurate and timely. Individual chapters or sections could stand alone. Black-and-white graphics are interspersed, usually illustrating aspects of anatomy. A glossary of medical terms is included. The *American Medical Association Complete Guide to Men's Health* is recommended for public libraries.—**Mary Ann Thompson**

355. Belmonte, Frances R. **Women and Health: An Annotated Bibliography.** Pasadena, Calif., Salem Press and Lanham, Md., Scarecrow, 1997. 203p. index. (Magill Bibliographies). $35.00. ISBN 0-8108-3385-9.

Women's health has finally emerged as a discipline in its own right. This annotated bibliography of approximately 300 books published during the past 30 years demonstrates the evolution of women's health from obstetrics and gynecology to care for the whole woman and the study of her interactions with society. The author, a substance abuse counselor and theologian, takes an interdisciplinary approach.

The chapters cover broad subject areas: descriptions of women, care of women, care by women, self-education and self-help, costs and benefits, and addictions. Each chapter has an introduction that attempts to set the parameters of its contents. Unfortunately, these are so full of jargon that it is hard to decide what the focus is. The actual citations offer only author, title, publisher, and date. The annotations, ranging in length from a one-third to a one-half page, offer brief summaries and some commentary by the author. Author, title, and subject indexes complete the work. The indexes are important because the chapter titles are so vague. The classic title *The New Our Bodies, Ourselves* (Peter Smith, 1996) could appear in several chapters; it is located in the self-education and self-help chapter.

Even though this work may be somewhat valuable for historical purposes in women's studies collections, it is not a necessary purchase for most libraries. The heavy use of jargon and vague organization make it minimally useful at best.—**Barbara M. Bibel**

356.   Dashe, Alfred M. **The Man's Health Sourcebook.** 2d ed. Lincolnwood, Ill., National Textbook, 1999. 288p. illus. index. $17.95pa. ISBN 0-7373-0109-0.

As the title implies, this text discusses men's health issues and should be read by both men and women, just as the author recommends. It includes a preface, introduction, glossary, index, illustrations, and tables. Unfortunately the reference section is limited and Internet and Web addresses are not provided.

In the preface and introduction the author explores recent trends and issues relevant to today's health care system. This includes the author's opinions in regard to the current status, insights, and future trends as seen from the eyes of a practicing physician. Both of these sections are informative and beneficial as they describe the sociological and health care changes taking place in our world.

The main body of the text is divided into two sections. The first section is a general overview of issues such as healthy living, how to choose a physician, and when to call a doctor. This section should be reassuring for those individuals who are either evasive or procrastinate when it is time to visit their physician. In fact, men who have not had a recent physical exam may find this text to be a motivator to take the first step.

The second section provides an overview of selected medical issues relevant to males. Topics include a basic review of the male anatomy, cardiovascular system, respiratory system, skin and hair, gastrointestinal system, endocrine system, male sexuality, male sexual health, the aging process, substance abuse, and mental health. At the end of each topic the author provides the reader with a useful summary of topic highlights.

Within the text are several tables, charts, and illustrations. The tables and charts are presented in a clear and concise manner. Although the illustrations are black-and-white, they are relevant, effective, and correspond with the text. Medical terminology is included and is either defined within the text or in the glossary.

This text contains information that can be of benefit to both sexes. It can be used as a general reference source and in conjunction with a physician's physical examination. A text of this nature is a valuable source of information and would be appropriately available in a variety of environments, including private physician offices, clinics, and home and school libraries.—**Paul M. Murphy III**

357.   **Men's Health Concerns Sourcebook.** Allan R. Cook, ed. Detroit, Omnigraphics, 1998. 738p. index. (Health Reference Series, v.38). $78.00. ISBN 0-7808-0212-8.

Men's Health Concerns Sourcebook is part of a 38-volume Health Reference Series by Omnigraphics. This sourcebook contains basic information about health issues that affect men. It helps men identify, prevent, detect, treat, and cope with their most common health threats, such as heart disease, stroke, cancer, and AIDS. It also contains facts on impotence, contraception, circumcision, snoring, and other topics. The book includes a gender focus: top 10 causes of death in men, family planning decisions, circumcision, sleep disorders, diet, and fitness. It has an excellent index. Materials have been collected from both governmental and nongovernmental groups. This comprehensive resource and the series are highly recommended for large public libraries for their health and reference collections. [R: BL, 1 Dec 98, p. 698]—**Theresa Maggio**

358.   **The Women's Complete Healthbook.** Roselyn Payne Epps and Susan Cobb Stewart, eds. New York, Delacorte Press/Bantam Doubleday Dell, 1995. 708p. illus. index. $29.95. ISBN 0-385-31382-9.

This peerless reference book was written by women doctors, many of them specialists, for women patients and health care consumers. As medical research on women's problems is recent and quite incomplete, the authors of the separate chapters provide much information from their practices and personal experience, as well as what is generally know about a disease or condition, including up-to-date medical information. Because each contributor writes from her own point of view, there is some intentional repetition of information, so the user can also review it from another approach (e.g., osteoporosis is discussed in the excellent overview chapter on aging, as well as under the musculoskeletal system).

Material is organized into chapters under four main headings: "Being a Savvy Consumer of Healthcare"; "Keeping Yourself Healthy"; "Reproductive Healthy"; and the longest section called "The Health Body: Symptoms, Diagnosis, and Treatments." Each chapter begins with an outline of its topics, so it is easy to locate specific information. The detailed index is also helpful. There are many clear figures and charts. An appendix describes common diagnostic tests. A list of associations keyed to the chapters provides access to further resources.

The aim of this large handbook is to provide an authoritative resource that empowers women who make health care decisions for themselves and their families. Its scope, clarity, and quality is incredible. It reflects most favorably on the American Medical Women's Association, who presented it. All kinds of libraries should find it valuable, and it is recommended for widespread individual purchase.—**Harriette M. Cluxton**

359a.   **Women's Health Concerns Sourcebook.** Heather E. Aldred, ed. Detroit, Omnigraphics, 1997. 567p. illus. index. (Health Reference Series, v.27). $78.00. ISBN 0-7808-0219-5.

This book is an example of an increasingly popular type of publication—a reprint collection of health information articles by government and nonprofit agencies. The advantage is that useful articles from a variety of sources are conveniently gathered together, arranged by topic, and indexed for maximum accessibility. The disadvantage, of course, is that what was once free now costs $78. This volume covers conditions and disorders either exclusive to or more common in women, from everyday issues of female health, such as menstruation, birth control, and menopause, to more unusual diseases, such as lupus, breast cancer, and anorexia. (Pregnancy, certainly one of the central health events in most women's lives, is not covered in this book, but will be the subject of a future volume.) The articles are arranged by topic in 24 chapters. Most are from patient-information publications by the National Institutes of Health, the Federal Drug Administration, or the Department of Health and Human Services. A few of the articles are as old as from 1983, although most are two to six years old. Most are written in an easy-to-read, simple manner, with diagrams and charts to aid in understanding. The information in most of these articles tends to be fairly general and basic. For some patients the articles will be just enough information, but for those determined to research a topic in depth, this will be just an introduction and starting point. [R: BR, Jan/Feb 98, p. 51]—**Carol L. Noll**

5 Nursing

BIOGRAPHY

359b. American Nursing, Volume 3: A Biographical Dictionary. Vern L. Bullough and Lilli Sentz, eds. New York, Springer Publishing, 2000. 307p. illus. $69.95. ISBN 0-8261-1296-X.

The "biographical history of American and Canadian nursing" is completed in this volume containing 132 biographies that "serves as a key to documenting the changes in attitude toward professional women during the last part of the twentieth century" (p. xiii). The first 2 volumes were reviewed in ARBA 89 (entry 1575) and ARBA 93 (entry 1659). Individuals include both living and dead, but were selected because of their significant impact on the nursing profession as seen in their leadership, administrative record, innovative practices, publications, articulation of theories, or because they were role models, broke barriers, and otherwise gained recognition for their contributions to the field. In the first volume, all those selected were believed to be dead; the second cited a few born before 1915 who were still living; and this last volume has many who were alive at publication, although all are at least 75 years old due to the 1925 cutoff date of birth.

Entries are written in a narrative style with an emphasis on a characterization of the individual in nursing and general American history as well as her or his qualifications for inclusion. Supportive personal and career information, publications (books, book chapters, and articles), selected references, and the contributor's name are found in each entry. Most entries also include a picture, and average 3 or 4 columns (1,200 to 1,500 words) in length. The credentials of the editors and the contributing editors to this volume are cited on a frontispiece page. A summary demographic and historical analysis of the individuals chosen for biographical study is found in the introduction. For ease in searching, a list of those nurses found in volumes 1 and 2 is printed at the end of this volume. (Volumes 1 and 2 included a listing of the first nursing schools attended by the biographees; this volume does not.) There is no keyword or subject index so use of the book(s) as a history of American nursing requires reading or scanning all volumes. However, the complete set serves to highlight 512 women (and 11 men) who are not apt to be found in any other twentieth-century biographical compilation since nursing, as other feminized professions, has been a neglected source of biographical study.—**Laurel Grotzinger**

DICTIONARIES AND ENCYCLOPEDIAS

360. The Gale Encyclopedia of Nursing & Allied Health. Kristine Krapp, ed. Farmington Hills, Mich., Gale, 2002. 5v. illus. index. $850.00/set. ISBN 0-7876-4936-8.

The term "encyclopedia" can conjure up a negative image for the professional, but this five-volume set for nursing and allied health negates that stereotype. The set includes more than

850 alphabetized entries that cover diseases and disorders, tests and procedures, equipment, anatomy and physiology, the health care professions, and the health care delivery system. Each item follows a standardized format for its particular category. For example, all disease entries discuss the definition, causes and symptoms, diagnosis, treatment and prognosis, health team roles, and prevention. Each topic concludes with a short reference list of books, journals, Internet sites, and relevant organizations. The references are current, most cited within the last two to three years. The contributors include representatives from all the health sciences. In addition, the entries were reviewed for accuracy and timeliness by an advisory board of prominent scientists and health care professionals. Volume 5 concludes with a comprehensive cross-index and a directory of nursing and allied health's professional organizations.

The editor notes that the encyclopedia is aimed at the beginning student, thus it is written in a style between the lay reader and the health care professional. Despite its purpose as a tool for beginners, the seasoned professional will find the reference to be helpful as a quick, accurate check across a comprehensive list of topics. The price most likely will discourage individual purchasers, but this set is highly recommended for health science libraries. [R: LJ, 15 Mar 02, p. 72; Choice, April 02, p. 1397]—**Mary Ann Thompson**

361.   Snodgrass, Mary Ellen. **Historical Encyclopedia of Nursing.** Santa Barbara, Calif., ABC-CLIO, 1999. 354p. illus. index. $75.00. ISBN 1-57607-086-7.

The term "nursing" is not used here as the name of a particular profession, but rather to include the personal and medical care given to all ages of people, in all places and time, under many circumstances, by religious and other organizations, and especially by individuals (many of whom are untrained). It is a social history of healers and health care from the earliest times to modern times. The emphasis is on the contributions of individuals, not labor movements, political acts, or educational efforts. Longer, more thoughtful survey articles, such as those on nursing in ancient times or in major wars, are mixed in alphabetically with biographies and brief discussions of trends. For example, "Gender Issues in Nursing" is followed by "Mother Angela Gillespie" of the Navy Nurse Corps. Many letters and memoirs were consulted as well as the usual biographies and histories of nursing and recollections of fellow workers. Sources are listed carefully in the longer items, and there is an extensive bibliography and a list of "Works By and About Healers." The section on the art of midwifery, covering changing attitudes toward it and its practitioners through the centuries, is particularly interesting.

The content is well researched and the author has succeeded in compiling a great deal of historical material about nursing (both good and bad), with a personal style and viewpoint that makes this excellent encyclopedia a worthwhile reference book.—**Harriette M. Cluxton**

DIRECTORIES

362.   **Delmar's A-Z NDR-97: Nurse's Drug Reference.** By George R. Spratto and Adrienne L. Woods. Albany, N.Y., Delmar, 1997. 1415p. illus. index. $29.95pa. ISBN 0-8273-7726-6. ISSN 1089-165X.

NDR-97 provides up-to-date information on the newest and most widely used prescription and over-the-counter drugs and the proper monitoring of drug therapy by the practitioner. Although one of the most important features of the book is the presentation of nursing considerations in a nursing process format, the summary for each drug is presented in clear, concise language that many laypeople will find easy to understand.

The initial chapter gives detailed information on how to use the book. Chapter 2 is an alphabetic list of therapeutic or chemical drug classes with general information for the class and a list of the drugs in the class covered in chapter 3. Each entry in chapter 3 consists of 2 parts: general drug information and nursing considerations. The general drug information includes the Food and Drug Administration pregnancy category, drug schedule, actions, uses, contraindications, side effects, drug interactions, laboratory test interference, and the usual dosage and administration information. The nursing considerations guide the practitioner in applying the nursing process to pharmacotherapeutics to insure safe practice. Suggestions for assessment, intervention, patient education, compliance, and outcomes identification are briefly summarized for each drug. Other useful features of the book include a list of common soundalike drug names, commonly used abbreviations and symbols, commonly used laboratory test values (e.g., normal serum values), and a table of drug compatibility. The index is extensively cross-referenced and simplifies drug location by pairing trade and generic names with the generic name in bold typeface. Purchasers of the book may also register for access to updates online (Delmar@Once). Monthly drug updates, weekly postings of related articles, and a question-and-answer forum are some of the features available electronically.

Because it is the official drug reference of the National Student Nurses' Association, health sciences libraries supporting schools of nursing and hospital nursing staff should have a copy of *NDR-97* on the shelf for the unique combination of comprehensive drug information and nursing interventions. Large public libraries may consider adding this item to the reference collection for the concise, easy-to-read information many laypeople require when searching for information on prescription drugs.—**Vicki J. Killion**

363. **Delmar's Therapeutic Class Drug Guide for Nurses 1997.** By George R. Spratto and Adrienne L. Woods. Albany, N.Y., Delmar, 1997. 1453p. illus. index. $29.95pa. ISBN 0-8273-7727-4. ISSN 1089-1641.

This is not a pharmacology text, and it does not concern itself with the chemical composition of drugs (like *Physicians' Desk Reference*). The guide succeeds admirably in providing a rich source of information about current therapeutic drugs, and it emphasizes the nursing considerations essential to their effective use. The directions to nurses appear at the end of each article and are arranged under assessment, interventions, client/family teaching, and evaluation.

Each section treats a separate classification of therapeutic drugs, with a general discussion of the class and a list of drugs included (e.g., "Cardiovascular Drugs" covers antiarrhythmic agents, antianginal agents, antihypertensive drugs, antihyperlipidemic agents, and drugs for congestive heart failure and peripheral vascular disease). Chapters list appropriate drugs in each category by generic name, with information arranged under general statement, action/kinetics, uses, contraindications, special concerns, side effects, drug interactions, laboratory test interferences, dosage, and nursing considerations. This format allows for quick access to specifics and for extensive subject coverage. Trade names with a tiny maple leaf indicate that the trade name is available only in Canada. Other abbreviations and symbols are commonly used in the text; a reference list and directions on using the guide appear in introductory pages.

There is a brief visual identification guide. Several appendixes give valuable supplemental information, such as common laboratory test values, pregnancy categories, and a "drug preview" of material received from the manufacturers too late for inclusion in this year's guide. Nurses in all specialties should find this book a valuable resource. The address for obtaining Internet updates is provided.—**Harriette M. Cluxton**

364. **Internet Resources for Nurses.** Joyce J. Fitzpatrick and Kristen S. Montgomery, eds. New York, Springer Publishing, 2000. 250p. index. $27.95pa. ISBN 0-8261-1371-0.

Anticipating a time when the Internet will be at every clinician's fingertips, the authors hope that this book will enhance professional nursing practice by serving either as an introduction to the resources available or as a handy resource guide. Specific content areas were chosen for their usefulness to clinical nurses. Nurses with interest and expertise in these areas searched the Internet for the top 6 to 10 Websites and provided a brief description and evaluation of each site.

The first section is a collection of clinical Websites by subject content. The second section is labeled "Professional Web Sites" and includes chapters on government agencies, professional organizations, education, research and grant resources, and nursing classification systems. Within each chapter the Website entries are in alphabetic order and provide the URL, a brief description, and a very brief evaluation that includes most of the standard criteria for evaluating Websites (i.e., authority or source, purpose or objectivity, content, currency, and design). A well-referenced chapter on evaluating health care information on the Internet is found at the end of the book. The appendix is an alphabetic list of the Websites evaluated (with the URLs) and their location within the book. The index is an integrated subject and name index.

Many of the Websites are not unique to nursing and are important sites for most health care professions. The added value is the inclusion in most of the evaluations of the relevance of the site to clinical nurses. Health sciences librarians are probably already aware of these Websites and have created dynamic links to them from their library's Web page. But nursing students, educators, and practitioners will find this guide helpful in locating relevant and reliable information of interest to them on the Internet. [R: Choice, Mar 01, p. 1246]—**Vicki J. Killion**

365.   **The Nurses' Guide to Consumer Health Web Sites.** Joyce J. Fitzpatrick, Carol Romano, and Ruth Chasek, eds. New York, Springer Publishing, 2001. 227p. index. $33.95pa. ISBN 0-8261-1455-5.

Wading through the World Wide Web for any type of information can be formidable. Adding the criteria that the information must be accurate and current only increases the challenge. In meeting this challenge, Fitzpatrick, Romano, and Chasek's reference on health-related Internet sites is a welcome addition to the nursing and consumer health literature. The editors have invited other nursing authorities to review and recommend up to six Internet sites in their particular area of expertise. Specific criteria used to review the sites are described. The book is written for nurses, but the intended audience is ultimately the nurses' patients or clients. The recommended sites, however, would also be helpful for almost any health care professional.

The book is organized into four major sections: "Megasites" (covering multiple topics), "Medications," "Negotiating the Health Care Delivery System," and "Special Topics" (including such areas as specific age groups, diseases, prevention, therapies, and treatments). Chapters are concise and easy to read and use. Particularly helpful is the note indicating whether the site's information is available in languages other than English. The reference concludes with a topical index as well as an alphabetic index of the Web addresses. The book is a convenient guide to reliable health information on the Internet. Because most of the recommended sites are based in permanent institutions or the government, the book is less likely to become quickly outdated. The book could easily be a direct resource for the consumer, so it is recommended for public and health care libraries and health care professionals' bookshelves. [R: LJ, 15 Oct 01, p. 68]—**Mary Ann Thompson**

366.   **PDR Nurse's Handbook.** 1999 ed. [CD-ROM]. By George R. Spratto and Adrienne I. Woods. Albany, N.Y., Delmar, 1999. Minimum system requirements (Windows version): Pentium processor or 486/66 processor. Four-speed CD-ROM drive. Windows 3.1, Windows 95, or Windows NT 4.0. 16MB RAM. Monitor with 8-bit color at 640x480 resolution. Sound Blaster-compatible sound card. Minimum system requirements (Macintosh version): 68040 or Power Macintosh. Four-speed CD-ROM drive. Macintosh OS 7.1. 16MB hard disk space. Monitor with 24-bit color at 640x480 resolution. $39.95. ISBN 0-7668-0639-1.

As the title suggests, this CD-ROM is a version of the *Physicians' Desk Reference* (56th ed.; see entry 412) designed for the drug information needs of nurses. Users can do a name search by trade or generic names and then the nursing focus is displayed about halfway down the article in a section called "Nursing Considerations." Other sections cover the generic name, a pregnancy category, the trade name, classification, *see also* references, and how the drug is supplied. Entries also discuss aspects of the drug such as its content, action and kinetics, uses, contraindications, special concerns, side effects, treatment, drug interactions, lab test interferences, dosage, administrative and storage concerns, assessment, interventions, client and family teaching, and an evaluation.

In addition, there is a feature for common sound-alike drugs that lists the names of drugs that sound like the drug users may be looking for. There is also an audio pronunciation feature with a voice giving the correct pronunciation of the drug name and a visual representation feature that shows a photograph of the pill, just as the *Physicians' Desk Reference* does. The photos of the pills are nice and large. Finally, a link is provided to the publisher's Website for this book.—**Lambrini Papangelis**

367. Spratto, George R., and Adrienne L. Woods. **PDR Nurse's Drug Handbook, 2002.** Montvale, N.J., Medical Economics Data, 2002. 1502p. illus. index. $32.95pa. ISBN 0-7668-3546-4.

The initials PDR represent the gold standard in drug information for the majority of health care professionals. This updated edition for nurses does not disappoint. The major part of the reference is an alphabetized listing of generic drugs with the requisite information particularly needed by nurses. A helpful new addition to these entries is the inclusion of potential drug/herbal product interactions. The book goes on to offer many other helpful pieces of information. It begins with a chapter on therapeutic drug classifications (alphabetized), providing general information organized in a format similar to individual drug entries. A section of more than 200 photographs of the most commonly prescribed drugs is an invaluable visual guide for the care provider. A total of 12 appendixes are included, highlighted by drug/food interactions and a section on wound care products. To increase its shelf life, a Website is provided for drug updates and new drugs. The book is extremely easy to use, with multiple cross-references and indexes as well as bold or red large font print to highlight names and discussion categories. Obviously, the language of the book requires medical knowledge or background, so it is most appropriate for health care professionals. This resource is highly recommended for nurses and libraries serving health care providers.—**Mary Ann Thompson**

368. **Springhouse Nurse's Drug Guide.** 4th ed. Springhouse, Pa., Springhouse Publishing, 2002. 1436p. index. $34.95pa. ISBN 1-58255-124-3. ISSN 1088-8063.

Drug guides for student nursing and nursing practitioners are a much-used resource in nursing schools, hospitals, and internships. *Springhouse* is one of the newer titles (first published in 1997), but has already produced a 4th edition in order to provide "accurate, essential information in a user-friendly format" (p. ix). The guide is published as an easy-to-handle, compact paperback that is clearly designed to locate information quickly as opposed to several other guides for drugs (e.g., the *Physicians' Desk Reference*). Inserted in the back cover is a mini-sized CD-ROM, *PharmDisk 4.0*, that is compatible with both Windows and Macintosh operating systems. The CD-ROM has an interactive self-test that "makes learning important content fun" (p. x). Reference is also given to a special Website for new developments.

The handy volume includes a basic "how to use" section; a guide to common abbreviations; four introductory chapters that give an overview of drug use (drug therapy and nursing, dosage calculation data, administration of drugs, and how to avoid medication mistakes); a section on drug classes (indication, actions, reactions, contraindications); and the bulk of the text (an alphabetic list of drugs by their generic designation). There are 10 useful appendixes, which are followed by a detailed index that includes brand and generic names, drug classification, diseases and related drugs, herbal remedies, and drugs pictured in full color. These are found in an easily identified section in the middle of the book.

The key information on each generic drug listed in the body of the *Drug Guide* includes pronunciation; brand names; the pharmacologic and therapeutic class; pregnancy risk category; indication and dosages; how supplied (e.g., capsules, tablets, injections); pharmacokinetics; pharmacodynamics; adverse reactions; interactions; contraindications and precautions; and a valuable "Nursing Considerations" section that includes assessment, nursing diagnoses, planning and implementation, and a patient teaching and evaluation.

The 2000 edition of *PDR for Nurses Handbook* and others are compact volumes that match *Springhouse* in ease of use. Also worth noting are *Davis's Drug Guide for Nurses* (see ARBA 92, entry 1692), *Delmar's A-Z NDR-97: Nurse's Drug Reference* (see entry 362), and *Mosby's Drug Guide for Nurses* (Mosby). The *Springhouse Nurse's Drug Guide* clearly competes well in a special market (nursing students, nurses, other health professionals, and any adult who administers or takes medications), which demands an excellent resource that gives understandable, clearly organized, accurate, and essential information on drug use.—**Laurel Grotzinger**

HANDBOOKS AND YEARBOOKS

369. Bua, Robert N. **The Inside Guide to American Nursing Homes.** New York, Warner Books, 1997. 1282p. $24.99. ISBN 0-446-67308-0.

This is an excellent yet affordable reference book to nursing homes in the United States. Its key features include rankings and ratings based on quality of care, insider tips on how to pay for nursing home care, comparison charts organized by state and county, and a 10-step program to help readers pick the best nursing home for their family. The publication is divided into 2 parts. The 1st section introduces the history of the rankings and ratings system as well as various aspects of the nursing home environment and health care decision-making and advance directives. The 2d section is devoted to the rankings and ratings for every certified nursing home in the United States. It is composed of the comparison charts, "best" nursing homes, most frequently violated nursing home standards, and state-by-state rankings and ratings. This publication is unique in its coverage and so inexpensive that almost any library could afford to purchase it.—**Theresa Maggio**

370. Copel, Linda Carman. **Nurse's Clinical Guide to Psychiatric and Mental Health Care.** Springhouse, Pa., Springhouse Publishing, 1996. 378p. index. $24.95 spiralbound. ISBN 0-87434-720-3.

It is a pleasure to review such a book as *Nurse's Clinical Guide to Psychiatric and Mental Health Care*, which so ably fulfills its stated purpose. According to the preface, the book was written as a guide for practicing nurses and students in designing individualized plans of care for psychiatric patients. This purpose is executed by taking the various pathological conditions (e.g., delirium) from the *Diagnostic and Statistical Manual of Mental Disorders* (4th ed., American Psychiatric Press, 1996) and listing the various North American Nursing Diagnosis Association (NANDA) nursing diagnoses for each. Goals for the client (Copel refers to patients as "clients") are then spelled out (e.g., "The client will maintain a safe and optimal level of functioning") .

Following the statement of goals, therapies, medications, and family care are treated. Copel covers the gamut of disorders and aberrations encountered by nurses in the mental health field, including attention deficit/hyperactivity disorder, Alzheimer's disease, partner abuse, and even rape. She has also included chapters on the special needs of homeless people with mental illness, of abuse victims, and of persons with HIV/AIDS. Her description of AIDS is beautifully clear and concise. Also refreshing to see is spiritual well-being discussed as a goal in the HIV/AIDS chapter.

Copel writes at the professional level; some terms, such as *dyspnea* and *diaphoresis*, are defined in the text, but some, such as *anoxia* and *extrapyramidal*, are not. The book is handy (the size of a thick paperback), and, owing to its spiral binding, has a back cover that folds around to provide a spine when it is placed on a shelf. It is highly recommended for nursing collections.—**Lambrini Papangelis**

371. Cowles, C. McKeen. **Nursing Home Statistical Yearbook, 1995.** Tacoma, Wash., Cowles Research Group; distr., Baltimore, Md., Johns Hopkins University Press, 1995. 246p. index. $45.00. ISBN 0-8018-5378-8. ISSN 1085-0309.

In this book's introductory essay, one of the leaders of the American Health Care Association briefly describes the rapidly changing nature of the United States' long-term care industry. He continues by recommending that the consumers, health providers, and policy-makers involved with nursing homes use this reference tool when making decisions concerning these facilities. Regrettably, the highly technical nature of this volume's statistical tables, which are not accompanied by explanatory text, challenges this recommendation.

The data used to create the complex statistical tables have been taken from the July 3, 1995, version of the Health Care Financing Administration's Online Survey Certification and Reporting database, and the author has illuminated the duplicate records from this database and spot-checked the validity of entry information. These data are organized into six broad categories: acuity or case mix, special patient needs, unique health problems of patients, deficiencies found in nursing homes, number of nursing homes and their capacities, and staffing information. This information is arranged, primarily, by state, and there is no coverage of individual nursing homes or of chains of these facilities.

While this reference work may be of some limited value to long-term care policy-makers, the statistical complexity of the tables and the overall format will be of little or no assistance to health providers and will frustrate potential nursing home users. Individuals seeking information about specific long-term care facilities should use *The Directory of Nursing Homes* (see ARBA 96, entry 1731) published annually by HCIA. —**Jonathon Erlen**

372. **Handbook of Clinical Nursing Research.** Ada Sue Hinshaw, Suzanne L. Feetham, and Joan L. Shaver, eds. Newbury Park, Calif., Sage, 1999. 696p. index. $89.95. ISBN 0-8039-5784-X.

For the past two decades, the nursing scientific community's goal was to generate a body of knowledge that would guide nursing practice in optimizing health care. This first handbook for the clinical nursing research addresses the major areas in which there is significant and reliable research that can be used to guide nursing practice, explores the depth of knowledge to date, and provides specific direction to advance the science of nursing for the future. It establishes a baseline for the evolving discipline and is intended for multiple audiences, including all degree programs in nursing, faculties, clinicians, and other health care professionals with similar issues.

In part 1 of the handbook, a theoretical analysis of the core of the discipline is examined and the methodological perspectives and issues in nursing research are addressed. It provides context for understanding the scientific processes underlying the various research areas. Part 2 presents syntheses of defined areas of clinical research (i.e., health needs of diverse racial and ethnic populations, clinical therapeutic strategies, health and illness in older adults).

As the first attempt to review and critique the state of clinical nursing research, the editors have been most successful in bringing together the foremost scholars, researchers, and educators.

Comprehensive in scope, this book deserves a place in every major academic medical library and nursing school.—**Vicki J. Killion**

373.   Janoulis, Brenda H., and Jason F. Janoulis. **Nursing Licensure Guidelines, 1998: State Information Manual for Nursing in the United States of America.** Atlanta, Ga., St. Barthelemy Press, 1998. 145p. $150.00 spiralbound. ISBN 1-887617-57-4.

Compiled from each state's nursing practices act, rules and regulations, and licensure applications and from Canadian provincial and territorial registration and licensing guidelines, this reference provides answers to the pertinent questions of licensure by examination or by endorsement. Licensure criteria and requirements for both registered nurses (RNs) and licensed practical nurses (LPNs) are listed alphabetically in a two-column question-and-answer format by state or province. Directory information for the specific licensing board is printed at the top of the page. Current fees, instructions to foreign nursing graduates, and special notes are included in the criteria.

A list of abbreviations, a statement on the issuance of licenses, information about the National Council Licensure Examination (NCLEX), a directory of the various boards of nursing, and a listing of nursing agencies and associations are also available. The authors have pulled into one source current information that will benefit the new nurse graduate and facilitate career moves for the practicing RN or LPN. Libraries supporting schools of nursing or large medical centers will find this resource useful.—**Vicki J. Killion**

374.   **PDR for Nurses Handbook.** 1999 ed. Montvale, N.J., Medical Economics and Albany, N.Y., Delmar, 1999. 1419p. index. $32.95pa. ISBN 0-7668-0913-7.

Although in most cases nurses do not prescribe drugs to a patient, they are usually the ones who must administer them, teach patients and families about them, and recognize adverse side effects and drug interactions. Therefore, knowledge of the ever-increasing pharmacopoeia is essential to any nurse. This new edition of the standard drug handbook for nurses is an invaluable reference on drugs, their uses, and their effects, all with particular consideration of the nurse's role in patient care.

Unlike the original weighty PDR for physicians, this is a true handbook, of a size to be carried around for quick reference. Yet it is packed with information. Previous editions were arranged by drug manufacturers; however, this new edition is arranged by the generic (or chemical) names of drugs, although with access to trade names through the index. There are three chapters. The first describes the best way to use the handbook. The second is an alphabetic listing of particular types of drugs. There are listings, for example, for such therapeutic classes as antihistamines, diuretics, and anticonvulsants. For each entry, there is a list of the individual drugs that appear in chapter 3 and a general discussion of the mode of action, uses, contraindications, side effects, and effectiveness of this type of medication. Under nursing considerations for each class of drugs there are tips on administration, storage, assessment of results, and patient education concerns.

Chapter 3 lists thousands of individual generic drugs, with detailed information on all the above topics and more. Of particular importance are the side effects sections, with life-threatening effects given in bold, and the overdose management section that gives symptoms and treatments. Other drugs that interact with each entry are listed, and the type of interaction is described. There is a lot of information here in very accessible form. The 10 appendixes include the elements of a prescription, the FDA Pregnancy Categories for drugs, and formulas for intravenous rate calculation. The index lists trade names and general subjects. A visual identification guide has full-color, actual-size pictures of 200 of the most common pills and capsules.

Of course, any handbook such as this is instantly out of date, with new drugs and new uses of old drugs being discovered every day. However, the publishers have provided a Website (http://www.nursespdr.com), which effectively solves that problem. There, in addition to daily pharmaceutical news and links to other drug sites, one can find monthly updates to the handbook, with listings for newly introduced drugs as well as new uses or therapeutic combinations of old drugs and newly recognized side effects. The combination of this convenient, information-packed handbook and constant updating through the Internet makes this a powerful tool for nurses and other health professionals.—**Carol L. Noll**

375.   **PharmFacts for Nurses.** Springhouse, Pa., Springhouse Publishing, 1996. 728p. illus. index. $34.95pa. ISBN 0-87434-803-X.

The administration of medication is one of a nurse's most important responsibilities. The rapid development of new drugs and increasingly complex delivery systems make the task more demanding than ever and require a highly comprehensive resource. This title organizes drug information into four sections. The first is "Drug Essentials," which explores common fallacies, legal considerations, errors, and conversions and calculations. The "Drug Alerts" section covers cautions and warnings, side effects and interactions, and the treatment of overdose. Part 3, "Drug Administration Tips and Techniques," describes the methods of delivery. Finally, the "Drug Therapy" section briefly discusses the most common medications used in common conditions and addresses the needs of special patients. Black-and-white photographs, which are rather small, and line drawings illustrate techniques, and tables serve to compress voluminous information into readily accessible form. A comprehensive index provides instant access to particular drugs or medical conditions.

This title is aimed at nursing professionals and will be of limited use to lay readers. The chapter on common conditions provides some information, but public libraries will do better with the American Hospital Formulary Service's annual *Drug Information.* Nursing schools and medical libraries, however, will want the title under review.—**Susan B. Hagloch**

376.   Sparks, Sheila M., Cynthia M. Taylor, and Janyce G. Dyer. **Nursing Diagnosis Pocket Manual: A Timesaving Guide to Better Patient Care.** Springhouse, Pa., Springhouse Publishing, 1996. 494p. index. $21.95 spiralbound. ISBN 0-87434-827-7.

This pocket manual is a condensation of the *Nursing Diagnosis Reference Manual* (3d ed., Springhouse Publishing, 1994). Designed to serve in a clinical setting, it gives brief guides to the physiological and psychosocial problems that nurses may legally diagnose and treat. This manual offers updated methods for physiological care, but also recommends approaches to geriatric, pediatric, psychosocial, and family-centered care. When appropriate, alternative medical approaches are described as acceptable treatments.

The manual offers 139 care plans approved by the North American Nursing Diagnosis Association (NANDA). Each plan puts forth a diagnostic statement with etiology, definitions, assessments to validate the diagnoses, defining characteristics including known risk factors, associated disorders, expected outcomes, interventions arranged according to time frame, and evaluation guidelines.

The appendixes contain a complete table of NANDA taxonomy, some selected reference works, and a clear and accurate index. This manual is highly recommended for nursing practitioners. —**Mary Hemmings**

6   Nutrition and Diet

DICTIONARIES AND ENCYCLOPEDIAS

377. **Encyclopedia of Human Nutrition.** Michele J. Sadler, J. J. Strain, and Benjamin Caballero, eds. San Diego, Calif., Academic Press, 1999. 3v. illus. index. $799.00/set. ISBN 0-12-226694-3.

Nutrition is finally getting recognition as an important biomedical discipline. Diet is a major factor in promoting health and preventing and treating disease. This encyclopedia, compiled by an international group of distinguished academics, research scientists, and food industry professionals, looks at both the scientific and the social aspects of nutrition.

The signed articles in this 3-volume set are alphabetically arranged. The volumes are consecutively paged. Each one contains the complete table of contents and index for the set. Each also has two appendixes. The first appendix consists of data from the Food and Drug Administration's Pesticide Residue Monitoring Program (1995). The second appendix is a group of charts and tables with weights and measures, growth charts, nutritional allowances, nutritional content of foods, and height and weight and other body dimensions.

The articles cover a broad range of subjects: individual nutrients; foods; social issues related to nutrition; nutritional therapy for diseases and conditions; anatomy and physiology; and diverse subjects such as nutrition education, food folklore, and nutrition policies in developed and developing countries. The articles are each 7 to 15 pages long. The longer articles are divided into sections. Some of the material is revised and updated from relevant sections of *The Encyclopedia of Food Science, Food Technology, and Nutrition* (Academic Press, 1993). The coverage of the social and political aspects of food and nutrition is a strength that sets this work apart from other sources, such as *The Concise Encyclopedia of Food and Nutrition* (see ARBA 96, entry 1524).

With its broad coverage of the nutrition field and its clear writing, *The Encyclopedia of Food and Nutrition* is highly recommended for academic and health science collections. Large public libraries with sufficient funds may want to consider it also. Purchase of the print edition includes a subscription to the online version of the encyclopedia. [R: LJ, 15 Mar 99, pp. 68-70; Choice, May 99, p. 1595]—**Barbara M. Bibel**

378. Lagua, Rosalinda T., and Virginia S. Claudio. **Nutrition and Diet Therapy Reference Dictionary.** 4th ed. New York, Chapman & Hall, 1996. 491p. $69.95; $37.95pa. ISBN 0-412-07051-0; 0-412-07061-8pa.

This 4th edition is still an excellent reference tool. The main text is the dictionary, with word descriptions; subentries; and *see*, *see also*, and *see under* cross-references. When a word has more than one meaning, the most accepted meaning is listed first, and other meanings continue to be listed in order of usage. The definitions are all related to nutrition in its various applications and are clearly and concisely written.

The 50 appendixes cover the nutritional contents on foods, vitamins, the food pyramid, U.S. nutrition labeling, the classification and utilization of carbohydrates, proteins, lipids, the digestive enzymes, selected hormones, the reference values for blood constituents and lipids, the fiber content of foods, and other nutritional data too numerous to name here. Three exceptional appendixes include the religious food practices chart, the public health nutrition programs and surveys in the United States and the administering agency, and the list of agencies and organizations with nutrition-related activities. This book also is a collection development resource for librarians, because one appendix lists sources of nutrition information broken down into the categories of books, journals, miscellaneous newsletters, pamphlets, videos, and tapes.

This book is highly recommended not only to medical libraries but to academic libraries where nutrition is taught as a major and as a part of other majors. The dictionary is also recommended to public libraries as an excellent source of information on the topic.—**Betsy J. Kraus**

379.   Lieberman, Shari, and Nancy Bruning. **The Real Vitamin & Mineral Book.** Garden City Park, N.Y., Avery Publishing, 1997. 342p. index. $12.95pa. ISBN 0-89529-769-8.

This book is an excellent source of information on vitamins and minerals that are necessary for the human body to function properly, and how highly processed food does not supply these nutrients when eating the recommended servings of the basic food groups. The book is divided into 4 parts for easy use. The 1st part is an introduction to these nutrients and explains the basics behind the recommended daily intakes (RDIs) and the optimum daily intakes (ODIs). Part 2, chapters 6-20, gives the details on the fat-soluble vitamins and water-soluble vitamins. Each chapter covers a description of the vitamin, its functions and uses, its relationship to cancer, the organs or parts of the body it affects, symptoms if the body is deficient, how supplements affect the body, ODIs, and the toxicity and adverse affects. Part 3, chapters 21-32, covers the minerals that are necessary building blocks and gives the same information as for vitamins. Part 4, chapters 33-40, discusses other necessary nutrients that are not covered by the previous chapters, with the same information furnished. The last 99 pages consist of in-depth references for the preceding chapters and an extensive index.

This book is well written and easy to understand. It would be useful in any public, academic, or medical library that deals with nutrition. The work is highly recommended for its content and its cost.—**Betsy J. Kraus**

380.   Murray, Michael T. **Encyclopedia of Nutritional Supplements: The Essential Guide for Improving Your Health Naturally.** Rocklin, Calif., Prima Publishing, 1996. 564p. illus. index. $19.95pa. ISBN 0-7615-0410-9.

Written to help users make sense of the voluminous information available on nutritional supplements, this book includes detailed profiles of all the major ones—vitamins, minerals, essential fatty acids, accessory nutrients, and glandular extracts—and tells how they can help one live longer, feel better, and fight the effects of aging. A concluding section counsels which nutritional supplements to take for a host of conditions, including high cholesterol, depression, and fatigue. A doctor of naturopathy, Murray, also the coauthor of *An Encyclopedia of Natural Medicine* (see ARBA 93, entry 1634), advocates supplementing with nutrients that the body needs anyway instead of or in addition to taking synthetic drugs. Murray's advice to everyone regarding supplements is a one-two-three punch of taking a multivitamin daily, supplementing with extra antioxidants, and taking a daily tablespoon of flaxseed oil, which is rich in essential fatty acids.

The 1,388 references to nutrition articles in medical journals are evidence of fine documentation (there are 95 references to carnitine alone), yet they are located at the back of the book endnote-style, a choice of format that makes the book more readable. The references at the end of each chapter constitute minibibliographies that could make a search of the journal literature on a topic unnecessary.

The book is written at a level that straddles the academic and the popular, making it suitable for academic or public libraries. It is considerably more scholarly than *The Complete Book of Natural & Medicinal Cures* (see ARBA 95, entry 1670). It is in softcover, which is not optimal for an encyclopedia, but which was probably the right choice because nutrition will probably change tremendously in the next five years, making a new edition necessary.—**Lambrini Papangelis**

381. Reavley, Nicola. **The New Encyclopedia of Vitamins, Minerals, Supplements, & Herbs.** New York, M. Evans, 1998. 792p. index. $19.95pa. ISBN 0-87131-897-0.

The New Encyclopedia of Vitamins, Minerals, Supplements, & Herbs is a gold mine of information on what the human body needs to fuel itself to maintain optimal health. The American public is inundated with new "miracle" vitamins and supplements that promise to enhance our health and longevity. It is nearly impossible for the layperson to keep up with the latest discoveries in how nutrition and health are related. This easy-to-use volume will provide many answers to commonly asked questions about nutrition.

The book begins with a question-and-answer section that features many common concerns among consumers, such as "Is it possible to get enough vitamins and minerals from food?" "Are vitamin and mineral supplements necessary?" and "Who might need supplements?" It is then broken down into chapters, including "Vitamins," "Minerals," "Other Nutrients," and "Herbal Medicines." Each vitamin, mineral, or supplement is listed alphabetically in its chapter, and a "quick guide" describes its role in fueling the body, sources of the nutrient, and daily recommendations, among other facts. The last section, "Health Problems," discusses the role of nutrients in fighting such health concerns as cancer, HIV/AIDS, insomnia, and many more. The book concludes with a glossary, list of references, and comprehensive index.

This book is extremely user-friendly and contains a lot of information that readers will be seeking on the subject of vitamins and nutrition and how they relate to human health. It is written for the layperson seeking quick information; however, the entries are interesting enough that many users will probably find themselves reading up on more than what originally they were looking for. This volume will be a valuable addition to the reference shelves of any public library.—**Shannon Graff Hysell**

382. Ronzio, Robert A. **The Encyclopedia of Nutrition & Good Health.** New York, Facts on File, 1997. 486p. index. $45.00. ISBN 0-8160-2665-3.

Health care reform has already occurred, regardless of the actions of health care professionals, the health care industry, and politicians. The information explosion has helped more people to take control of their own health. *The Encyclopedia of Nutrition & Good Health* is a reliable source of information about one's body, health, and nutrition.

This source contains current information on foods and food technology; food labels; vitamins; minerals; and major nutrients, such as fats, carbohydrates, and proteins. The encyclopedia includes a discussion of food-related conditions, including eating disorders, dieting and weight loss, food sensitivities, and aging. Special diets, such as Pritikin, are summarized. The volume contains more than 2,500 entries with cross-references and a comprehensive subject index. The encyclopedia is well organized and alphabetically arranged. It evaluates every available nutritional supplement, from vitamin A to zinc, omega-3 fatty acids to ginseng. Bibliographic references are provided after most entries. The evaluations are objective with a few obvious exceptions, such as the link between caffeine and certain symptoms and the ill effects of crash dieting.

This is an unusually well-balanced guide to the facts about nutrition and good health. *The Encyclopedia of Nutrition & Good Health* will find an important place in the resources of physicians, nutritionists, naturopaths, chiropractors, and laypeople with an interest in taking charge of their own nutrition.—**Marilynn Green Hopman**

383.   Sharon, Michael. **Nutrients A to Z.** London, Prion Books; distr., North Pomfret, Vt., Trafalgar Square, 1999. 344p. index. $14.95pa. ISBN 1-85375-325-4.

Diet and nutrition have increasingly become hot topics of interest to the general public. The public is bombarded with new information both promoting and diminishing the benefits of vitamins, supplements, and foods. This work is designed for the layperson who is looking for simple definitions to understand better what specific vitamins do, how to get them naturally, and how much is needed to remain healthy.

The book's short preface and introduction explain how the entries were chosen and where to find the vitamins and special foods discussed in the entries. The book then goes on to alphabetically list vitamins, minerals, herbs, and foods that contribute to human health. The entries are generally one to two paragraphs in length and give information such as the nutrient's or food's history, what its benefits or deficiencies are, and where it can be found. The words throughout the entries that are in bold typeface can be found elsewhere in the book under their own entry. The book concludes with a thorough index.

This book provides adequate information on a wide variety of nutritional concerns. It will answer many questions that users will have. For libraries looking for a more complete guide to nutrition, *The New Encyclopedia of Vitamins, Minerals, Supplements, & Herbs* (see entry 381) may be a better choice because of its more thorough explanations of how nutrients affect human health.—**Shannon Graff Hysell**

DIRECTORIES

384.   Dauphinais, Marc. **The Incredible Internet Guide to Diets & Nutrition.** Edited by James R. Flowers Jr. Tempe, Ariz., Facts on Demand Press, 2000. 328p. illus. (Incredible Internet Guides). $15.95pa. ISBN 1-889150-14-2.

This directory to Websites featuring articles and information about diet and nutrition is easy to use and will complement any fitness and nutrition library collection. Dauphinais admits that he is not a dietician, nutritionist, or even a physical trainer; he is merely an interested consumer concerned with health and fitness. As a result this book is beneficial more for the layperson then those in the field of nutrition.

The book is broken down in to eight main sections presenting the following topics: understanding nutrition, adopting a healthy weight, weight loss programs, vegetarian lifestyles, preventative nutrition, fitness, issues of food safety, and combating fraud online. Each topic is further broken down into subtopics, which list relevant Websites. The Websites in these sections are not annotated but some of the sites feature black-and-white images of the site so that readers can get a feel for what is presented. The final section, which comprises one-half of the volume, is titled "Diets & Nutrition Site Profiles." These are annotated lists of some of the Websites featured in the volume. They present a brief description as well as let readers know if the Website has chat rooms, mailing lists, message boards, sells items, and so on. Because there is no index it is a little difficult to find information on a specific topic. Because this work focuses more on the popular sites associated with nutrition rather than the scholarly sites, this work is better suited for public libraries.
—**Shannon Graff Hysell**

HANDBOOKS AND YEARBOOKS

385. Balch, James F., and Phyllis A. Balch. **Prescription for Nutritional Healing.** 2d ed. Garden City Park, N.Y., Avery Publishing, 1997. 600p. index. $19.95p. ISBN 0-89529-727-2.

The 2d edition of *Prescription for Nutritional Healing* is a comprehensive in-home guide of nutritional information for optimum health and fitness. It provides drug-free remedies for more than 300 ailments and disorders, including 50 additional health problems from the last edition. Up-to-date findings in the field of nutrition, the latest research on herbal medicine, and traditional remedies are discussed. The first section of the book, "Understanding the Elements of Health," explains types of nutrients, food supplements, and herbs. Part 2, "The Disorders," describes common health problems from backaches to cancer. Each entry has an excellent description of the problems and often gives information in a table for easy comparison. Helpful nutrients, herbs, and general recommendations for treatment are followed by a section of considerations and further information. Often, sources of further reading and addresses of treatment agencies or associations are given. Part three is a guide to traditional methods of treatment. The book has an index, manufacturer and distributor information, a list of health organizations, and health and medical hot lines.

Written by a medical doctor and a certified nutritionist, this guide provides alternative treatments and information for patients with serious illnesses or for average people who want to design their own nutritional program for better health. This book is designed to help individuals with differing health care needs, and its easy-to-use format makes it an important health resource.
—**Natalie Brower-Kirton**

386. **Diet and Nutrition Sourcebook.** 2d ed. Karen Bellenir, ed. Detroit, Omnigraphics, 1999. 650p. index. (Health Reference Series). $78.00. ISBN 0-7808-0228-4.

This book is beautifully done for its stated purpose. It is a consumer's reference book on all things nutritional and dietetic. The writing is excellent. It is at a level that most adults without advanced degrees can read. The sections are very complete and present two sides of a controversy, if there is one (e.g., olestra). The backgrounds and developments of some dietary substances are given (aspartame), regulatory concerns are discussed (food supplements), basic health information is given in relation to diet (asthma), terms are understandably defined (lipoproteins), and some easily confused concepts are explained thoroughly (salt and sodium). One major part of the book even goes into nutritional research.

The book is authoritative. The basis of the writing is a large variety of documents from federal agencies, university medical and nutrition departments, and professional organizations for nutrition and dietetics. There are many bibliographies throughout the book.

The last part of the book is made up of five chapters that give additional help and information. There is a very good glossary of terms, a large section on federal nutritional support programs, online information sources, a sizable list of books for further reading, and a resource list of CDs, books, and computer programs.

The book's format makes it easy to find information. There are large broad categories that are broken down into more specific chapters. The index, however, is really good, making this a valuable reference tool. A test of the page locators indicates that they are accurate, there is liberal use of *see* and *see also* references, there are a substantial number of double postings, and there are qualifiers that explain acronyms. Common terms like "overweight" send users to the more scientific terms (obesity).

This reference document should be in any public library, but it also would be a very good guide for beginning students in the health sciences. If the other books in this publisher's series are as good as this, they should all be in the health sciences collections.—**Lillian R. Mesner**

387.   **Diet Information for Teens: Health Tips About Diet and Nutrition.** Karen Bellenir, ed. Detroit, Omnigraphics, 2001. 399p. index. (Teen Health Series). $48.00. ISBN 0-7808-0441-4.

Diet Information for Teens is broken down into six main sections. The 1st section discusses the basics of food and nutrition. It details information on the various vitamins and minerals. The 2d section covers choices and guidelines relating to diet. It includes information on caffeine, provides help in understanding food labels, and explains "The Food Guide Pyramid." The 3d section discusses planning and preparing meals. Healthy recipes are included in this section that teenagers would probably enjoy. It also includes information on breakfasts, sandwiches, snacks, and food safety. The 4th section is about controlling weight. Information in this chapter covers healthy and unhealthy ways to gain or lose weight. The 5th section discusses eating disorders. It includes symptoms for the various disorders along with describing them, the different sources of treatment, and the ways that these disorders can be prevented. The 6th section is where readers will find additional sources of information. A bibliography on cookbooks is included that teenagers might find interesting. There is also a reference to two cookbooks that can be accessed on the Internet.

Diet Information for Teens is full of helpful insights and facts throughout the book. Smaller sections of helpful information include "It's a Fact!," "Weird Words," "Quick Tip," and "Remember!" They are easy to spot as users flip through the book, as they are printed in different shapes and darker color to help them stand out. Healthy habits are important for teenagers to develop so that they will stay with them as they become adults. This book does a very good job detailing healthy, and not so healthy, habits and it would be an excellent resource to be placed in public libraries or even in personal collections. [R: SLJ, June 01, p. 162; BR, Sept/Oct 01, p. 74]—**Brenda Leeds**

388.   **Fitness and Exercise Sourcebook.** 2d ed. Kristen M. Gledhill, ed. Detroit, Omnigraphics, 2001. 646p. index. (Health Reference Series). $78.00. ISBN 0-7808-0334-5.

"Fitness impacts every area of a person's life. It plays a role in the maintenance of health, disease prevention, life expectancy, and the quality of life." So begins the 2d edition of the *Fitness and Exercise Sourcebook*, an extensive compilation of writings from governmental agencies, nonprofits, and periodicals on health and fitness. Arranged into 40 chapters in 6 parts—"General Fitness and Exercise," "Fitness and Your Diet," "Fitness for Specific Groups of People," "Exercise and Specific Medical Conditions," "Specific Activities," and "Additional Help and Information"—this sourcebook is comprehensive, easy to understand, and authoritative.

The text provides very good explanations of health and fitness basics, such as fitness testing and benchmarking; physical activity and its relationship to healthy living; the relationships between fitness and diet; physical activity and well-being at different ages; and the affects of exercise on arthritis, asthma, HIV, and diabetes. Perhaps the most interesting parts of the sourcebook are on various activities that can be done for fitness, and fitness for specific activities such as bicycling, skiing, and inline skating. Many of the chapters touch on how-to aspects of exercise, and illustrations or photographs would have helped to clarify and enhance the text. But the extensive bibliographies, the excellent and lengthy glossary, and the very useable index make up for the lack of visual enhancement. This work is recommended for all general reference collections.—**Thomas K. Fry**

389.   Gastelu, Daniel, and Fred Hatfield. **Dynamic Nutrition for Maximum Performance: A Complete Nutritional Guide for Peak Sports Performance.** Garden City Park, N.Y., Avery Publishing, 1997. 404p. illus. index. $19.95pa. ISBN 0-89529-756-6.

This dietary guide for both professional and amateur athletes or fitness enthusiasts is divided into 4 parts. Part 1 covers nutrients, their roles in fitness and health, and what foods contain them; part 2 discusses anatomy, digestion, and metabolism; part 3 guides users through such activities as building muscle and carbo loading; and part 4 supplies plans specific to individual sports. An introductory section on how to use the book stresses the importance of slowly incorporating new techniques into a fitness regimen and following the advice of a health care provider above all. Helpful tables, charts, and boxes provide information supplementary to the text. Mathematical formulas for determining daily caloric requirements, metabolic rates, and body fat percentages are also useful.

The information combines both time-tested ideas of fitness and nutrition with the latest scientific data and the personal experiences of the two authors (a sports nutritionist/wrestler and a world champion power lifter, respectively). Some of the information may be controversial. The authors appear to espouse carbohydrate consumption over protein, stating that athletes who consume too much meat will suffer from decreased performance and a struggle with body fat. Although many people would agree with this, some nutritionists and weight loss experts would not. Although the book does not seem to overtly promote a vegetarian diet, the preference seems to be there. Proteins are discussed in terms of the amino acids of which they are made; the authors stress that animal protein contains the proper proportions of amino acids, but that vegetarians can have the same quality of protein by combining legumes with grains. Vegetarians will welcome a fitness guide that does not dismiss their dietary choices.

Part 4 will excite the most interest. Featuring 28 sports nutrient plans, each sport is discussed in terms of energy sources, where the energy comes from, dietary guidelines, recommended nutrients, and recommended supplements that may be unique for the activity. For less common sports, a table guides users to comparable sports. For example skateboarding leads to fitness activities (which also incorporates running, aerobics, boating, cheerleading, and many other activities), and water polo directs to swimming. Supplemental materials at the end of the volume include logs for personal use, reference daily intakes for nutrients, illustrations of the muscles of the body, a glossary of unfamiliar or unknown terms, and a bibliography that points the way to further reference sources.

This book would be useful for consultation. The information appears to be accurate and explanatory enough to cover differing sides of issues. However, the true value of this book would come from reading it cover to cover, making it more useful for public and especially individual libraries.—**Melissa Rae Root**

390.   **Obesity Sourcebook.** Wilma Caldwell and Chad T. Kimball, eds. Detroit, Omnigraphics, 2001. 376p. index. (Health Reference Series). $48.00. ISBN 0-7808-0333-7.

This book is part of the extensive Health Reference Series published by Omnigraphics. The cover of this volume states that the purpose is to provide "basic consumer health information . . . about obesity." It does just that. The book is divided into five sections: general information about obesity; associated diseases; managing obesity; special populations (for example, children, the elderly, and minorities); and an extensive resource directory. The book is written in a simple style with concise chapters (usually 2 to 5 pages). The content has been extracted from reliable health resources—generally Internet sites associated with the government or voluntary organizations. The reference clearly and simply explains the positives and negatives of the many different means for treating and managing obesity. In reading the book from cover to cover one finds unnecessary repetition of certain ideas and concepts. A few chapters are too lengthy and others are too short. A layperson might be interested in specific information evaluating the more common weight loss programs (e.g., Weight Watchers) but this is not included. In the end, however, the book synthesizes the reliable medical literature on obesity into one easy-to-read and useful resource for the general public. [R: BL, 15 April 01, p. 1582]—**Mary Ann Thompson**

7 Occupational and Physical Therapy

391. **Quick Reference Dictionary for Occupational Therapy.** 3d ed. Karen Jacobs and Laela Jacobs, eds. Thorofare, N.J., Slack, 2001. 547p. $24.00pa. ISBN 1-55642-495-7.

The 3d edition of the *Quick Reference Dictionary for Occupational Therapy* reflects the continued complexity of the roles of occupational therapists (OTs). Definitions include the many medical and anatomical terms OTs must master, the terminology of the field, and computer terms useful to the technological savvy OT. The editors have extensive experience as practicing occupational therapists and thoroughly cover topics required for basic competence in the field. The dictionary would be especially helpful to occupational therapy students or recent graduates beginning their first employment.

A number of appendixes supplement the dictionary, providing the "quick reference" cited in the title. These appendixes comprise half of this pocket-sized volume. They include anatomical diagrams, standards for common physical tasks, information on relevant laws and legislation, Braille and American Sign Language (ASL) alphabets, commonly used words in several languages (including ASL), prescription drug information, state licensure board contact information, professional society information, and psychological disorder diagnoses from the DSM-IV. All appendixes are listed in the table of contents, but the lack of an index hinders the "quick reference" claim of the title. Infrequent users of this resource will find it difficult to quickly find needed reference appendixes from the table of contents. However, this problem is a minor flaw in an otherwise useful resource.—**Lynne M. Fox**

392. **Quick Reference Dictionary for Physical Therapy.** Jennifer M. Bottomley, ed. Thorofare, N.J., Slack, 2000. 574p. $24.00pa. ISBN 1-55642-426-4.

This work is much more than a dictionary. Packed into its compact paper binding is a wealth of ready-reference material for physical therapists. The dictionary itself only takes up about one-quarter of the book. The rest consists of exhaustive appendixes that define acronyms; reprint the Guidelines and Ethical Statements, Mission and Goals of the American Physical Therapy Association (APTA); and list the governing members of APTA. State licensure regulations and the history of this specialty are also included, with abstracts of the relevant legislation. The World Health Organization's official definitions of *impairment*, *disability*, and *handicapped* are also included, as is a section on the most common diseases and pathologies that may lead to or affect physical therapy, complementary rehabilitation, and alternative therapies.

Common frames of reference for therapists, such as range of motion and weights and measures, are listed, along with the documentation required for claims review and a representative pharmacopoeia. Print and Website resources are provided, as are lists of organizations and networks. Well organized and presented, this reference provides an excellent resource for physical therapy professionals. Libraries serving such clientele will wish to include it, although most physical therapists will probably want their own copy.—**Susan B. Hagloch**

8 Pharmacy and Pharmaceutical Sciences

DICTIONARIES AND ENCYCLOPEDIAS

393.   **Dictionary of Substances and Their Effects.** [CD-ROM]. Norwood, Mass., SilverPlatter, 1996. Minimum system requirements: IBM or compatible 386. CD-ROM drive with Microsoft CD-ROM Extensions 2.1. Windows 3.1. 4MB memory (8MB for Windows for Workgroups, Windows 95, Window NT, and OS/2). 14MB hard disk space. $1,795.00/stand-alone version.

These data represent information on more than 4,000 physiologically or ecologically active chemicals. Included are the basic uses, physiochemical properties, and toxicology/adverse effects. Also provided are short bibliographies. Chemicals selected for inclusion are listed on the dangerous substances and pollutant lists from the European Union, the United States, and Canada. Also evaluated were the legislative requirements of the European Union, the United States, and Japan. Information extends to the details of legislation, limit values, and references.

This compilation does not provide risk assessment, but offers pieces of information associated with the identification of chemical hazards. Examples include occupational exposure, ecotoxicity, mammalian toxicity, teratogenicity, and environmental fate. The authors indicate that this resource will benefit persons who are involved in a human or environmental risk assessment. —**Sue Lyon Mertl**

394.   **Drugs: Synonyms and Properties.** 2d ed. G. W. A. Milne, ed. Brookfield, Vt., Ashgate Publishing, 2002. 1108p. index. $165.00. ISBN 0-566-08491-0.

Most drugs developed commercially by international pharmaceutical companies have several trade names assigned to them for marketing purposes. In addition to these nonsystematic names, the drug will also have a chemical name that allows for precise identification of the chemical involved. Over the drug's life span, an average of 5 to 6 aliases is typical, resulting in confusion not only for the consumer who usually has only a trade name, but also for the scientist who may have the chemical name but no information on the drug's ownership, licensing status, or therapeutic uses. Providing comprehensive coverage of the 10,000-plus drugs currently in common use worldwide, the key component of this reference is the extensive index of over 30,000 drug synonyms and trade names.

Organized alphabetically by the therapeutic category, the entries in part 1 are listed alphabetically by the most commonly used name of the drug (usually the U.S. adopted name) and include the Chemical Abstracts Service (CAS) Registry Number and the Existing Commercial Chemical Substances (EINECS) number. The molecular formula, chemical name, synonyms, therapeutic use, physical properties, toxicity, and the manufacturer/supplier complete the entry.

Part 2 contains the CAS Registry Number index, the EINECS Number index, and the name and synonym index, which is where the user should begin a search if a drug name or synonym is known. Part 3 is the "Manufacturer and Supplier Directory."

This dictionary represents the starting point for a user with only a drug trade name or a drug chemical name; however, the number of drugs included increases the success rate of locating synonyms and essential information for the drug in question. Health sciences libraries, especially those that support schools of pharmacy and medicine, will find this resource invaluable. [R: LJ, 1 April 02, p. 92]—**Vicki J. Killion**

395.   **Encyclopedia of Pharmaceutical Technology.** 2d ed. James Swarbrick and James C. Boylan, eds. New York, Marcel Dekker, 2002. 3v. index. $850.00/set. ISBN 0-8247-2825-4.

This encyclopedia lives up to its own billing as "a unique, comprehensive compilation that brings together knowledge from every specialty encompassed by pharmaceutical technology." The 3-volume set presents graduate-level information on about 200 topics ranging from "Absorption Enhancers" to "Zeta Potential." All basic topics in physical pharmacy, biopharmaceutics, and pharmacokinetics are described. With over 3,000 pages, some narrow topics comprise as few as 4 pages, while broader ones take up 30 pages. Most notable is the contribution of about 130 contributing authors, most of whom are experts in their field. Also notable is a bibliography with each monograph. Hence, the *Encyclopedia of Pharmaceutical Technology* will be a valuable resource for one who wishes to quickly become familiar with specific topics in pharmaceutics. A limitation is its $850 list price. For libraries with an emphasis to serve researchers in pharmaceutical technologies, particularly academic libraries, the convenience of this unique encyclopedia is worth the price, particularly since several topics in the pharmaceutical technologies are difficult to search via MEDLINE and even International Pharmaceutical Abstracts (IPA). However, for more general health science libraries, MEDLINE, IPA, and their current collections (e.g., Remington: The Science and Practice of Pharmacy, Physical Pharmacy) mean that this encyclopedia may not be essential, even though it is an up-to-date, expertly written convenience.—**Bruce Stuart**

396.   Graedon, Joe, and Teresa Graedon. **The People's Pharmacy Guide to Home and Herbal Remedies.** New York, St. Martin's Press, 1999. 428p. index. $27.95. ISBN 0-312-20779-4.

The goal of *The People's Pharmacy Guide to Home and Herbal Remedies* is to educate consumers on the available herbal supplements, how they affect the human body, and who should and should not be taking them. The authors stress that because the Federal Drug Administration does not monitor herbal supplements, they are often not used correctly or can be taken in doses that are dangerous to consumers. The book begins with the authors' favorite home remedies, many of which will be new to readers. It then discusses dangerous herb-drug reactions that commonly occur. After a short introduction and explanation of how to use the book, the authors discuss healing herbs and home remedies. These are listed in alphabetic order and include everything from relief from allergies to soothing bug bites to treating varicose veins. Throughout this section are well-written anecdotes from the authors and sidebars of questions and answers. After this section there is a 16-page section of references listed.

The second half of the book focuses specifically on herbal supplements and remedies. Each herbal therapy has a description of the active ingredients, its uses, the adequate dose, special precautions, adverse effects, and possible interactions. This section contains information that will be new to many readers and that may prevent future medical complications. The book concludes with a list of Websites containing additional herbal supplement information and a subject index, with topics that are treated in depth printed in bold typeface.

This book is intended for the general public and will therefore be most beneficial for public libraries. Medical libraries with patrons outside of the medical profession may also want to purchase it; however, those catering to medical professionals will benefit more from a resource such as *Natural Medicines Comprehensive Database* (see entry 406), which is a more scholarly choice. [R: LJ, Dec 99, pp. 104-106]—**Shannon Graff Hysell**

397.   Hocking, George Macdonald. **A Dictionary of Natural Products: Terms in the Field of Pharmacognosy.**... Medford, N.J., Plexus Publishing, 1997. 994p. $139.50. ISBN 0-937548-31-6.

According to the definition found within this dictionary, *pharmacognosy* is "that branch of pharmacy relating to medicinal substances from the plant, animal, and mineral kingdoms in their natural, crude, or unprepared state, or in the form of such primary derivatives as oils, waxes, gums, and resins." The above statement represents an excellent summary of what this dictionary is about. The majority of the more than 18,000 terms in this work consist of scientific and common names of plants and animals; scientific terms for the families and genera of the plants and animals; drugs acquired from animals and plants; pharmaceutical preparations; animal products, such as antitoxins, sera, and the like; terminology used in pharmacognosy and phytochemistry; and botanical terms associated with the field.

The length of the information given for the types of terms contained within the work varies from several sentences to several pages. For example, in considering the amount of information given when a genera is listed, all appropriate scientific names of the organisms within the genera are considered, along with the type of medicinal product they produce as well as the uses of said product. Many entries of this type can run one or more pages. It should also be noted that a number of abbreviations are used as part of the information given in order to save space. The key to the abbreviations can be found in the beginning of the book; however, most abbreviations can be determined by their context within the definitions. References are identified by means of numbers within the definitions, and a list of these references can be found in appendix A.

This dictionary represents copious, detailed information on medicinal products, their uses, and the biological organisms responsible for the products. The dictionary is extremely well researched, with a total of 2,798 references cited. A bibliography of general reference works on pharmacognosy and economic botany; a list of serials in the field of pharmacognosy; a list of terms describing properties and therapeutic uses of drugs, pesticides, and so forth; diagrams of types of inflorescences and of flowers; a description of a classification scheme; and a list of the scientific names of plants that produce natural rubber can be found at the end of the work. It is highly recommended for college, universities, and large public libraries.—**George H. Bell**

398.   Mathiowitz, Edith. **Encyclopedia of Controlled Drug Delivery.** New York, John Wiley, 1999. 2v. illus. index. $595.00/set. ISBN 0-471-14828-8.

This multi-authored, 2-volume set on controlled drug delivery is an advanced reference text. The audience for this source will most likely be graduate students, biomedical researchers or scientists, medical professionals, and certain business managers. The author has also recently coauthored a text on bioadhesive drug delivery systems. However, this is the first encyclopedia on controlled drug delivery that includes topics such as history from 1975 to date, pros and cons of controlled versus traditional delivery systems, descriptions of types of controlled drug release, pharmaceutical applications, stabilization and characterization of proteins, methods, characterizations, marketing, economics, gene therapy, and polymer technology. Each drug delivery system has keywords listed and an outline and bibliography. Even though there is no table of contents, the thorough index allows readers to search for narrower terms than the broad categories. The timely knowledge provides needed information on new approaches in treating conditions such as cancer, heart disease, alcoholism, infectious diseases, and others. Agents for contraception, orthopedics, and vaccination are discussed. Polymer substances such as polyanhydrides, chitosan polyesters, hydrogels, and bioadhesives are described. Techniques such as gel permeation and X-ray photo-electron spectroscopy are commented on. Gene therapy, blood substitutes, food ingredients, and tissue engineering are explained. Various methods of administration, such as parenteral, intravitreal, oral, rectal, ocular, nasal, buccal, vaginal, and the central nervous system, are discussed. Controlled drug releases, such as osmotic pumps, pendent-chain systems, membrane systems, nanoparticles, and liposomes, are detailed. Patents, regulatory issues, manufacturing approaches, in vitro and in vivo methods, pharmacokinetics, and others are described.

With the large amount of information on controlled drug delivery systems presented here, this text fills a void for those who wish to understand more about how the controlled drug can target a specific body part and what its medical and economic impact is on the health industry. And this text is costly; many academic centers might consider this as a major purchase.—**Polin P. Lei**

399.   **Mosby's GenRx: The Complete Reference for Generic and Brand Drugs.** 8th ed. [CD-ROM]. St. Louis, Mo., Mosby's GenRx, 1998. Minimum system requirements: IBM or compatible 486. CD-ROM drive. Windows 3.1. $69.95.

Mosby's GenRx is a CD-ROM database of drug prescribing information. Its scope encompasses prescription drugs only. Both generic and brand-name drugs are included. The database aims to be comprehensive, and indeed, with its drug name index, supplier profiles, keyword index, listings by pharmacological and therapeutic class, indications for use, imprint index (photographic images of pill markings), and drug interaction tool, is capable of replacing a number of print reference works. These might include *Mosby's Medical Drug Reference* (1999 ed.; Mosby, 1998) and *Mosby's Nursing Drug Reference and Review Cards* (1999 ed.; Mosby, 1998). This reviewer does not recommend canceling one's standing order for *Physicians' Desk Reference* (56th ed.; see entry 412) yet, however, as the articles in PDR are long and full of desirable detail.

The database represents a beautiful marriage of reliable drug information and modern computer searching. However, a user who is not a professional searcher, such as a physician or pharmacist, would not get the full benefit of this CD-ROM. But for libraries, this resource can be thoroughly recommended.

This CD-ROM comes in a cardboard sleeve with no instructions as to how to install it on one's computer. But if not including a pamphlet helps keep the price down, this reviewer is in favor of it, because drug information needs to be updated frequently and one will want to get the new edition every year. The product does come with a postage-paid card to send back to the publisher to be eligible to receive technical support.—**Lambrini Papangelis**

400.   **Mosby's Over-the-Counter Medicine Cabinet Medicines.** By Richard P. Donjon. St. Louis, Mo., Mosby, 1997. 127p. index. $12.95 spiralbound. ISBN 0-8151-8053-5.

Mosby's Over-the-Counter Medicine Cabinet Medicines is a guide that tells what you need to know about the over-the-counter medicines you take. The book is divided into various subject areas, including allergies, asthma, colds, flu and coughs, constipation, diarrhea, diet aids, headache, hemorrhoids, nausea and vomiting, pain and fever, quitting smoking, skin problems, sleep aids, and vaginal infections. Each section describes what it is and the symptoms; medicines and products that relieve symptoms, including side effects; interactions and precautions; use in children; use in the elderly; and use in pregnancy and nursing. It also has commonly asked questions about the topic. The publication includes a product index. The book could be more extensive as it is only 127 pages. Most public libraries should purchase this volume for their consumer health collections.—**Theresa Maggio**

401. **The Pill Book.** 10th ed. Harold M. Silverman, ed. Westminster, Md., Bantam Dell Publishing Group, 2002. 1216p. illus. index. $6.99pa. ISBN 0-553-58478-2.

The stated purpose of this book is "to provide educational information to the public" covering the most widely prescribed medications by physicians. The editor also states that it is not an exhaustive list of prescription drugs. The information in the book is based on FDA-approved information only. This edition covers 35 new drugs recently approved by the FDA in addition to adding several dozen more entries excluded from the previous edition (2000). Again, the color insert pages of actual size pills are provided for the consumer. Each entry lists the generic name of the drug with a phonic pronunciation in parenthesis and includes the following categories: brand name, type of drug, what the drug is prescribed for, general information, cautions and warnings, possible side effects, drug interactions, usual dose, overdosage, special information, and special populations. The entries are written concisely in a readable style and in easy-to-understood terms. The index is an alphabetic listing of generic and brand name drugs. At the end of the main text is a short chapter titled "Drugs Against Bioterrorism," 20 questions one should ask either their physician or pharmacist, safety information on taking Rx drugs, and the top 200 prescribed drugs in the United States. Families who have to take a lot of prescription medications will also find it useful to keep at home; the cost is very reasonable for the information provided. Medical staff will find this a helpful guide for quick, concise drug information that is not biased by drug company literature. The new edition is highly recommended to public libraries, medical libraries, and especially to libraries doing patient education.—**Betsy J. Kraus**

402. Stein, C. Michael. **Arthritis Medicines A-Z: A Doctor's Guide to Today's Most Commonly Prescribed Arthritis Drugs.** New York, Three Rivers Press, 2000. 324p. $14.00pa. ISBN 0-609-80507-X.

Although this title has the subtitle of "A Doctor's Guide to Today's Most Commonly Prescribed Arthritis Drugs," it may well be more appropriate for the victims of arthritis or their caretakers. The definitions are easy to understand and answer questions that a lay person would have instead of those of a physician with access to more advanced resources. The book is arranged in alphabetic order by each drug's generic name. Listed under each drug is its brand name, its drug family, what type of arthritis it is prescribed for, how it works (a more detailed description more suitable to those in the health field), things to avoid while taking the drug, side effects and physical things to look out for, interactions with other drugs, any important information, common dosage, and additional comments. Each of the 85 drugs listed here is given a thorough description. The book concludes with a glossary of abbreviations and acronyms and an index.

This will be a useful and inexpensive resource for public libraries and consumer health libraries. Users should keep in mind that the information presented here is current as of 2000.—**Shannon Graff Hysell**

DIRECTORIES

403. **The CenterWatch Directory of Drugs in Clinical Trials.** 2d ed. Farmington Hills, Mich., Gale, 2001. 737p. index. $149.00. ISBN 1-930624-18-2.

A subsidiary of the Medical Economics Company, publishers of the renowned *Physicians' Desk Reference* (56th ed.; see entry 412), CenterWatch continues the tradition of producing a valuable resource with *The CenterWatch Directory of Drugs in Clinical Trials*. The preface states that this work is not exhaustive, but it does provide information on more than 1,900 drugs in clinical trials and details on the latest drug delivery systems under study. Access to the weekly updated online database of the directory is an added value with the purchase of the print version. The language is technical and requires some knowledge of medical terms, so the primary audience is health care providers, medical students, upper division and graduate students, and educated laypersons.

The book is divided into medical specialty areas, each with a brief introduction of the specialty and the diseases/conditions involved. The information for each drug includes name, manufacturer, description, indication, and research phases. There are excellent indexes, both adult and pediatric, of manufacturers names, therapeutic indication, and scientific and trade names. A list titled "Useful Websites" is included in the appendix. A valuable and informative resource, this title is recommended for health science and university libraries. [R: Choice, Mar 02, p. 1212]—**Lynn M. McMain**

404.   Garrison, Robert, Jr., and Michael Mannion. **Pharmacist's Guide to Over-the-Counter and Natural Remedies.** Garden City Park, N.Y., Avery Publishing, 1999. 368p. index. $6.95pa. ISBN 0-89529-850-3.

The purpose of this book is to give important information on over-the-counter (OTC) and natural remedies and to explain how they can be used beneficially for treating conditions not requiring prescription drugs. The information provided is clearly and concisely written for understanding by the majority of readers. This book is divided into 2 main sections. Part 1 lists "fifty common herbs and their potential interactions with regular drugs" alphabetically and other broad general information on these remedies, such as what type of labeling information to look for, the units of measurement, and "vitamin and mineral intakes." Part 2 is an alphabetic list of common conditions. Each entry describes the condition, the OTC remedies, the natural remedies, and if there are specific precautions to note. Appendix A is a list of organizations to contact for further information on any of the conditions or remedies listed. Appendix B is a personal medical form, which includes a place to list all medications, making it easier for someone to note if there might be interactions among medications, OTCs, and natural remedies. There is a list of references for further reading and an alphabetic index of all conditions and natural remedies. Cross-references are included in the index. This book is highly recommended for all library collections because more people are looking for alternative treatments.—**Betsy J. Kraus**

405.   Mindell, Earl, and Virginia Hopkins. **Prescription Alternatives: Hundreds of Safe, Natural, Prescription-Free Remedies to Restore and Maintain Your Health.** 2d ed. Lincolnwood, Ill., National Textbook, 1998. 562p. index. $19.95pa. ISBN 0-87983-989-9.

Written in clear, understandable language, the theme of this work is to be aware of alternative ways of treating medical disorders rather than becoming part of what the author suggests is the "drug treadmill." The source is organized into 2 parts. Part 1 consists of laying the foundation for good health, and part 2 considers prescription drugs and their natural alternatives. Such areas as being aware of the pill-popping mindset; how to avoid prescription drug abuse; the interaction of drugs with food, drink, supplements, and other drugs; and how to read drug labels and information inserts are some of the issues that are considered in part 1

Part 2, which makes up the majority of the work, considers various types of medical problems, the drugs that are usually prescribed to alleviate the problem, and the alternative remedies to prescription drugs. Each of these medical problems is arranged in a chapter-by-chapter format. For example, chapters on diabetes drugs and their natural alternatives and drugs for pain relief and their natural alternatives are present. Other medical areas considered are digestive tract problems, insomnia, eye diseases, osteoporosis, cold, cough, and asthma. For each medical area considered, general information regarding the malady, prescription drugs given for the malady, along with their side effects and natural alternatives for treating the disease, are given. All of this information

is written for a layperson in an informal style and does not follow the conventional type of reference book. More than 1,000 simple, safe, nature-based remedies are presented, along with explanations on how to monitor the body as one switches from drugs to natural health. A list of recommended readings, a list of references reflecting each of the chapters presented, and a subject index complete the work. This work is recommended for all high school, public, and college libraries. Persons interested in this topic may wish to purchase the guide for their own home libraries.
—**George H. Bell**

406.   **Natural Medicines Comprehensive Database.** 2d ed. Stockton, Calif., Therapeutic Research Faculty, 1999. 1310p. index. $92.00. ISBN 0-9676136-2-0.
     The *Natural Medicines Comprehensive Database* is a monumental compilation of nearly every "natural" medicine distributed in the United States today. For this works purpose "natural" refers to all herbal and non-herbal supplements, some of which may not be collected from natural sources but are still categorized along with natural products. The need for this particular resource arose from the influx of natural products into the general market in the past several years and the inability of either pharmacists or laypersons to keep up on the new research and uses for a particular natural product. This book is designed to answer many of the questions that come with using a natural supplement as well as give readers new information on the products.
     The book is arranged in alphabetic order and each supplement listed provides information on the product in 15 categories. These categories include providing the name of the product, any names the product may also be known as, its scientific name, what the product is often used for (regardless of whether it is effective in this area or not), its safety and a recommendation of who should not use the product, its effectiveness, the possible mechanism of action and active ingredients, adverse reactions and allergies, what other drugs it may interfere with, the typical dose or how the product is administered, and a section for comments from the publisher about the product. Each entry is generally a page to a page and a half in length. Entries provide references which are provided in the 80-page reference section at the back of the book. The publisher admits that many of the sources list contradicting information on these natural products so the editors take the evidence into consideration to reach a consensus decision on the effects and reliability of the drug. There is also a general index, a brand name listing, an interaction listing, a therapeutically effective products list, and a nutrient depletion chart at the end of the volume. Readers will find much of this information in these charts of value.
     This resource is also available in a Web version that is updated daily. The Web version allows health professionals to interact and discuss new findings about natural drugs. It provides a forum for questions, answers, and relevant citations to be posted. The price for this service is $92 per year. This work is an invaluable resource for those in health-related fields or those in the profession of providing information to them. Medical libraries, academic libraries, and many large public libraries will find this a much-used resource.—**Shannon Graff Hysell**

407.   **PDR Electronic Library 2000.** [CD-ROM]. Montvale, N.J., Medical Economics Data, 2000. Minimum system requirements: IBM or compatible PC. Double-speed CD-ROM drive. Windows 95 or higher. 8MB RAM. 10MB hard drive space. VGA color monitor. $195.00 (individuals); $595.00 (institutional).
     When considering this work, remember that the *PDR Electronic Library CD-ROM* consists of the *Physicians' Desk Reference* (2000 ed.; American Medical Association, 2000), the *Physicians' Desk Reference for Nonprescription Drugs and Dietary Supplements* (21st ed.; see entry 414), and the *Physicians' Desk Reference for Ophthalmic Medicines* (30th ed.; see entry 255). Many libraries already have the *Physicians' Desk Reference* in the print version. At its price, the print version might be a better choice for some libraries, since drug information changes a lot and

libraries will want to purchase the new edition every year as it comes out. In fact, the cost of the three titles in print is considerably less than the cost to institutions at $595 for the CD-ROM. At these rates, libraries might want to add the *Physicians' Desk Reference Companion Guide* (56th ed.; see entry 413) in the print version. It might be a helpful addition, and it is not included on the CD-ROM.

If libraries prefer to search by computer, the CD-ROM allows users to search by product, manufacturer, category, indication, contraindication, side effect, photograph, and structure. Once users are on the page of the drug they are interested in, they can look at its description, chemical structure, clinical pharmacology, indications and usage, contraindications, warnings, precautions, drug interactions, and adverse reactions. Information is also provided about abuse of the drug, overdose, dosage and administration, and how the drug is supplied, along with a product photograph. Interested buyers should note that this CD-ROM uses Internet Explorer as a browser, and when users wish to find a keyword in the text by clicking under "Edit" on the Internet Explorer menu bar they cannot do so. But users can find a keyword in the text by clicking on "Word Search" within the *PDR Electronic Library*.

It should also be noted that dental preparations are not covered extensively on this product. Finally, there is another feature included that covers drug interactions. This feature is separate from the three PDR works listed above and has to be clicked on separately.—**Lambrini Papangelis**

408.   **The PDR Family Guide to Prescription Drugs.** 5th ed. New York, Crown, 1997. 797p. illus. index. $23.00pa. ISBN 0-609-80153-8.

The Physicians' Desk Reference (PDR) is a standard reference source that has been providing information about prescription drugs for 50 years. It is written in technical language for health professionals. *The PDR Family Guide to Prescription Drugs* (see ARBA 94, entry 1879) is an abridged version of the PDR written in lay language. It provides information on more than 1,000 commonly prescribed medications.

The book has 2 sections. The main part consists of drug profiles. The drugs are listed alphabetically by both generic and brand name, with the profile appearing under the most familiar term. Thus, information about nitroglycerin appears under *nitroglycerine*, whereas the profile of diphenhydramine appears under *Benadryl*. Drugs with several brand names appear under the one with the highest sales figures. *See* references direct users to the information. Each entry explains indications for use, a key point about the drug, how to take the medication properly, side effects, contraindications and special warnings, possible interactions with foods or other drugs, safety during pregnancy and breast-feeding, recommended dosage, and signs of overdose. A color drug identification guide helps users identify stray pills.

The 2d section contains disease overviews. These are brief explanations of common ailments and their treatments. Heart disease, arthritis, allergies, and common childhood infections are among the conditions covered. These articles are superficial, but they do contain some useful information, such as warnings about the effects of drugs on the elderly. Two appendixes offer guidelines for safe medication use and a list of poison control centers.

The PDR Family Guide to Prescription Drugs is a source that belongs in circulating and home collections rather than reference collections because it contains a limited amount of simplified information. *The Physicians'* Desk Reference (see entry 412) itself, *Mosby's GenRx* (see entry 399), or the *Complete Drug Reference* (Consumer Reports, annual) are better choices for the reference desk.—**Barbara M. Bibel**

409.   **PDR for Herbal Medicines.** 2d ed. Montvale, N.J., Medical Economics Data, 2000. 858p. illus. $59.95. ISBN 1-56363-361-2.

Herbal medicine's growing popularity has created a need for reliable information about medicinal plants. Because these preparations are not regulated by the Food and Drug Administration (FDA), they are not subjected to rigorous tests and clinical trials. The 1st edition of the *PDR for Herbal Medicines* (1998) was one of the few sources that offered scientific information about herbal products. The 2d edition has several new features that make it even more useful.

Using the findings of the German Regulatory Authority's herbal watchdog agency, Commission E, the editors have compiled information based on an intensive examination of peer-reviewed literature. Commission E has studied approximately 300 common botanicals. An exhaustive literature review conducted by the PhytoPharm U.S. Institute of Phytopharmaceuticals provides data on 400 more herbs not studied by the Commission E reports.

Organized like the other members of the PDR family, the book begins with a series of indexes. The alphabetic index lists the herbs by their common, brand, and scientific names. In this edition, the common name is used as the main entry in both the indexes and the monographs, creating a more user-friendly work. Manufacturers are listed for brand names. The therapeutic category index organizes herbs alphabetically by their drug class: analgesics, hair growth stimulants, revitalizing agents, and so on. A bold dot next to the name means that Commission E has deemed it effective. The indications index lists symptoms and conditions alphabetically in bold typeface. Under each one, herbs used as proven or traditional remedies appear. The side effects index is an alphabetic list of reactions in bold typeface with the herbs that cause them listed underneath (e.g., apathy-marijuana). The drug and herb interaction guide is an important feature. Alphabetic lists of drugs and herbs are coupled with lists of products that may interact with them. This edition has four new indexes, including a homeopathic indications index and the Asian indications index that group herbs by their therapeutic uses within these disciplines. The Asian indications index includes both Chinese and Indian traditions, indicated by a "C" and an "I" respectively. The safety guide lists herbs that must be avoided while a woman is pregnant or nursing and herbs that should be used only under professional supervision. The manufacturers index provides contact information for the suppliers of products appearing in the monographs. The herb and product identification guides provide color photographs of over 400 herbs and of selected herbal preparations and their packaging.

The herbal monographs comprise the main body of this source. They are detailed profiles of 700 medicinal herbs, including trade names, description, actions, indications, contraindications, adverse effects, overdose, dosage, and literature citations. Most of the literature is in German. A glossary and a directory of U.S. poison control centers complete the work.

PDR for Herbal Medicines fills a genuine need in reference collections. It complements sources such as the *Encyclopedia of Medicinal Plants* (see entry 202), which has more illustrations and cultural and historical background information about herbal medicine. *Herbal Drugs and Phytopharmaceuticals* (Medpharm/CRC, 1989) contains technical and manufacturing specifications. *PDR for Herbal Medicines* provides the necessary information for using herbs safely. It belongs in all medical and public library reference collections. [R: LJ, 1 Mar 99, pp. 74-76; BL, 1 Mar 99, pp. 1252-1253]—**Barbara M. Bibel**

410.   **PDR for Nutritional Supplements.** Montvale, N.J., Medical Economics Data, 2001. 575p. index. $59.95. ISBN 1-56363-364-7.

Arranged in the same manner as the other PDR volumes, this work provides the latest medical findings on hundreds of nutritional supplements in order to make informed judgments on the use of these supplements. According to the foreword, this reference "weighs the available scientific evidence, makes the appropriate conclusions, and presents the pertinent facts in a clear, accessible manner." For each nutritional supplement monograph listed, the trade names, a description (molecular structures are provided in many cases), actions and pharmacology (including mechanism of action and pharmacokinetics), indications and usage, research summary, contraindications, precautions, adverse reactions, interactions, overdosage, and dosage and administration are given. In addition, a useful bibliography is presented at the end of each monograph. In short, more than 200 monographs, several pages in length and covering nearly 1,000 nutritional products, are presented. Products such as amino acids and oligopeptides, fatty acids and other lipids, metabolites and cofactors, nucleic acids, proteins, glycosupplements, phytosupplements, hormonal products, and probiotics are included.

Indexes found in the front portion of the volume include a supplement name index, a brand name index, a category index, an indications index, a side effects index, an interactions guide, a companion drug index, and a manufacturers index. In addition to the indexes, a series of tables showing a comparison of related multi-ingredient products, common lab test values, poison control centers, and drug information centers can be found completing the reference source. This reference is highly recommended for all public libraries (large and small) and college and university libraries. Many large high school libraries would also find this work useful. In addition, many health conscious people may also wish to purchase this for their own home. [R: LJ, 1 Sept 01, pp. 168-170; BL, Aug 01, pp. 2172-2173; AG, Sept 01, p. 62]—**George H. Bell**

411. **PDR Generics 1998.** 4th ed. Montvale, N.J., Medical Economics Data, 1998. 2869p. illus. index. $79.95. ISBN 1-56363-253-5.

Designed to provide clinicians with the most comprehensive information on virtually every generic drug product currently on the market, *PDR Generics 1998* is the collaborative effort of the editorial boards of the Medical Economics Company and Micromedex, Inc. Arranged alphabetically by generic name, four different indexes provide easy access: brand and generic name, product category, indications, and international drug name. Prescribing information for each drug includes FDA-approved uses as well as recognized off-label uses. Dosage and administration, indications and usage, adverse reactions, contraindications, and precautions are provided in detail. Additional information on available supplies, pricing, and therapeutic equivalency emphasizes the targeted market for this volume—the health care professional or clinician.—**Vicki J. Killion**

412. **Physicians' Desk Reference 2002.** 56th ed. Montvale, N.J., Medical Economics Data, 2002. 3635p. $89.95. ISBN 1-56363-411-2.

The *Physicians' Desk Reference* (PDR) is standard equipment in physicians' offices, clinics, and hospitals throughout the United States. Every student in any discipline of health care quickly learns the incomparable value of the PDR. Produced by Medical Economics Data, a part of Thompson Healthcare, this 3,000-page annual drug reference provides essential information on the efficacy, possible adverse effects, clinical pharmacology, recommended use, and dosages of literally thousands of commonly used drugs. The first three sections of the volume are divided into color-coded indexes: manufactures index (white), brand and generic name index (pink), and product category index (blue). The remaining three sections are a "Product Identification Guide" (gray), the "Product Information," and "Diagnostic Product Information." "Keys to Controlled Substances Categories," "Keys to FDA Use-in-Pregnancy Ratings," and a national directory of poison control centers are included just before the "Product Information" section, while U.S. Food and Drug Administration telephone numbers and sample "Adverse Event Report" forms are appended at the end of the book.

Each of the indexes provides valuable information. The manufacturers index furnishes contact information and a list of products for individual pharmaceutical companies. The brand and generic name index is a particularly helpful cross-reference, allowing the location of an individual drug by either its brand or generic name. The "Product Identification Guide," organized alphabetically by manufacturers, supplies a full-color, actual-size photograph of tablets and capsules, while inhalers and other dosage formats are shown smaller. This pictorial guide is an invaluable asset to those who may need to identify an unlabeled medication. The heart of the PDR is the "Product Information" section. Organized alphabetically by manufacturers, there is in-depth information on the clinical pharmacology; indications for use; contraindications; warnings and precautions; adverse reactions; the signs, symptoms, and treatment for over dosages; dosage and administration; and how the drug is supplied. The only caveat is, all of the information in the PDR is supplied by the pharmaceutical manufacturer and may therefore have a bias. This fact notwithstanding, this a classic and very useful book, recommended for all academic and public libraries.—**Lynn M. McMain**

413. **Physicians' Desk Reference Companion Guide 2002.** 56th ed. Mukesh Mehta, ed. Montvale, N.J., Medical Economics Data, 2002. 1736p. index. $64.95. ISBN 1-56363-416-3.
     This work, which offers the reader 9 separate sections, provides a wide variety of ways to accessing the information found within the *Physicians' Desk Reference* (PDR; 2002 ed., see entry 412), the *PDR for Nonprescription Drugs and Dietary Supplements* (23d ed.; Medical Economics Data), and the *Physicians' Desk Reference for Ophthalmic Medicines* (30th ed.; see entry 255). The first of these sections, which composes approximately two-thirds of the reference, is the interactions index. This section is alphabetically arranged by the brand name or, when applicable, the generic name of the drug. Listed below each entry are interactions that can occur when taking the medication. Page numbers are also included for each entry in this section, as well as in all other sections, that refer the reader to the 2002 editions of the PDR and the *PRD for Ophthalmic Medicines*, as well as the 2001 edition of the *PDR for Nonprescription Drugs and Dietary Supplements*.
     The "Food Interactions Cross-Reference" provides an alphabetic list of food items (alcohol included) that are said to interact with specific medications. Medications are listed under each of the food items listed. The side effects index that follows presents an alphabetic list of every side effect reported in the "Adverse Reactions" section of the product descriptions in the PDR and its companion volumes. Under each side effect heading are the lists of drugs that have the potential to produce the side effect. A 4th section, an indications index, provides an alphabetic list of every indication cited in the PDR and its companion volumes. Under each of the headings, drug names are listed that can be administered for this type of affliction.
     Other sections in the work are the "Off-Label Treatment Guide" that identifies medication routinely used, but never officially approved, for nearly 1,000 indications; the contraindications index that is an alphabetic list of every medical condition cited as a contraindication in the PDR and its companion volumes; the international drug name index; the "Generic Availability Guide" that allows readers to determine which forms and strengths of a brand name drug are available generically; and, finally, the "Imprint Identification Guide" that allows readers to identify solid oral medications by imprint alone. A list of poison control centers, arranged by state, completes the reference volume. This guide is highly recommended for university, college, and public libraries, as well as anyone else with an interest in this type of material. If, however, readers already have the *PDR Electronic Library* (2000 ed.; see entry 407) that allows users to retrieve information in the same way that this book is arranged in and more, then they may wish to pass on this work. —**George H. Bell**

414. **Physicians' Desk Reference for Nonprescription Drugs and Dietary Supplements 2000.** 21st ed. Montvale, N.J., Medical Economics Data, 2000. 888p. illus. $48.95. ISBN 1-56363-341-8.

Arranged alphabetically by name of drug company, this classic work provides a wealth of information on over-the-counter drugs as well as dietary supplements. The information is prepared by the drug manufacturer and edited and approved by the manufacturer's medical department, medical director, or medical consultant. Such information as active ingredients, inactive ingredients, warnings, drug interaction, directions for use, and how the drug is supplied is given for each drug listed. The amount of information given for the dietary supplements, however, can vary from one listing to another. A description of the supplement is given for each one listed. Additional information such as active ingredients, recommended dosage, ingredients, warnings, and so on can vary from one supplement listing to another.

Because the arrangement of these products is by drug manufacturer, it is best to become familiar with the indexes. These indexes appear at the front of the work rather than at the end and include over-the-counter drugs as well as dietary supplements. There is a product name index (e.g., Alka-Seltzer, Sleepinal, and Neosporin), a product category index (e.g., acne preparations, pain relievers, antibiotics, and antacids), and an active ingredients index (e.g., acetaminophen, caffeine, glycerin, and lanolin). There is also a companion drug index of over-the-counter products that may be used in conjunction with prescription drug therapy in order to reserve drug-induced side effects, relieve symptoms of the illness, or treat sequelae of the initial disease. The sugar-free products index provides a list of the products that are sugar free by therapeutic category, such as analgesics and cough, cold, and allergy preparations. The alcohol-free products index provides a list of products that are alcohol free by therapeutic category. The lactose and galactose free products index is arranged alphabetically by product name and the product identification guide index provides full-color photographs of the product package and tablets or capsules.

A listing of poison control centers, drug information centers, and state boards of pharmacy can be found at the end of the volume. It should also be noted that access to much of the information contained within the *Physicians' Desk Reference* and its main companion volumes is free of charge. This information can be found on the Web at www.pdr.net. Registration for this information is required and there is a fee for additional information.

This work is very highly recommended for all small and large public, high school, college, and university libraries. Many people who are interested in this type of information may also wish to purchase a copy of this work for their own library.—**George H. Bell**

415.   **Physicians' Guide to Nutriceuticals.** 2d ed. Douglas L. Ringer, ed. Omaha, Nebr., Nutrition Data Resources, 2000. 437p. $49.95. ISBN 0-96656-652-1.

The *Physicians' Guide to Nutriceuticals* (PGN) is described by the publisher as an educational tool providing detailed information on quality products without the advertising hyperbole. Dietary supplements, herbal medicines, nutraceuticals (the generally accepted spelling rather than the editors' choice of *nutriceuticals*), and other forms of consumable natural products are being purchased by ever increasing numbers of people seeking to improve and prolong their health. The resulting multi-billion dollar industry bombards consumers with product advertisements for every possible health enhancement that the reluctantly aging baby boomer can imagine. PGN attempts to represent companies that make quality products that are safe and effective using formulating techniques and manufacturing practices backed by hard science and cutting-edge technology. The list of companies is very short.

The education section consists of seven articles introducing the reader to some basic theory and regulatory information on the natural products industry. The company index lists directory information and products for the 25 companies participating in this edition. A product name index and a universal (health condition or natural product name) index directs the reader to the main part of the book, the product information section. Each product listed contains the manufacturing company profile, description, ingredients, intended usage, warnings, interactions, references, how the product is supplied, and how it can by purchased. The section on clinical studies is information provided by the participating company on its specific marketed product. A glossary of more than 500 terms and a short list of vitamins and minerals and their corresponding Recommended Daily Allowance (RDA) and biological function complete the text.

As with all natural product preparations, the consumer is warned that the FDA has not evaluated the information supplied by the manufacturer and that the product is not intended to diagnose, treat, cure, or prevent any disease. The clinical studies conducted by the manufacturers show that many of the trials were conducted on very small groups of patients for limited time periods.

In the past there have been few resources available that list ingredients for nonprescription products, especially natural products preparations. This text is useful for that reason. Public libraries may consider adding PGN to their collections because of the current popularity of self-medication with natural products. Libraries supporting pharmacy schools should consider adding it for the unique information it offers, but also for the opportunity it provides the student for evaluating the type of information upon which consumers are relying. —**Vicki J. Killion**

416.   Snow, Bonnie. **Drug Information: A Guide to Current Resources.** 2d ed. Chicago, Medical Library Association and Lanham, Md., Scarecrow, 1999. 752p. index. $70.00; $46.00pa. ISBN 0-8108-3320-4; 0-8108-3321-2pa.

This 2d edition is arranged so it can be used either as a textbook for a class or as a reference tool for librarians. The book is described as being a "problem solver" and not just a list of useful tools or Internet sites. The 16 chapters cover where to find information on everything from nomenclature, laws and regulations, searching protocols, evaluating sources, specific areas of drug information such as side effects or patient information, business and statistical data for drugs, market research areas, and regulatory sources. Print, CD-ROM, and online sources are covered. Appendix A covers the core drug collection for a hospital library and also lists a separate collection for public libraries. Appendix B covers online sources listed by subject category. The other appendixes cover full-text online newsletters, professional and trade associations, practicum exercises, and abbreviations. The book also includes a glossary and an extensive index. Due to the wealth of information, this is a tool any librarian should have. It is a must for hospital libraries and pharmaceutical libraries. —**Betsy J. Kraus**

HANDBOOKS AND YEARBOOKS

417.   Allison, Kathleen Cahill. **EveryWoman's Guide to Prescription and Nonprescription Drugs.** New York, Broadway Books, 1997. 770p. illus. index. $19.95pa. ISBN 0-553-06906-3.

During the past 10 years, efforts have been made to include more women in clinical drug trials. Prior to that time, researchers were reluctant to include women of childbearing age and postmenopausal women because of the differential effects of the menstrual cycle. This exclusion, plus the physiological differences between men and women, resulted in inappropriate dosages and unexpected drug toxicity for many women. In an effort to help women become informed consumers, the editors of this book have created a resource that emphasizes the information women should know about their prescription and nonprescription drugs: Will the medication interact with birth control pills, will hormone replacement therapy affect the medication, can it be taken if pregnant or attempting pregnancy, can it be taken if breast-feeding, will bone density be reduced, and will it affect the menstrual cycle?

The 1st section of the book provides general information on drug testing, types of drugs, interpreting the prescription, routes of administration, and alternative remedies. The chapter on drug safety stresses the communication women must have with the physician and the pharmacist, potential side effects, adverse drug reactions, and drug interactions. In the chapter on choosing drugs for a healthier lifestyle, readers are cautioned about abusing nonprescription products for smoking cessation, weight loss, sun exposure, and constipation. Drug profiles for 200 drugs representing more than 1,000 generic and brand-name drugs, are provided in the 2d section of the book. The profiles are from the database created by the U.S. Pharmacopeial Convention, an independent, not-for-profit organization that sets the official standards of strength, quality, purity, packaging, and labeling of medical products sold in the United States. Each profile includes information on the drug's purpose, information the patient should communicate to the physician or pharmacist, use and administration, precautions, and possible side effects. As the title suggests, the focus is on women's health and well-being. The drug index lists both brand and generic names; the general index provides access to the appropriate drug outline by disease name or symptom.

Although the drug information is written from a woman's point of view, so to speak, it is available in other resources. The value of the book resides in the first few chapters, in which women are encouraged to be informed consumers and learn more about the drugs they use. Women's health issues are extremely important, and this book offers valuable information while fulfilling a current and popular need in many libraries' consumer health collections. [R: RBB, 1 Mar 97, p. 1188]—**Vicki J. Killion**

418.   **Ashgate Handbook of Antineoplastic Agents.** G. W. A. Milne, ed. Brookfield, Vt., Ashgate Publishing, 2000. 170p. index. $125.00. ISBN 0-566-08382-5.

Chemotherapy is one of the most potent weapons currently in use against cancer. This volume includes information on all of the major chemical agents used to fight tumors of all types. The main entries are divided into two sections: antineoplastic agents and cytoprotectant agents. Arranged alphabetically by name, each entry includes the Chemical Abstracts Service (CAS) registry number for the compound, the corresponding Merck Index number and the European Inventory of Existing Commercial Chemical Substances (EINECS) number. The molecular structure of the compound is also provided as well as the chemical name of the compound. In each entry is a list of the synonyms, trade names, and other also-known-as names. Separate indexes are provided for CAS registry numbers, EINECS numbers, and names and synonyms. The third part of the book is a directory of pharmaceutical and chemical manufacturers, arranged alphabetically by company name, with contact information.

The editor, Milne, was a senior researcher at the National Institute of Health and is the current editor of the American Chemical Society's *Journal of Chemical Information and Computer Sciences*. He is also the joint recipient of the 1999 Skolnik Award of the Chemical Information Division of the American Chemical Society. This volume will be a vital addition to pharmacology and oncology libraries and of peripheral interest to general professional medical collections. —**Susan B. Hagloch**

419.   **Ashgate Handbook of Cardiovascular Agents.** G. W. A. Milne and E. J. Zeman, eds. Brookfield, Vt., Ashgate Publishing, 2001. 484p. index. $225.00. ISBN 0-566-08386-8.

Following the same format as *Ashgate Handbook of Endocrine Agents and Steroids* (see entry 420), this work provides chemical information and molecular structures on all the major drugs that directly affect the cardiovascular system. A total of 1,937 drugs are included. These drugs are currently listed in the *U.S. Pharmacopia*, as well as in another Ashgate publication entitled *Drugs: Synonyms and Properties* (see entry 394). The names of the drugs are alphabetically arranged by generic drug name under each of six main sections. These sections include "Vasoactive Agents," "Antihypertensive Agents," "Antianginal, Antiarrythmic, and Cardiotonic Agents," "Antihypercholesterolemic Agents," "Blood Formation and Coagulation Agents," and "Water and Electrolyte Balancing Agents."

A typical entry, such as the record for *Nadolol*, include the CAS registry number, Merck Index number, and European Inventory of Existing Commercial Chemical Substances (EINECS) number. The drug's molecular formula, structural formula, chemical name, synonyms, therapeutic use, physical properties, toxicity, and the manufacturer/supplier are also included. It should be noted that not all entries contain all of the various pieces of information. A CAS registry number index, an EINECS number index, and a drug name/synonym index can be found near the end of the volume.

It should also be noted that there is one problem with the reference source. In examining the drug name/synonym index, the drug Lipitor was absent. Lipitor is the brand name for Atorvastatin and is widely prescribed for lowering cholesterol. Atorvastatin is an entry in the main body of the work, but if a reader was not aware of Lipitor's generic name, the drug name/synonym index would not have helped. In fact, the term Lipitor, as a synonym, is not mentioned in the body of information dealing with Atorvastatin.

This is a highly specialized reference work and, as such, is recommended for university, pharmaceutical, chemical, and other specialized libraries dealing with this topic. It should be noted that the online version of *The Combined Chemical Dictionary*, an amalgam of the Chapman and Hall dictionary sets, contains much of the information presented within this volume, save for supplier/manufacturer information.—**George H. Bell**

420.   **Ashgate Handbook of Endocrine Agents and Steroids.** G. W. A. Milne, ed. Brookfield, Vt., Ashgate Publishing, 2000. 250p. index. $150.00. ISBN 0-566-08383-3.

This work provides chemical information and structures on all the major drugs that are, or have been, used in endocrine pharmacology. A total of 818 endocrine agents and steroids are included. The names of the drugs are alphabetically arranged under each of the eight sections. These sections include pituitary and hypothalamic agents, adrenocortical agents, androgens and anabolic steroids, calcium metabolizing agents, estrogens and progestins, glucose regulating agents, thyroids and antithyroids, and general steroids.

A typical entry includes the Chemical Abstracts Service (CAS) registry number, the *Merck Index* number (12th edition), the European Inventory of Existing Commercial Chemical Substances (EINECS) number, the molecular formula, the structural formula, the chemical name, synonyms, its therapeutic use, physical properties, toxicity, and the manufacturer or supplier. It should be noted that not all of the entries contain the same amount of information as stated above. For example, drug entries representing small polypeptides contain, in many cases, the amino acid arrangement or molecular formula rather than the structural formula. Structural formulas can be found for each of the steroids listed. In some cases, for both steroids and non-steroids, physical property information is absent or not as complete as the typical entry. A CAS registry number index, an EINECS number index, and a drug name and synonym index can be found near the end of the volume. A manufacturer and supplier directory, arranged alphabetically by company name, completes the volume.

This is a highly specialized reference work is recommended for university, pharmaceutical, chemical, and other specialized libraries dealing with this topic. It should also be noted that *The Combined Chemical Dictionary on CD-ROM*, which is an amalgam of the Chapman and Hall dictionary sets, contains much of the information presented within this volume, save for supplier and manufacturer information.—**George H. Bell**

421.   **Burger's Medicinal Chemistry and Drug Discovery.** 5th ed. Manfred E. Wolff, ed. New York, John Wiley, 1995-1997. 5v. index. $975.00/set. ISBN 0-471-57556-9 (v.1); 0-471-57557-7 (v.2); 0-471-57558-5 (v.3); 0-471-57559-3 (v.4); 0-471-57560-7 (v.5).

This series is divided into 5 hardback volumes. Volume 1 eloquently explains the scientific and legal aspects of drug discovery processes, product development issues, 3-dimensional chemical structure information, and various drug discovery technologies. The remaining volumes are devoted to important individual drug classes. Chapters are structured by disease category (e.g., antihypertensive agents); therapeutic modality (e.g., beta-blockers); or a combination of the two.

Individual chapters contain up-to-date information in each of the basic sciences, including molecular biology, biochemistry, and pharmacology. Every contributor provides a masterful synopsis of the huge quantities of available data. For older drugs, a historical perspective is included that focuses on the product's contribution to improved quality of life and decreased health care costs. Extensive bibliographies conclude each chapter, and indexes appear within each volume (with a cumulative index in volume 5). This reference series is an essential addition to the libraries of medical and allied health professionals, medicinal chemists and biopharmaceutical industry professionals, and certain members of the legal community.—**Sue Lyon Mertl**

422.   **Clin-Alert 2000.** Joyce Generali, ed. Lancaster, Pa., Technomic Publishing, 2000. 427p. index. $94.95pa. ISBN 1-56676-962-0.

The purpose of the *Clin-Alert* newsletter is to summarize and provide newly published information on significant adverse drug events and drug interactions. Typically an abstract to the original article appears in the semi-monthly issue within two or three weeks of the original publication date. A list of keywords for the issue is printed on the front page and an annual index is included in the last issue of the year.

What does *Clin-Alert 2000* provide that cannot be found in the newsletter? The book collates data from the past two years. The abstracts are arranged by drug class and there are five different indexes—drug, FDA and manufacturer alert, first published reports, legal action, and drug interaction.

The prospective audience is pharmacists or physicians, but given the critical nature of the information (i.e., adverse drug effects), readers will need to refer to the primary literature. The collected abstracts do provide a convenient method to keep current with the literature, but a search in the MEDLINE database is just as effective and more efficient.—**Vicki J. Killion**

423.   **Drug Topics Red Book 2000.** Montvale, N.J., Medical Economics Data, 2000. 900p. index. $59.95. ISBN 1-56363-357-4. ISSN 1072-1142.

Pharmacists extensively use this annual catalog produced by Medical Economics Data, the publishers of the well-known *Physicians' Desk Reference* (56th ed.; see entry 412). A thorough table of contents, divided into 10 sections, leads to important pricing information as well as sections on emergency and clinical facts regarding both prescription and nonprescription drugs. There are also sections on professional pharmacy and health care organizations, federal and state drug reimbursement programs, drug manufacturer and wholesaler contact information, over-the-counter and nondrug product listings, and product identification photographs. The section on prescription products lists prescription drugs alphabetically by the prevailing drug name, with cross-references from generic name to trademarked name. This latest edition includes two new sections on practice management and professional development and complementary and herbal products. There is no specific product information such as actions, side effects, and contraindications, so this book is not as useful to consumers, but it remains an essential tool for pharmacists. Other health care professionals, particularly those who prescribe and those who administer prescription medication in a clinical setting, will also find this a valuable resource, as will students in health care programs. —**Lynn M. McMain**

424. Ehrenpreis, Seymour, and Eli D. Ehrenpreis. **Clinician's Handbook of Prescription Drugs.** New York, McGraw-Hill, 2001. 979p. $34.95pa. ISBN 0-07-134385-7.

According to the author's preface, "It can be quite time consuming and frustrating to search for important information on individual entries in a large comprehensive volume such as the *Physicians' Desk Reference.* Thus, our main objective in creating this book was to provide the most essential information on all commonly prescribed drugs in a concise, accurate and easy-to-read manner." The authors should be congratulated on doing just that. This work, alphabetically arranged by the generic name, offer such essential information as mechanism of action, indications/dosage/route, adjustment of dosage, onset of action, peak effect, duration, warnings/precautions, advice to patients, adverse reactions, and parameters to monitor among other informational items.

There is a brand name index in the front of the volume. It is important to be aware of this brand name index because many users of this book can easily miss an entry by going into the bulk of the work with the brand name, rather than the generic name. Tables, such as general information on common amino glycosides; first, second, third, and fourth generation cephalosporins; antifungal agents; and oral contraceptives can be bound at the end of the compendium. This work is highly recommended for libraries on a budget (i.e., those libraries that would prefer not to spend their money on high costing drug monographs). It is also highly recommended for health care workers and for home use.—**George H. Bell**

425. Friedman, J. M., and Janine E. Polifka. **The Effects of Drugs on the Fetus and Nursing Infant: A Handbook for Health Care Professionals.** Baltimore, Md., Johns Hopkins University Press, 1996. 648p. $49.95pa. ISBN 0-8018-5345-1.

This reference text is well written and presented in an easy-to-read format. Readers should be advised that the text uses medical terminology and deals with such topics as "teratogen." The work deals directly with medications, their effects on the fetus, and complications associated with the use of certain medications while pregnant or nursing an infant. Although medical terminology is used, the authors do define some of these terms so that the adult reader can follow the material. Having a medical background may be of benefit when using the text.

The introduction explains the purpose and goals and offers suggestions on how to apply the material in a clinical setting. The body of the text reviews hundreds of medications and their effects on the fetus, potential complications with breast feeding, and developmental issues associated with the use of medications. The medications are summarized with the following information: defining the drug and how it works, what the drug is used for, and its dosage. Teratogenic risk is also discussed in detail. Additional topics, such as reports of fetal malformation, impact on breast feeding, and pregnancy complications, are also included. A reference list for each medication is present, which allows the reader to consult other resources.

As indicated in the handbook, a majority of this information has been obtained through various computer systems or programs, such as TERIS, MEDLINE, TOXLINE, and DART. This text may be most useful to those in the medical field (especially obstetrics) or those interested in learning more about the effects of medications on pregnancy, fetal development, and the nursing of infants.—**Paul M. Murphy III**

426. Friedman, J. M., and Janine E. Polifka. **The Effects of Neurologic and Psychiatric Drugs on the Fetus and Nursing Infant: A Handbook for Health Care Professionals.** Baltimore, Md., Johns Hopkins University Press, 1998. 369p. index. $49.50pa. ISBN 0-8018-5962-X.

Health care professionals face a number of challenges when a woman receiving medication for a mental health condition or abusing substances becomes pregnant. *Effects of Neurologic and*

Psychiatric Drugs on the Fetus and Nursing Infant is an indispensable resource for health professionals in maternal and fetal or infant care. Experts in teratology and toxicology prepared the entries based on a thorough review of existing medical literature. Controlled and common illicit substances are included. Herbal preparations or alternative treatments with possible teratogenic effects are not included. Arrangement is alphabetic by drug or substance name. Cross-references are given from product names to main entries by agent. Entries include risk ratings and an evaluation of the amount and quality of existing research on effects. Short reviews cite relevant studies and include references lists of significant research. Special attention is given to the impact of maternal drug use on nursing infants. This title is recommended for libraries with an interest in maternal and fetal or infant care, due to the convenience and authority of information provided.—**Lynne M. Fox**

427.   Fudyma, Janice. **What Do I Take? A Consumer's Guide to Nonprescription Drugs.** New York, HarperPerennial/HarperCollins, 1997. 177p. $13.00pa. ISBN 0-06-273422-9.

For those people whose bursitis is acting up again, or who need some relief and cannot find the time to schedule a doctor's appointment, this small but informative monograph is the book to consult. By turning to the bursitis/tendinitis page, a number of over-the-counter products are listed and rated by pharmacists. Ratings of each product (based on a 1-to-10 scale) consider the following categories: "Most Effective," "Speed of Relief," "Minimal Side Effects," and "Percentage of Pharmacists Who Most Often Recommend." The participating pharmacists, who are members of the American Pharmaceutical Association, were selected based on three or more years of practice, and were chosen from diversified geographic locations. The results of the ratings represent a 90 percent confidence level, plus or minus 8 points. In the case of bursitis, a total of 11 over-the-counter medications are rated.

For each affliction listed, in addition to the rating scale some general information on the affliction, on the medications themselves, and when it is best to see a doctor are outlined. A total of 57 afflictions are presented with ratings of 400 over-the-counter products. Other afflictions include heartburn, coughs, ringworm, eye redness, fever, and so on. Aside from the alphabetic list of afflictions, a 2d section contains an alphabetic list of the products discussed. For each product listed, dosage form, active ingredients, and warnings are presented. The work concludes with a two-page glossary. This guide is recommended for all public libraries as well as for individual purchase.—**George H. Bell**

428.   Graedon, Joe, and Teresa Graedon. **The People's Guide to Deadly Drug Interactions: How to Protect Yourself....** New York, St. Martin's Press, 1995. 434p. index. $25.95. ISBN 0-312-13243-3.

The People's Pharmacy (rev. ed., St. Martin's Press, 1996) authors expand their concern for consumers into the arcane world of substance interactions: food/drug, vitamin/drug, vitamin/mineral, drug/alcohol, and drug/drug (both prescription and over-the-counter). Three types of interactions are discussed: additive (one substance increasing the effectiveness of another), antagonistic (one canceling the effectiveness of the other), and unpredictable. Graphs, charts, and a heedful narrative are used to inform readers of thousands of potentially deadly chemical combinations. Sample interactions range from those commonly documented, such as grapefruit juice and calcium channel blockers, to others that are only remotely possible. Half the book is composed of a convenient listing of drugs, by type and by name, with possible interactions charted. It is this feature that should appeal to reference desk staff.

So that they may propose that timely mechanisms do not exist for determining the potential for drug interactions and for notifying doctors of such dangers, the authors do not discuss the communication that routinely takes place between pharmaceutical companies and the medical community. Yet such written notifications routinely crossed this reviewer's desk as a hospital librarian. The book makes many unsubstantiated criticisms of both the private and governmental wings of the health care community; studies are referred to but not cited and statistical evidence is rarely used to support conclusions. Contradictions also undermine the credibility of the text—for example, "Since the FDA does not have a system for gathering interaction data. . . ." (p. 2), and "Reports of dizziness attacks and heart palpitations began trickling in to the Food and Drug Administration (FDA)" (p. 5). A subtler flaw is raised by the authors' view that an improbable and minor risk is as worthy of concern and attention as a likelier, major risk. Treating all contraindications equally dilutes the jeremiad's impact.

Unexpected substance interactions do occur, and reasonable caution should be exercised in the consumption of foods, medicines, and supplements. However, it is difficult to take seriously a purported reference source that opens with the statement "Would you want to play Russian Roulette?" (p. 1). The book's graphs and charts offer a good deal of valuable information. It is unfortunate that the tone of the narrative is inclined to be pejorative, distrustful, and alarmist. Reference librarians are advised to preface their quoting of the book with the phrase, "In the opinion of the authors. . . ." [R: RBB, Jan 96, p. 890]—**Ed Volz**

429.   Kirschenbaum, Harold L., and Michelle M. Kalis. **The Pharmacy Practice Handbook of Medication Facts.** Lancaster, Pa., Technomic Publishing, 2000. 783p. index. $64.95pa. ISBN 1-56676-762-8.

This reference guide is designed for health professionals who prescribe, dispense, or evaluate patients treated with prescription drugs. There are many such compendia available on the market, including *The Physicians' Desk Reference* (2000 ed.; American Medical Association, 2000) and *Drug Facts and Comparisons*, among others. This handbook is distinguished by its compact size (5 by 7 inches) and succinct format. All prescription drug products available on the market through 1998 are listed alphabetically by generic name under 22 therapeutic classes (e.g., cardiovascular agents, lipid lowering agents, blood modifiers) and by drug subclass (e.g., calcium channel blockers, Alpha-1 blockers). The handbook provides a table for each drug that lists common brand names, normal adult dosage ranges, major adverse effects and cautions, key patient counseling points, and miscellaneous issues. The handbook also includes 19 appendixes, with information on everything from medical abbreviations and temperature conversions to a Spanish/English dictionary for pharmacists. Although no substitute for the more complete drug compendia, this guide does an excellent job of condensing pertinent information to caregivers who need a quick reference source. On the negative side, any guide like this becomes quickly dated as new drugs go on the market and others are recalled. There is no indication the handbook is designed to be a serial.
—**Bruce Stuart**

430.   Kuhn, Cynthia, Scott Swartzwelder, and Wilkie Wilson. **Buzzed: The Straight Facts About the Most Used and Abused Drugs from Alcohol to Ecstasy.** New York, W. W. Norton, 1998. 317p. illus. index. $14.95pa. ISBN 0-393-31732-3.

Drug education is often incomplete. We tell our young people to "Just Say No," and cite horror stories of relatively rare cocaine deaths and marijuana "addiction." In addition, many of the drugs that young people encounter go by names we do not know or are themselves arcane and little known outside the youth scene. This excellent resource lays out the plain unvarnished facts in language that high school and college students can understand. Part 1 examines broad categories of drugs: alcohol, caffeine, herbal drugs, entactogens, hallucinogens, inhalants, marijuana, nicotine, opiates, sedatives, steroids, and stimulants. It describes how each is introduced into the system (e.g., ingest, inhale, inject), the effects on the body, common terms used for the substance, overdose, interactions with other drugs and, where applicable, the different effects of different forms.

Each substance is thoroughly examined with no inflated scare tactics. Part 2 covers the basics of brain function and drug function in general as well as legal issues. A bibliography is appended and an excellent glossary of slang terms is provided. This resource will be useful for public library reference departments, but be sure to buy several circulating copies too.—**Susan B. Hagloch**

431. Litt, Jerome Z. **Drug Eruption Reference Manual 2000.** millennium ed. Pearl River, N.Y., Parthenon, 2000. 662p. illus. $149.00pa. ISBN 1-85070-788-X.

Adverse drug reactions in the form of cutaneous (skin) eruptions are increasing as more new drugs appear on the market. This manual describes and catalogs the adverse cutaneous side effects of more than 700 prescription and nonprescription drugs currently on the market in the United States. More than 16,000 references and sources from journal articles, books, and observations from dermatologists are cited.

Listed alphabetically by generic name, each entry also includes trade (brand) names, trade names from other countries, indications, drug category, and drug half-life. The reactions section is classified into four categories: skin, hair, nails, and other (referring to mucous membrane, teeth, muscle, and various other reactions). The references to the literature are listed under each appropriate reaction pattern. Three additional sections complete the text: adverse reactions to popular marketed herbals and botanicals, descriptions of the 29 most common reaction patterns, and a list of drugs responsible for 95 common reaction patterns. Color photographs illustrating the common reaction patterns are also included.

This manual is intended for practicing health care professionals, in particular for dermatologists and physicians treating hospitalized or ambulatory patients. Hospital libraries and academic health sciences libraries will want to add this state-of-the-art annual compendium. [R: Choice, Oct 2000, p. 306]—**Vicki J. Killion**

432. McLaughlin Jr., Arthur J., and Stuart R. Levine. **Respiratory Care Drug Reference.** Gaithersville, Md., Aspen, 1997. 383p. index. $45.00 pa. ISBN 0-8342-0788-5.

This guide is intended to provide health care professionals treating patients for respiratory or cardiovascular problems with a convenient, concise, easy-to-read, and portable guide to the information needed to treat patients. Drugs covered include not only those intended to alleviate respiratory symptoms, but other drugs the patients may have been prescribed or which they have bought over the counter.

Part 1 is a useful guide to various categories of drugs. Information in this section includes an overview of their pharmacology, uses, precautions, and possible adverse reactions, as well as advice to give patients and a list of individual drugs in that category included in the book. Part 2 is an alphabetic listing of generic drugs. Under each is a prominent box giving respiratory care considerations for that drug, as well as information on the drug's uses, dosages, administration routes, and availability. The index includes both generic and trade names. Appendixes include lists of drugs on the Drug Enforcement Agency Schedule of Controlled Substances, U.S. Food and Drug Administration pregnancy risk categories, and frequently used drugs in the treatment of pulmonary and cardiovascular conditions as well as a resource bibliography. Because the book's language is less technical and information on respiratory considerations easier to find than in standard sources such as the *Physicians' Desk Reference* (56th ed.; see entry 412), it will be a useful resource for those suffering from respiratory diseases as well as health care professionals, although, of course, it is not a substitute for consulting a physician.—**Marit S. Taylor**

433. Shepard, Thomas H. **Catalog of Teratogenic Agents.** 9th ed. Baltimore, Md., Johns Hopkins University Press, 1998. 593p. index. $125.00. ISBN 0-8018-6075-X.

Even seemingly harmless substances can cause malformations in the fetus. The *Catalog of Teratogenic Agents* is a guide to the agents, the studies that determined whether malformations could occur, and the quantities of the agents that cause malformations. This new edition contains 250 entries not listed in the prior edition and the revision of other entries. The catalog is a standard reference text that can be found in many medical and hospital libraries. It is included in electronic form in the Micromedex database that is used as a reference tool by many pharmacists and hospital emergency departments. Arrangement is by agent name, and each entry includes a brief description of recent studies, outcome of the studies, and a list of references. There is an extensive index to the authors of the studies consulted in the preparation of the entries and an agent index for quick location of information. Most medical and hospital libraries find this work indispensable. University libraries with chemical toxicology collections, genetic counselors, and medical institutions without access to Micromedex should find the *Catalog of Teratogenic Agents* an essential purchase. Pregnant women with advanced questions about the effect of substances on the fetus may also find this reference useful. However, the intended audience is professionals with knowledge of chemistry and fetal development.—**Lynne M. Fox**

BIBLIOGRAPHY

434.   **Bibliographic Guide to Psychology 1998.** Thorndike, Maine, G. K. Hall/Macmillan, 1999. 452p. $295.00. ISBN 0-7838-0228-5. ISSN 0360-277X.

G. K. Hall has once again compiled a comprehensive annual subject bibliography devoted to select psychology materials that were cataloged in 1998 but may have been published between 1990 and the present. The guide is made up of recent publications cataloged by The Research Libraries of The New York Public Library (NYPL), which share two or more Library of Congress subject headings from MARC psychology records. Other materials included have been cataloged by the Library of Congress in the same time period and retrieved from the LC MARC tapes with a "BF" classification.

Alphabetically arranged in a dictionary format, all main entries supply full bibliographic information, conveniently including call numbers and subject tracings. Another way to access information is to use the added entries, such as titles, editors, and compilers, which are also supplemented with cross-references to proper LC headings. These valuable features enhance the guide's usefulness not only as an authoritative reference source of recently published psychology materials, but also as a research tool for students and other research-oriented patrons. It is recognizable as a collection development tool, providing the means to maintain current awareness of noteworthy resources within the field. Having such complete technical information easily accessible, catalogers and acquisitions librarians will also find it worthwhile to consult. Visually pleasing, the entries are in bold typeface and include all languages and formats. Major subject areas include such topics as child psychology, applied psychology, temperament, character, personality, the occult sciences, and parapsychology, to name a few.

Unfortunately, the omission of the NYPL holdings indicator and Classmark for appropriate records as promised in the preface is a definite flaw. The overall quality of the guide, which is intended for librarians, students, and researchers, meets previous high standards established in G. K. Hall's series. This resource is appropriate for libraries serving research needs, but it may have limited appeal due to its increased cost.—**Marianne B. Eimer**

435.   Wilson, C. Dwayne, and Bernard Lubin. **Research on Professional Consultation and Consultation for Organizational Change: A Selectively Annotated Bibliography.** Westport, Conn., in cooperation with NTL Institute for Applied Behavioral Science, Greenwood Press, 1997. 135p. index. (Bibliographies and Indexes in Psychology, no.10). $59.95. ISBN 0-313-28034-7.

As corporate and organizational worlds are revolutionized, the literature on organizational leadership, organizational change, and organizational behavior is expanding. There are now several graduate programs specifically focused on organizational change. A volume identifying the literature on consultation and organizational change is welcome; this bibliography studies two decades of research on consultative practice and its influence on individuals and groups in organizations and how their participation creates organizational change. Leaders who are in business and industrial settings, educational settings at all levels, legal and criminal justice settings, hospital care and health care settings, mental health and psychiatric settings, and leaders in any organizational consultation environment will have a ready source to find the information they need. The bibliography will be a helpful place to seek out what consultation services bring to an organization in the midst of change and challenges from internal and external forces. This is a bibliography of research reports, and it is an efficient volume for a manager or an organizational leader. The volume aids access for those users who require information on consultation for decision-making in organizational and practice-related issues, and it provides resources to researchers who want to uncover new facts regarding consultation practice.

This comprehensive yet succinct, well-organized volume provides administrators with systematic, relevant, and valuable knowledge that will enable them to promote individual, group, and organizational change. It is a valuable volume for professionals in the consultation field and in the field of guiding organizational change, because it provides and sets the stage for direction for further study. Major bibliographic indexes were manually reviewed; therefore, most of the items listed are available through various library services. The major indexing services—ERIC, PsycLit, PAIS, Dissertation Abstracts, Sociofile, and Social Science Index—were also consulted for sources of data. This is a fine work of carefully selected materials in the area of organizational change via consultants. The volume is a must for every advanced student of organizational behavior and especially in the area specialty of consultation for change.—**Gerald D. Moran**

BIOGRAPHY

436. **Biographical Dictionary of Psychology.** Noel Sheehy, Antony J. Chapman, and Wendy A. Conroy, eds. New York, Routledge, 1997. 675p. index. $130.00. ISBN 0-415-09997-8.

Biographical Dictionary of Psychology serves as a current update and expansion of information previously published in Greenwood Press's *Biographical Dictionary of Psychology* (see ARBA 85, entry 666); *A Guide to Psychologists and Their Concepts* (see ARBA 76, entry 1504); and *Women in Psychology: A Bio-bibliographic Sourcebook* (see ARBA 91, entry 918). This resource incorporates biographical information on 500-plus psychologists and individuals who have contributed to the field of psychology. The scope is international and runs from the late 1700s through the late 1900s. The methodology used by the editors in choosing entries included surveying several reference sources in the psychology literature. From that review, additional lists were created and ranked; then experts in the field were consulted and the list was reduced to its current number. It is noted that some individuals chose not to respond, so the editors were not able to produce a substantial entry, and therefore the individual was not included.

Each entry includes name; date and place of birth, and date and place of death if appropriate; nationality; main area of interest according to the American Psychological Association standards; education; principal appointments, honors, and awards; principal publications; and suggested references for further reading. The most confounding part of the entries is the lack of entries on the women who are part of the number of husband-wife teams of psychologists who have similar research interests, complement, and in most cases, enhance their husbands' research. There is not a separate or even supplemental statement about their contributions. In many cases, in the husband's entry, these contributions are not even acknowledged. Aside from this observation, the entries are clearly written using three-quarters to a full page. The only other piece of information missing is current institutional affiliation. [R: RBB, 15 Oct 97, pp. 425-426]—**Mila C. Su**

437. **Portraits of Pioneers in Psychology, Volume 3.** Gregory A. Kimble and Michael Wertheimer, eds. Washington, D.C., American Psychological Association, 1998. 363p. index. $79.95pa. ISBN 1-55798-479-4.

The preface of *Portraits of Pioneers in Psychology* states that the set presents "informal portraits of some of the giants in the history of psychology." The editors' purpose for this book is to provide collateral source material for undergraduate and graduate courses in the history of psychology. There are 20 portraits in the book ranging in length from 16 to 24 pages. Following the preface, the editors include a section containing brief sketches of the authors and editors.

The subjects of the biographies run the gamut from those whose names are instantly recognized by almost anyone, such as Alfred Binet and B. F. Skinner, to others to whom this reviewer was introduced for the first time in this volume. Because a different author or authors write each review, the writing varies from chapter to chapter, as does the organization of each chapter. Each chapter contains information about the personal life of the psychologist, his or her professional life, and a description of the contributions he or she made to the field of psychology. Some of the biographers did not know their subject personally because they died in the late nineteenth or early twentieth century. Others were coworkers, students, or relatives of the subjects. Myrtle McGraw's chapter contains her life story in her own words, a window into the thought processes of an important influence in modern psychology.

This reference book provides the information the editors intended it to: supplementary information on seminal figures in the history of psychology. Although the entire set would be more useful in a reference collection, volume 3 can stand alone if necessary. It will be useful for student researchers or anyone interested in the history of psychology. [R: Choice, Sept 98, p. 224] —**Nancy P. Reed**

DICTIONARIES AND ENCYCLOPEDIAS

438. **Baker Encyclopedia of Psychology and Counseling.** 2d ed. David G. Benner and Peter C. Hill, eds. Grand Rapids, Mich., Baker Book House, 1999. 1276p. (Baker Reference Library). $59.99. ISBN 0-8010-2100-6.

This is the 2d edition of a work born out of an awareness of the need for a comprehensive treatment of psychology from a Christian point of view. Not only do articles present psychology in its own terms, but many also contain a biblical or theological perspective. This new edition gives more attention to pastoral care and counseling than the 1st edition, and includes a large number of new articles that explore issues of particular interest to clergy, Christian counselors, and mental health practitioners.

Included in this edition are articles covering psychological fields of specialization and professional organizations; people who have contributed to the field of psychology; systems and theories; human development; learning, cognition, and intelligence; sexuality, marriage, and family; social behavior; personality; psychopathology; and pastoral psychology and counseling. The signed articles are arranged alphabetically and most conclude with reference or reading lists. Article contributors include academicians and practitioners who specialize in psychology, psychiatry, social work, and pastoral care. Each was chosen for his or her involvement in the current discussion of the relationship between psychology and Christianity. Aids for use of the book include guide words at the top of each page, headings for articles and subdivisions of articles in bold type-face, and a category index. [R: Choice, Nov 99, p. 506]—**Dana McDougald**

439.   Campbell, Robert Jean. **Psychiatric Dictionary.** 7th ed. New York, Oxford University Press, 1996. 799p. $59.95. ISBN 0-19-510259-2.

In preparing the present volume, Campbell has made use of the 4th edition of the American Psychiatric Association's *Diagnostic and Statistical Manual of Mental Disorders* (DSM-IV) (1994), the 10th revision of the *International Statistical Classification of Diseases and Related Health Problems* (ICD-10) (World Health Organization, 1994), and the World Health Organization's lexicons on mental disorders. Some of the 12,311 entries are fascinating; for instance, *insanity* is now obsolete as a medical term (it is still used in its legal sense). Also, a distinction exists between the word *fantasy* (spelled with an "f" and referring to conscious constructions) and the word *phantasy* (spelled with a "ph" and referring to unconscious constructions). Some of the entries go beyond prose definitions to include tables, such as the "Table of Manias and Philias" that is part of the "mania" entry.

It is refreshing to see the author, a Cornell medical school professor as well as director of a New York City hospital, demonstrate open-mindedness toward the supernatural. The word *shaman* is defined as "[a] practitioner whose ability to heal comes from trancelike experiences and inspiration from a supernatural spirit-partner with whom he works in curing sick people" (p. 666). One thing the reader will not find in this work is entries for individual drugs, neither under their brand names (e.g., Prozac) nor under their generic names (e.g., fluoxetine). This is not a failing, because drugs do not really have definitions per se, and anyhow, there would be too many to include even if they did. Campbell does refer to fluoxetine, however (among other drugs listed in the "antidepressant" entry).

One of the stated aims of this work is to provide a dictionary that is comprehensible to the nonspecialist, and Campbell achieves that aim. For this reason, this work is recommended for libraries supporting degree programs in psychology, counseling, and social work. As for selection by medical school libraries, the dictionary is a must; however, it does not replace the DSM-IV or the ICD-10.—**Lambrini Papangelis**

440.   **The Corsini Encyclopedia of Psychology and Behavioral Science.** 3d ed. W. Edward Craighead and Charles B. Nemeroff, eds. New York, John Wiley, 2001. 4v. index. $600.00/set. ISBN 0-471-23949-6.

Psychologists, psychiatrists, and behavioral scholars have known about the usefulness of the *Encyclopedia of Psychology* for decades. It is known for its concise, unbiased, and factually based articles; a go-to source when someone wanted a no-nonsense, fast, ready-reference source. This is the 3d edition of this valuable source and in honor of its former editor, the set has been renamed *The Corsini Encyclopedia of Psychology and Behavioral Science.*

Craighead and Nemeroff, the present editors, have done a masterful job in keeping to the philosophy of Raymond Corsini: that the work must first of all be of immediate value and not become a museum piece. They have extensively re-edited the work, removing up to a third of the texts concerning moribund or outdated topics. They have updated about two-thirds of the prior edition and replaced the excised third with new topics.

Under the editorship of Corsini, the encyclopedia has always championed an international flavor of topics and this tradition is carried on in this edition as an international array of scholars give their intelligence to this set. Perhaps what is most amazing is the restraint shown by the editors. This encyclopedia, resting on its famous laurels, could have easily become a bloated and turgid exercise in grandiose exposition. However it instead emphasizes a Spartan utility and keeps its articles tightly written, succinct summaries. This work is strongly recommended even for libraries possessing the earlier editions. [R: LJ, 15 Feb 01, p. 156; AG, Feb 01, p. 49]—**Glenn Masuchika**

441.   Corsini, Raymond J. **Dictionary of Psychology.** Philadelphia, Taylor & Francis, 1999. 1156p. $124.95. ISBN 1-58391-028-X.

The author of *The Encyclopedia of Psychology* and *The Concise Encyclopedia of Psychology* (John Wiley, 1994 and 1996, respectively) has produced another outstanding reference work in this discipline. The preface states that the dictionary was developed from interviews with about 100 randomly selected psychologists who were asked what they wanted and did not want in a dictionary of psychology. Based on this, it includes more than three times the number of headwords, illustrations, biographies, and appendixes of any other dictionary of psychology in English. Its 30,000 entries include words and concepts from every area of psychology, including clinical, social, experimental, and physiological psychology. Commonly used, psychologically oriented phrases like "glass ceiling" and "worst scenario"; historical expressions like "sacred disease" for epilepsy; and some slang, foreign, and obsolete terms are included.

Its 10 appendixes comprise prefixes, suffixes, and affixes; DSM-IV categories; the Greek alphabet; medical prescription terms; systems of treatment; tests and measurements; symbols; leaning theory symbols; Rorschach descriptors; and mini-biographies of deceased persons important to the history of psychology. Headwords are presented in their natural order and definitions are short (averaging 31 words). Developed for psychologists and students of psychology and likely to become the standard scholarly resource, this dictionary's clear language, user-friendly organization, and unparalleled comprehensiveness will also serve a wider range of users in academic and large public libraries.—**Madeleine Nash**

442.   **Dictionary of Biological Psychology.** Philip Winn, ed. New York, Routledge, 2001. 857p. $140.00. ISBN 0-415-13606-7.

Winn, associated with the School of Psychology at Scotland's University of St. Andrews, notes in the introduction to this excellent reference work that "in order to understand modern psychology, it is increasingly necessary to use an eclectic vocabulary drawn from . . . biology, information theory, computer science, the neurosciences . . . as well as the technical language of psychology and its various disciplines" (p. xiii). As a result, this broadly based dictionary was compiled to cover the multiple parameters of what the Library of Congress identifies as psychobiology. Although users must cope with British spellings, they largely occur at the end of a word and do not hinder alphabetical location. In addition, there is a comprehensive use of *see* references, and, within an entry, small capitals indicate terms defined elsewhere (e.g., an entry on *epigenesis* has *development* and *embryo* as additional entries to consult).

A quick search of reference sources revealed no other print reference dictionary that was focused on biological psychology or psychobiology although a *Biological Psychology Dictionary* by James W. Kalat was found at http://psychology.wadsworth.com. Kalat has also authored texts on biological psychology that are available in print. In addition, several significant and comprehensive dictionaries of psychology, notably Raymond J. Corsini's *Dictionary of Psychology* (see entry 441), are available. However, the Winn compilation is the essential resource dealing with the fact that "psychological processes are increasingly thought of as being biological in nature" (p. xiii), and students, postgraduates, and researchers must understand the terms found within the biological sciences.

All the key ingredients of a good reference source are found in this volume: an editorial board and list of contributors (mainly drawn from Canada, England, Scotland, and Wales with a smattering from the United States); a clear-cut "How to Use This Dictionary"; a list of references;

a glossary of abbreviations; a table of Greek letters; and a well-designed, highly readable A-Z dictionary with cross-references. The entries range from brief to extensive to long paragraph entries. Many of the entries over 50 words are signed and often include 1 or 2 references. There are a limited number of tables in the work (e.g., "The Cardiovascular System Simplified" on page 111 or "Sensory Receptors of the Skin" on page 721). No illustrations or diagrams are included. All in all, the work is highly recommended as an acquisition for all academic and special reference collections that serve the many faces of psychology. [R: AG, Sept 01, p. 62]—**Laurel Grotzinger**

443.   **Encyclopedia of Mental Health.** Howard S. Friedman, ed. San Diego, Calif., Academic Press, 1998. 3v. illus. index. $500.00/set. ISBN 0-12-226675-7.

The concept of mental health has changed a great deal. Current research demonstrates the intricate relationship of the mind and body. Biochemical imbalances play significant roles in schizophrenia and various mood disorders. Ordinary activities such as commuting and using a computer affect behavior. This new encyclopedia examines mental health using an interdisciplinary approach. It emphasizes health by looking at ways to promote wellness and prevent mental illness.

The encyclopedia editor and contributors are academics who are acknowledged experts in their fields. Their names and affiliations appear at the beginning of each article. Most of the material here is new, but some entries are reprinted from the *Encyclopedia of Human Behavior* (see ARBA 95, entry 778). This is noted at the end of the article. The 3 volumes contain alphabetically arranged articles that are 10 to 20 pages long. Each article begins with an outline and a glossary defining terms as they are used specifically within the context of that article. All articles have bibliographies. Each volume contains the table of contents for the entire set and instructions for using the encyclopedia. There is a detailed index in volume 3. Using the index ensures finding all relevant material on a given subject area because the articles cover broad topics. Cross-references also direct users to related material.

The articles cover a wide range of subjects: adolescence, commuting and mental health, human-computer interaction, mental hospitals and deinstitutionalization, brain scanning and neuroimaging, and psychopharmacology. Specific conditions and therapies are covered as well, including Alzheimer's disease, mood disorders, behavior therapy, and family therapy. A search for information about recovered memory turned up nothing in the table of contents. There is no specific index entry either. Bits and pieces show up under dissociative disorders, hypnosis, and child sexual abuse, but there is no article on this controversial topic.

This is, however, a fine encyclopedia with a great deal of excellent information on subjects of interest to both professional and educated lay readers. Academic, health science, and large public libraries will find it useful. [R: Choice, Sept 98, p. 92]—**Barbara M. Bibel**

444.   **The Encyclopedia of Psychiatry, Psychology, and Psychoanalysis.** Benjamin B. Wolman, ed. New York, Henry Holt, 1996. 649p. index. $135.00. ISBN 0-8050-2234-1.

This single-volume resource is a product of the same editorial team that produced the *International Encyclopedia of Psychiatry, Psychology, Psychoanalysis, and Neurology* (see ARBA 78, entry 1367), which won the Dartmouth Medal from the American Library Association. That 12-volume set was lauded for its comprehensiveness and currentness. The volume under review not only abridges the larger work but also revises and updates the entries, and it endeavors to cover the advancements of the past 20 years of the topics at hand. Neurology has been omitted from this encyclopedia but will be the topic of a separate volume.

Adhering to the A to Z format found in the larger encyclopedia, this volume provides articles on a variety of topics, from abortion to human immunodeficiency virus and acquired immunodeficiency syndrome to stimulus-response theories in social psychology. The entries are signed by one of the nearly 700 contributing authors, many of whom hold Ph.D.s or M.D.s. Scope of the articles covers studies conducted (with the year), important statistics, people active in that particular study, and related concepts. They cover basic ground without delving too deeply into complex ideas. Much of the biographical information is brief, so brief as to be of little value to most users. A useful bibliography complements the body of the encyclopedia. The index is functional, providing *see also* references to related terms.

The intended audience for this one-volume encyclopedia is professionals in the fields discussed and graduate students or postdoctoral scholars. For its ready-reference value, one can easily see that audience making good use of the volume. It is doubtful that professional psychiatrists or psychologists would have a need for this volume beyond ready-reference; the same holds true for students. The articles are not in-depth enough for the book to serve as a textbook or as an answer-all encyclopedia. However, for quick answers to questions involving psychology, psychiatry, and psychoanalysis, this somewhat reasonably priced encyclopedia will be helpful to that audience not having access to the full 12-volume set.—**Melissa Rae Root**

445.   **Encyclopedia of Psychology.** Alan E. Kazdin, ed. New York, American Psychological Association/Oxford University Press, 2000. 8v. index. $995.00/set. ISBN 1-55798-187-6.

The broad scope of the science of psychology presented a daunting challenge to the creators of this eight-volume encyclopedia. What should be included, how should these topics be handled, and how to present sufficient international coverage are only a few of the difficulties encountered by the senior editorial staff drawn from the American Psychological Association and Oxford University Press who labored jointly for eight years on this project. Their final product fully justifies all their efforts. More than 1,400 contributors, many the leading scholars in their specialties, produced over 1,500 entries, including some 400 biographies of major figures in psychology's history.

Entries vary in length from half a page to extensive, multipage coverage. Topics range in scope from narrowly defined subjects (e.g., deafness, cancer, xenophobia) to extremely broad conceptual entries (e.g., emotion, peace, creativity). Special attention is given to the historical aspects of the subjects covered, thus making this work an indispensable resource for the history of psychology. An additional useful feature is overview articles describing the development of psychology in specific countries or regions of the world. Partially annotated bibliographies are provided for every entry—a most helpful feature—with citations coming from both historical and current literature. The use of extensive cross-indexing in the text and a comprehensive master index in volume 8 provides easy access to this encyclopedia's treasury of information. As with any large-scale project the quality of the writing varies between entries and some articles contain factual errors. For example, the famous Roman era physician, Galen of Pergamon, is misdated and the section on informed consent omits the key legal case that established this legal doctrine in 1957. However, taken as a whole this reference tool is a reliable source.

The editors and contributors of this encyclopedia are to be congratulated for creating a reference work that will be of immeasurable assistance for anyone seeking information concerning both the history and current state of the science of psychology. These volumes are a valuable addition to the reference collection of all academic, healthcare, and large public libraries. [R: LJ, 15 Mar 2000, p. 72; BL, Aug 2000, p. 2190; Choice, Nov 2000, p. 511; RUSQ, Summer 01, pp. 381-382]—**Jonathon Erlen**

446.   **Encyclopedia of Psychology. http://www.psychology.org/.** [Website]. Free. Date reviewed: Nov 02.

This site, hosted by the Department of Psychology at Jacksonville State University, has two goals: to provide links to original research findings from respected practitioners in the various fields of psychology, and to provide a "hierarchical" database that links to information on the scientific aspects of psychology. Users can search by 8 categories, which list the number of links they connect to. These include: Career, People and History, Environment Behavior Relationships, Publications, Resources, Organizations, Underlying Reductionistic Machinery (biological factors related to psychology), and Paradigms and Theories. The larger categories, such as Environmental Behavior Relationships with 1,016 links, are broken down into smaller, more manageable categories (e.g., addiction, intelligence, marriage). The Web pages that this site links to are full of information and current research. The host asks for feedback from users for additional sites that should be added or modifications that need to be made. This will be a useful site for those doing research in the field of psychology at the undergraduate and upper-graduate levels.—**Shannon Graff Hysell**

447.   **Encyclopedia of Psychotherapy.** Michel Hersen and William Sledge, eds. San Diego, Calif., Academic Press, 2002. 2v. index. $450.00/set. ISBN 0-12-343010-0.

The use of the word "psychotherapy" in a reference title along with a classification as an encyclopedia is highly unusual. Although the term appeared in the late nineteenth century and emerged fully in the twentieth century, a search for encyclopedias of psychotherapy in WorldCat from OCLC retrieves only seven English titles. The volume under review is the sole item clearly described as an "encyclopedia of psychotherapy." Two or three titles use dictionary in their names, and the others presumably have the content if not a title designation. As a result, the volumes reviewed here claim the attention of all psychology reference librarians as well as the students, researchers, and clinicians in the field. Attention should also be given to the four-volume *Comprehensive Handbook of Psychotherapy* (see entry 461), which provides additional recent coverage that might also be considered encyclopedic. At the same time, it should be noted that psychotherapy, the use of psychological rather than physical measures, is a term associated with or implied in the use of many terms, including psychology practices, mental health care, treatment plans, psychiatric disorder management, clinical psychology, and others. ARBA has published numerous reviews of encyclopedias, handbooks, and dictionaries covering these terms in recent decades.

Without a doubt, there is a tremendous confluence of authority, research, and breadth of coverage in this encyclopedia. Hersen, Sledge, four associate editors, and a strong editorial advisory board have compiled and edited "a comprehensive reference to extant knowledge in the field" (p. xvii). As expected, the articles are arranged alphabetically, but the nature of the title would not be obvious since some describe a treatment, some refer to the patient treated, some are theoretical, and so on. Entries range from relatively short (2 to 3 pages) to lengthy (15 or more pages), and many include a glossary, description of treatment, case illustration, theoretical basis, applications and exclusions, empirical studies, summary, and further reading (e.g., "Competing Response Training") . Some articles, however, do not lend themselves to this approach; for example, "Behavior Therapy: Historical Perspective and Overview" includes a glossary, brief history, conceptual foundations, science and practice, and then a summary and further readings, or "Self-Help Groups" that covers an overview and history, a description of how self-help groups work, effectiveness, and the future. Still others, such as the entry on "Flooding," include brief commentaries on theoretical bases and empirical support. All include a glossary, a summary, *see also* references, and bibliographic citations. A few articles also have tables to display information, but there are no illustrations.

The contributors and their affiliations are identified in volume 2 just before a detailed subject index. The volumes are well designed and printed but given the breadth of the subject, coverage is inevitably weaker in some areas than others—and the motivation and organization of the articles varies from instructional to general informational to specialized purposes. [R: LJ, 15 Oct 02, p. 62]—**Laurel Grotzinger**

448.   **The Freud Encyclopedia: Theory, Therapy, and Culture.** Edward Erwin, ed. New York, Routledge, 2002. 641p. index. $165.00. ISBN 0-415-93677-2.

No other individual in psychology congers up an immediate image and opinion from the general public such as Sigmund Freud. His influence on mass culture and language cannot be disputed. In this single volume, 238 articles cover a fascinating array of topics on the history, science, and philosophy of psychology. Articles cover historical figures that have influenced, or were influenced by, Freud and psychoanalytic theories and concepts and their worldwide development. Arrangement is alphabetic, with article length averaging three to eight pages. A comprehensive index provides good access to article contents. Many articles make a discussion of primary source material, particularly in the article on Sigmund Freud, and contain bibliographies that make this work an excellent source for the students seeking further resources.

The unique feature of this encyclopedia is the combination of both the historical focus and the inclusion of a modern interpretation, or updating, of Freud's ideas in light of current research. Criticism is intelligent and balanced. This aspect is particularly evident in the article on dream theory. Specific examples of Freud's theory are contrasted against current findings, criticized but not discarded. Rather, they are updated to the benefit of both the old theory and the new research. Readers can find many of the same topics discussed in other excellent psychology encyclopedias, but none will have the same focus and depth.

A student wanting to do a paper on Freudian slips can find excellent, but very different, articles in this encyclopedia and in Kazdin's *Encyclopedia of Psychology* (see entry 445). Where the focus will be broader in scope with less historical information in Kazdin, the Erwin volume provides good historical information on Freud's theory, a discussion of his psychoanalytic approach, and current research. This encyclopedia is written at a level that may pose a challenge for the average undergraduate. The intended audience is not stated in the preface, but most articles appear to assume some prior knowledge of Freudian theory. It is an excellent resource for psychology majors, students of philosophy, graduate students, or researchers. [R: LJ, 1 Mar 02, p. 86; Choice, May 02, p. 1562]—**Lorraine Evans**

449.   **The Gale Encyclopedia of Mental Disorders.** Ellen Thackery and Madeline Harris, eds. Farmington Hills, Mich., Gale, 2003. 2v. illus. index. $250.00/set. ISBN 0-7876-5768-9.

Some 30 million people visit physicians and 2 million spend time in hospitals every year due to mental disorders. Many people visit a library to learn more about them. *The Gale Encyclopedia of Mental Disorders* provides a good overview of mental illness, psychotherapy, and other treatments. Medical writers, pharmacists, and mental health professionals wrote and edited the 400 signed, alphabetic entries in the set.

The entries cover disorders (anorexia nervosa, schizophrenia), diagnostic procedures and techniques (magnetic resonance imaging, Kaufman Short Neurological Assessment Procedure), therapies (behavior modification, electroconvulsive therapy), medicines and herbs (Paroxetine, St. Johns Wort), and related topics (advance directives, neurotransmitters). Entries for disorders include a definition, description, cause and symptoms, demographics, diagnosis, treatments, prognosis, and prevention. Those for medications contain the definition, purpose, description, recommended dosage, precautions, side effects, and interactions. Entries for herbs and supplements have a leaf icon next to the heading. All entries have a resource list of print and electronic sources and organizations to contact. Some 100 black-and-white photographs and charts illustrate the text. A color photograph gallery repeated in both volumes has enhanced versions of some of the photographs. There are ample cross-references, making it easy to locate drugs, which are entered by generic name. Boxes with definitions of key terms help readers understand the material. A full glossary is at the end of volume 2. Users will find a symptom list here also, which demonstrates patterns that are linked to various disorders.

Although there is some overlap with *The Gale Encyclopedia of Medicine* (2d ed.; see entry 158), *The Gale Encyclopedia of Mental Disorders* offers more detailed coverage of psychiatric disorders and their treatments. The articles are more accessible than those in a medical textbook or the DSM-IV-TR, but they still require a fairly high level of literacy. This is an excellent resource for public, academic, and consumer health libraries. —**Barbara M. Bibel**

450.   **Internet Mental Health. http://www.mentalhealth.com/.** [Website]. Free. Date reviewed: Sept 02.

Internet Mental Health was designed by Canadian psychiatrist Phillip Long to make much-needed mental health information available to those in the profession, mental health patients and their families, support groups, and students. The site provides information on disorders, such as schizophrenia, anxiety disorders, alcohol dependence, and many more. Each disorder is given an American description, a European description, a general description of how it can be treated, recent research and important past research, and downloadable pamphlets from mental health organizations and agencies (e.g., American Psychiatric Association). Users can also research common psychiatric medications on this site. Each medication description provides information on pharmacology, indications and counterindications, adverse effects, dosage and overdosage, and precautions to take when on the drug.

Users are provided with additional resources to consult (e.g., articles, books, booklets, news, newsletters, and stories of recovery) through the "Magazine" and "Research" links. The site also provides links to related Internet sites, generally those of official agencies and organizations (e.g., Anxiety Disorders Association of America). A list of one to three asterisks following the site indicates the sites popularity. Diagnosis programs are available by linking to Dr. Long's related site, MyTherapy.com, for a fee.

The information provided here is lengthy and authoritative. While written in easy-to-understand language, it will still be best understood by those with some upper-level education. This will be a useful place for those researching mental health disorders to begin their research.—**Shannon Graff Hysell**

451.   Kahn, Ada P., and Jan Fawcett. **The Encyclopedia of Mental Health.** 2d ed. New York, Facts on File, 2001. 468p. index. (Facts on File Library of Health and Living). $71.50. ISBN 0-8160-4062-1.

The 2d edition of *The Encyclopedia of Mental Health* (1st ed.; see ARBA 95, entry 780) adds new articles that relate to the contemporary issues and cross-cultural influences on mental health. This encyclopedia is for the layperson's use and reference. The entries are arranged alphabetically and more than a few have at least one cross-reference. There is a comprehensive index as well as appendixes, which contain a bibliography and a resource section that lists related organizations with addresses and telephone numbers for further research.

Many of the criticisms for the 1st edition review remain the same for the 2d edition. The appendix of organizations still has no listing for the National Association of School Psychologists or the National Association of Social Workers. The bibliography still has the notable omission of a category for school-related problems such as learning disabilities. The authors have dealt with the issue of the angry woman syndrome entry by leaving the entry out in the 2d edition, which is disturbing. Does this mean that this disorder does not exist or that the authors believed the solution to the issue was to delete the entry entirely?

The authors view the book's use as helping "readers put terminology into better perspective and be more empowered to sort through the vast language explosion in this area." Again, the authors succeed with providing their goals. This will be useful for a general definition for a topic on mental health. Public libraries and colleges will find this a useful resource for their users. [R: LJ, 1

April 02, p. 94; BR, May/June 02, p. 64; Choice, April 02, pp. 1397-1398]—**Sandhya D. Srivastava**

452. **Learning & Memory.** 2d ed. John H. Byrne, ed. New York, Macmillan Reference USA/Gale Group, 2003. 716p. illus. index. (Macmillan Psychology Reference Series). $130.00. ISBN 0-02-865619-9.

In the 2d edition of *Learning & Memory* Macmillan Reference has provided an excellent resource for the theoretical underpinnings of educational psychology, learning, and memory. As a thorough revision of the 1st edition, this resource has been updated to reflect the most up-to-date information about learning and memory and includes a number of new entries. The book contains a large amount of information in a single volume, and the entries were written by a distinguished list of contributors. These entries are well written and fairly easy to understand for an undergraduate-level reader.

The book is well laid out for ease of use. The indexing is complete, and there are plenty of *see* and *see also* notes to guide the user in his or her search for information. A bibliography at the end of each entry guides the reader to further information if needed. The illustrations and charts are clear and generally informative. The only things missing from this resource are color illustrations, which would have been useful for clarifying many of the entries. Overall, this book will be a useful addition for academic libraries, and the price is low enough that larger public libraries with patrons working on rather in-depth psychological reading could purchase it as well. [R: LJ, Jan 03, p. 92]—**Mark T. Bay**

453. Noll, Richard. **The Encyclopedia of Schizophrenia and Other Psychotic Disorders.** 2d ed. New York, Facts on File, 2000. 344p. index. $60.00. ISBN 0-8160-4070-2.

This informative encyclopedia provides an overview of the topic, aiming for a better understanding of schizophrenia and associated psychotic disorders. More than 2 centuries of historical, biographical, and clinical information is included about a disease that affects more than 2 million people in the United States and Canada, and which costs the United States more than $70 billion annually.

A brief history of schizophrenia precedes the entries, which were selected for their continuing usefulness, and which vary in length from a few lines to a page. Many contain *see* and *see also* references as well as references to DSM-IV and ICD-10 standard diagnostic manuals. Reference sources are included in each entry to encourage further research. Four appendixes have diagnostic criteria and directories of organizations associated with schizophrenia and with other mental illnesses. An index of names and subjects provides additional access.

As with many books covering such a wide topic, lack of detail in individual entries is offset by an extensive list of other resources. This reference work summarizes past research and promotes future inquiry into a prevalent, devastating brain disease. [R: LJ, Jan 01, pp. 90-92]—**Anita Zutis**

454. **Psychology and Mental Health.** Jaclyn Rodriguez, ed. Hackensack, N.J., Salem Press, 2001. 2v. illus. index. (Magill's Choice). $95.00/set. ISBN 0-89356-066-9.

On its own merits, *Psychology and Mental Health* is an easily accessible work for the general audience or high school or college students, with a focus on abnormal behavior, psychopathology, emotional disorders, and treatments. It is, however, largely a shortened reprint of *Magill's Survey of Social Science: Psychology* (1993) and *Magill's Medical Guide* (2d rev. ed.; see entry 165). There are minor updates to the bibliographies.

The 107 articles are in alphabetic order. Each topic is introduced by "Type of Psychology" and "Fields of Study" headings that categorize the subject within the larger discipline. The topic is defined and the principal terms are followed by the text of the article. Each article contains an annotated bibliography and cross-references. A category list, allowing a subject breakdown of the contents, and an index to subjects and names are provided. The format, structure, and article text is basically unchanged from the previous *Magill's Survey*. Updating consists of the addition of several newer references for each article. For the most part, updated references refer to books or manuals, not the most recent research findings. This is appropriate for a general audience, but not the individual requiring in-depth, current literature. This would be a good addition for the basic collection that does not already include the larger 1993 edition or more current and comprehensive psychology encyclopedias. [R: Choice, June 01, p. 1778]—**Lorraine Evans**

455.   Roesch, Robert. **The Encyclopedia of Depression.** 2d ed. New York, Facts on File, 2001. 278p. index. (Facts on File Library of Health and Living). $60.50. ISBN 0-8160-4047-8.

Since the National Institute of Mental Health estimates that 20 million Americans, ranging from children to senior citizens, are affected by depression (p. v), it is important for libraries to offer information about this illness to its patrons. This volume, which contains a wide variety of current information on depression in a dictionary format of almost 600 entries, fills the need very well.

The book features the latest information on the various aspects of the disease, options for treatment, leading scholars, and current research. One of the most interesting features is a fascinating look at famous individuals who have suffered from depression. For example, some theologians consider the biblical Job to be a victim of reactive depression (pp. 117-118). The entries are fully cross-indexed, with sources used cited where applicable.

The book boasts seven appendixes. Two of the most helpful are those that cover a list of psychiatric drugs and sources of information. This last appendix lists agencies and organizations in the United States, Canada, and the United Nations, and major English-language journals dealing with all aspects of depression. An extensive bibliography and full index complete the volume. This is a valuable book for any reference collection as it fills a need even in smaller medical collections. It is a recommended purchase for any public library. [R: BL, 1 Sept 01, pp. 150-152]—**Nancy P. Reed**

456.   Zuckerman, Edward L. **Clinician's Thesaurus.** 5th ed. New York, Guilford, 2000. 385p. index. $35.00pa. ISBN 1-57230-569-X.

The *Clinician's Thesaurus*, now in its 5th edition, continues to provide mental health professionals at all levels with an excellent guide through the client assessment and report writing process. The book's arrangement has varied since its 1st revision (see ARBA 91, entry 791). The current edition is divided into three major sections, with further subdivisions indicated by bold, underlined, numbered headings. The first section assists the user in conducting full mental health evaluations. The questions follow a logical sequence, use appropriate terminology, and allow the user to select items reflective of their personal style. The second section explores the terminology used in writing psychological reports. Again, the layout follows a logical sequence, guiding the practitioner from start to finish. Highlights include standard words and phrases, alternatives, and clear examples of how—and how *not*—to say things appropriately. The third section, entitled "Useful Resources," introduces two features new to the 5th edition: reproducible forms for writing treatment plans compatible with managed care and an updated list of psychotropic medications.

Other new features include reproducible mental status evaluation forms, a combined introduction and overview, and an annotated list of suggestions for further reading. The book also has a lay-flat binding for convenience and durability.—**Leanne M. VandeCreek**

DIRECTORIES

457. **The Complete Mental Health Directory, 2002: A Comprehensive Source Book for Individuals and Professionals.** 3d ed. Lakeville, Conn., Grey House Publishing, 2002. 687p. index. $190.00; $165.00pa. ISBN 0-930956-07-X; 1-930956-06-1pa.

458. **The Complete Mental Health Directory. http://www.greyhouse.com**. [Website]. Millerton, N.Y., Grey House Publishing. $215.00/year subscription; $300.00 (w/purchase of print directory). Date reviewed: May 02.

This directory, available both online and as a book, is invaluable for health professionals and people researching a particular mental health disorder. The directory covers 24 broad categories of mental disorders with particular disorders described in each. For example, the section on impulse control disorders includes kleptomania, pyromania, pathological gambling, and so on. After a brief description, associations, agencies, books, Websites, support groups, and hotlines are then listed for these disorders. Information on addresses, telephone numbers, prices, and the people in charge is very complete.

This resource could be used a number of ways. A health professional could use it to enrich his or her own knowledge, to help a patient, or as a referral tool for advising patients. Library professionals could use it as a selection tool for books and a research tool for Websites in the health field. Finally, high school and college students will find it very helpful for writing papers in psychology.—**Carol D. Henry**

459. Grohol, John M. **The Insider's Guide to Mental Health Resources Online.** 2002/03 ed. New York, Guilford Press, 2002. 309p. index. $21.95pa. ISBN 1-57230-754-4.

Now in its 4th edition, this guide for professionals is also invaluable for students and others with a strong interest in mental health. It describes hundreds of online mental health resources, including Websites, databases, and search tools, as well as communication vehicles like chat rooms, newsgroups, and listservs. Changes from the 2000/01 edition (see ARBA 2001, entry 767) include coverage of more than 40 new resources, updated reviews and critical ratings of sites from previous editions, and current URL and e-mail addresses. There continues to be an accompanying Website that provides ongoing updates to the current edition.

Grohol is a psychologist whose vast experience includes co-founding the search guide *Mental Health Net*, building the mental health center at *drkoop.com*, and creating *Psych Central* (his own highly regarded Website located at http://psychcentral.com). His selection of key resources and lesser-known sites gives the book its "insider" quality, while clear writing and good organization make the large amount of information understandable. The author's method of evaluating Websites is fully explained and includes a four-star rating system.

The book is arranged into three parts. The first is an orientation to the basic features of the online world, such as the Web, search engines, and search strategies. The second covers specific topics of interest, including finding treatment information online, networking with other professionals, and finding and downloading psychology-related software. The third part features online resources for patient education and self help. Four appendixes comprise a glossary of terms, resources for further reading, ways to get online, and basics of creating a Website. A general index and an index of Websites are also included. This book serves Internet novices and old timers equally well and is highly recommended for all libraries.—**Madeleine Nash**

460. Pagliaro, Louis A., and Ann Marie Pagliaro. **Psychologists' Psychotropic Desk Reference.** Bristol, Pa., Taylor & Francis, 1999. 704p. index. $59.95. ISBN 0-87630-964-3.

The *Psychologists' Psychotropic Drug Reference* (PPDR) provides essential information on a variety of prescription drugs commonly used in the treatment of psychological disorders. Intended for use by practicing psychologists and as a guide for psychology graduate students, it is a valuable ready-reference source of psychotropic drugs often prescribed in North America. The authors are careful to point out that current guidelines are cited for the prescription of the psychotropic drugs that should be considered supplemental to clinical psychotherapy treatment. Other medical personnel and well-educated family members will also appreciate the comprehensive treatment of each drug included.

Organized in a similar fashion to the *Physicians' Desk Reference* (56th ed.; see entry 412), the main section begins with an alphabetic list of drugs by generic name. Categories range from antidepressants to benzodiazepine and opiate analgesic antagonists. Each entry has several components on such topics as the therapeutic action of the drug, any possible adverse reactions, and toxicity symptoms, which might be confused with and worsened by psychological disorders. There is comprehensive coverage of clinically significant drug interactions, overdose amounts, and the resulting symptoms. Respected authorities in the field of psychology, university professors, or program directors have contributed to a useful category titled "Cautions and Comments." This section delineates increased risk factors in a patient's condition, which may alter the effect of the drug. Other conditions of prescribing each drug are explored, such as the usual dosage and method of administration, and the physical characteristics of the absorption of the drug.

An alphabetically arranged subject index, which includes brand names, is located at the back of the volume. A section devoted to references cited facilitates further research. One of the most helpful appendixes included gives the pharmacologic classification and listing of all drugs included in the PPDR. Also included are the U.S. Drug Enforcement Agency Schedule Designations and the Food and Drug Administration Pregnancy Categories. The final appendix lists the abbreviations and symbols found in the entries. The intended audience will find this and future editions an easy-to-use reference tool.—**Marianne B. Eimer**

HANDBOOKS AND YEARBOOKS

461. **Comprehensive Handbook of Psychotherapy.** Florence W. Kaslow and Jeffrey J. Magnavita, eds. New York, John Wiley, 2002. 4v. index. $600.00/set. ISBN 0-471-01848-1.

The theories and practice of psychotherapy have undergone significant changes in the past decades. New trends and current knowledge and practices in the field are explored in this four-volume work, whose comprehensive coverage ranges from psychodynamic to cognitive, behavioral, humanistic, and eclectic theories. Contributing authors have achieved recognition in their respective fields and are from around the world, a reflection of the globalization of the discipline itself. Graduate students, professors, clinicians, and researchers should all benefit from this work, which is also intended to stimulate new ideas in its readers, leading to future trends.

Individual volumes, topically arranged, are divided into sections and chapters. Many have charts and tables, and all include a chapter summary and an extensive list of references. Each volume concludes with an author index and a subject index.

This comprehensive work will hopefully be updated again before too many decades have passed. Perhaps an index to all of the volumes, facilitating comparison, will be included.—**Anita Zutis**

462. **Depression Sourcebook.** Karen Bellenir, ed. Detroit, Omnigraphics, 2002. 580p. index. (Health Reference Series). $78.00. ISBN 0-7808-0611-5.

This newest addition to the Health Reference Series displays the high quality and usefulness of the other titles in the long-standing Omnigraphics effort. This volume, following the series' standard format, contains reprints of government documents, with additional documents from other organizations, publications, and individuals. The articles, targeted for consumer health, contain information about all types of depression in different groups of people.

The first three sections cover the causes of depression, how depression affects the individual suffering from it, and the various treatments currently in use. Written in an easy-to-understand style and covering all facets of the subject, the book offers much valuable information in a readable style. For example, the question "How does depression differ from occasional sadness?", is answered clearly and succinctly in three paragraphs (p. 209). While not an in-depth description of the two states and their differences, it serves the purpose for which it is intended.

Covered in the latter part of the book are common health problems that are often accompanied by depression, such as diabetes or heart disease. Another section covers suicide, with a following one dealing with current research. Each chapter closes with a listing of resources for more information on the particular facet of depression covered in the preceding pages. The final section of the book boasts a complete glossary and five different listings of sources of more information and help. An index completes this comprehensive coverage of depressions geared to the average consumer. This volume is recommended for purchase.—**Nancy P. Reed**

463.   **Handbook of Child and Adolescent Psychology. Volumes 5-7.** Joseph D. Noshpitz, ed. New York, John Wiley, 1998. 3v. $125.00/set. ISBN 0-471-19329-1.

This set expands the old *Basic Handbook of Child Psychiatry* by two new volumes, plus a revision of the outdated volume 5. The new title reflects the growth within child psychiatry and the shifting concern from medical issues of development and syndromes of actual illness toward how children and adolescents can be enabled through early intervention and treatment, improvement in parenting, and cooperative efforts of other health care workers to achieve a better life and adjustment to our changing world.

The lists of contributors reads like a "who's who" of psychiatric clinicians and instructors, plus some other specialists in related fields, such as psychology, education, and pediatrics. Chapters are arranged under sections in each volume and are easily located through the detailed table of contents. Volume 5 deals with studies on assessment and evaluation of children, adolescents, and their families. Volume 6 considers basic science issues in the field and the current status of various treatment techniques. The concluding book, intriguingly called "Advances and New Directions," discusses the impact of sociocultural events, topics such as prevention and the process of consultation with other professionals, forensic issues, and handling emergency assessment and intervention, as well as professional issues in child and adolescent psychiatry.

This scholarly trio of books was carefully compiled and subjected to much revision and review, even by editors of the other volumes and the late editor Noshpitz. Bibliographies are extensive. It is a major contribution to the literature of child and adolescent psychiatry, containing much practical material useful to its practitioners, students, various mental health workers, and those who represent other cooperating professions. There are some articles in the final volume, such as those involving young persons who have witnessed violence (as in the current school shootings), that may be of interest to general readers, but some knowledge of mental health activities is really needed for understanding the vocabulary and discussions in these impressive volumes. —**Harriette M. Cluxton**

464.   **The Handbook of Child Psychology.** 5th ed. William Damon, ed. New York, John Wiley, 1998. 4v. index. $150.00/vol. ISBN 0-471-17893-4.

Now in its 5th edition, this handbook should still be considered a standard reference work in the field of developmental psychology. It reflects previously established scholarly traditions of utilizing editors who are renowned in their areas of expertise. It has evolved into a useful tool for undergraduates, graduates, practitioners, and researchers, and provides authoritative coverage and in-depth analysis of both theoretical and practical topics. Significantly expanded from the 4th edition, there are now contributions from 112 authors, most of whom are professors at institutions of higher education around the world. The scope of the work continues to be comprehensive, with concepts and practices having significance for students and practitioners also in such areas as education, psychiatry, sociology, pediatrics, history, medicine, and anthropology.

Comprising 4 volumes, the handbook documents the current status and future trends in the understanding of developmental psychology. Volume 1 is devoted to "Theoretical Models of Human Development," documenting the growth of developmental psychology into an interdisciplinary science; volume 2 details the current understanding of cognitive development, its history, and predictions of future directions in cognition, perception, and language; volume 3 provides state-of-the-art reviews of ongoing work dealing with social, emotional, and personality development issues; and volume 4 covers "Child Psychology in Practice," providing concrete examples for analysis.

A detailed table of contents at the beginning of each volume and an additional breakdown of subject matter in the beginning of each chapter provides an excellent topical approach. Chapters conclude with extensive scholarly references, supplying additional avenues for research. All volumes have both author and subject indexes listed in the back, providing easy access to data. This set is suitable for all academic libraries and special libraries with an interest in this area.
—**Marianne B. Eimer**

465.   **Handbook of Innovative Therapy.** 2d ed. Raymond Corsini, ed. New York, John Wiley, 2001. 754p. index. $85.00. ISBN 0-471-34819-8.

This is a revised edition of the original publication *Handbook of Innovative Psychotherapies* (John Wiley, 1981). While it adds to and updates several entries, this new edition retains the general layout of the 1st edition. There are 69 psychotherapeutic techniques currently in use presented in this volume, which are alphabetically arranged but also with an author and broad subject index. Criteria for inclusion in this volume are that the therapies are different or unusual, although not necessarily new.

Each entry consists of a brief outline of a specific therapy, followed by sections covering the history and current status of the therapy, a theoretical and methodological discussion of the therapy, a review of its possible applications, and a case study example. A summary of each therapy and a list of further references is also provided. Entries are written by authorities in that field of therapy, including both psychologists and psychiatrists. This volume will serve both as a handy introduction to students and as a quick refresher for practitioners. Many of the therapies included are already well covered by other standard reference works, making this volume more suitable for comprehensive research collections in psychology.—**Elizabeth Patterson**

466.   **Handbook of Psychology.** Irving B. Weiner, ed. New York, John Wiley, 2003. 12v. index. $1,800.00/set. ISBN 0-471-17669-9.

John Wiley is becoming well known for their advanced compilation of works in the area of psychology. In the past year alone, five handbooks in various areas of psychology have been released from this publisher, including *Handbook of Sport Psychology* (see entry 467), *Handbook of the Psychology of Women and Gender* (see entry 468), and *Handbook of Clinical Child Psychology* (2002). This 12-volume set provides an overview of the topics covered above as well as many others. Each volume is edited by a different scholar in the field and was compiled with the help of 25 contributing editors.

The set begins with volumes 1 and 2 addressing the history and research methods of psychology. The "History of Psychology" volume gives an overview of each discipline, including abnormal psychology, counseling psychology, and school psychology. Volumes 3 through 7 provide comprehensive information on 5 broad areas of the study: biological psychology, experimental psychology, personality and social psychology, developmental psychology, and educational psychology. The final five volumes address the practice of five areas of study: clinical psychology, health psychology, assessment psychology, forensic psychology, and industrial and organizational psychology. The scholarly essays are well written and all provide ample lists of references. Unfortunately, there are no cross-references, which would have served to interconnect the volumes. Each volume provides its own author index and subject index, but no cumulative index for the set is provided.

This set will be worthwhile for graduate students of psychology, psychologists looking for the latest research in their field, and psychologists needing information outside of their own specialty. University libraries and health care libraries needing a comprehensive overview of both the history of psychology and new research in all fields should consider its purchase if budgets permit.—**Shannon Graff Hysell**

467. **Handbook of Sport Psychology.** 2d ed. Robert N. Singer, Heather A. Hausenblas, and Christopher M. Janelle, eds. New York, John Wiley, 2001. 876p. index. $95.00. ISBN 0-471-37995-6.

Since the publication of the 1st edition of this work in 1993 there has been new research and increased interest in the area of sport psychology. The editors state in the preface that this work retains much the same format as the 1st edition but much of the information within has been updated and expanded on to reflect the field of sport psychology's focus on exercise psychology, expertise, and psychophysiology. They also reflect the expanding research on the effects of activity on psychological well-being and the effects of psychology on athletic performance.

More than 80 experts in the field of sport psychology contributed to this handbook, each of which is listed at the beginning of the work. This edition retains the same part titles as the last: "Skill Acquisition," "Psychological Characteristics of High-Level Performance," "Motivation," "Psychological Techniques for Individual Performance," "Life Span Development," "Exercise and Health Psychology," and "Future Directions." The articles are written with scholars in mind and often provide illustrative charts and a long list of references. The work concludes with an author index and a subject index. This work will be useful for graduate libraries that feature sports medicine and psychology programs.—**Shannon Graff Hysell**

468. **Handbook of the Psychology of Women and Gender.** Rhoda K. Unger, ed. New York, John Wiley, 2001. 556p. index. $75.00. ISBN 0-471-33332-8.

Women and gender studies have been in the research mainstream and the university curriculum for decades. A current, comprehensive research handbook on the psychology of women is long overdue. Rhoda K. Unger, distinguished in women studies and psychology, has compiled such a resource. *Handbook of the Psychology of Women and Gender* provides a review of the research in 27 thought provoking articles. The only comparable work is Denmark and Paludi's *Psychology of Women: A Handbook of Issues and Theories* (Greenwood Press, 1993). Unger's handbook provides a needed update and expands on this work. It will be an essential source for graduate students, faculty, and professionals, as it will be for undergraduates involved in capstone-level research. Many of the articles provide a deep level of analysis that scholars will find interesting and valuable but will likely be challenging for students. Five sections organize the chapters by categories: theoretical/methodological issues, developmental issues, social roles and social systems, physical and mental health, and institutions/power. The specific areas covered within these broad divisions are comprehensive, addressing issues and content areas of research on women and gender. Subsequent editions could provide chapters on women and the workplace and careers. While workplace issues are addressed in a number of articles, particularly Gilbert and Rader's article on work, family, and life, it is such a major aspect of a woman's life that it justifies greater focus. Likewise, a discussion of gender and the schools would warrant a chapter, if not more. Neither is there a specific discussion of female participation, or lack of, in male-marketed sports (e.g., skateboarding, snowboarding). Articles such as Kite's on changing gender roles and Good and Sherrod's article on the psychology of men certainly provide ideas that would help one speculate on the issue.

The volume and quality of analysis far outweigh any omissions, however, and simply provide content for future handbooks. An added bonus to this resource is that many of the chapters are written in a way that provokes ideas and questions in the reader's mind. This makes for interesting reading, an excellent tool for teaching, and an incubator for research ideas. Such qualities are not found in many handbooks. There is an index and a comprehensive list of references. Unger's handbook should be a part of any academic library or larger public library collection.—**Lorraine Evans**

469. **Handbook of Work and Organizational Psychology.** 2d ed. Pieter J. D. Drenth, Henk Thierry, and Charles J. de Wolff, eds. Bristol, Pa., Psychology Press/Taylor & Francis, 1998. 4v. index. $200.00/set. ISBN 0-86377-528-4.

In 1984, the *Handbook of Industrial and Organizational Psychology*, edited by the present editorial team and their former colleague Paul Willems, appeared as the first comprehensive European handbook in this field. Since then, the rapid development of the discipline led the editors to produce a revision. The result is not just an updated book, but a completely rewritten one, including a title change and an expansion from two to four volumes.

The introductory volume, *Introduction to Work and Organizational Psychology*, deals with the definition, history, research methods, and the role of the work and organizational psychologist. Volume 2, *Work and Psychology*, concentrates on the issues of the direct relationship of the worker to the organization, or the "human factors." *Personnel Psychology*, the 3d volume of the handbook, examines the differences of individuals and the consequences for the organization. The last volume, *Organizational Psychology*, concerns itself with how organizational and environmental characteristics affect the behavior of individuals and groups, and how those characteristics are in turn influenced by behavioral features.

All 4 volumes are arranged in standard chapters, each chapter beginning with an introduction and concluding with a list of references. Tables and figures are interspersed throughout the text. Each volume ends with an author and subject index. There is no cumulative index for the entire set, presumably because each volume works equally well as a stand-alone title and can, in fact, be purchased separately. With the multitude of new studies and research, the changes in organizational psychology have been extensive enough that this new work will be a much-needed addition to any academic or large public reference collection.—**Rachael Green**

470. **Mental Health Disorders Sourcebook.** 2d ed. Karen Bellenir, ed. Detroit, Omnigraphics, 2000. 605p. index. (Health Reference Series). $78.00. ISBN 0-7808-0240-3.

Using information on the subject of mental health and mental illness from a wide range of sources, including government agencies, professional organizations, and journals, the 2d edition of this reference tool is again written for the general reader. Primarily updating article information and URLs, it provides medical information about mental disorders and their treatments, specifically phrased in nontechnical terms, offering clear explanations to paraprofessionals, patients, and family members. Exploring both mental health and mental illness, the handbook provides information on early warning signs and symptoms of mental illness, identifying diagnostic tools, and even statistics about the incidence of mental illness. Composed of eight sections, each having its own chapters, such topics as anxiety disorders, depression, eating disorders, and bipolar disorders receive in-depth coverage. Beginning with an overview of the topic, the user finds definitions, organizations, and types of the disorder in every section. Along with specific disorders, the editor includes sections on treatment methods, both traditional and alternative, and medications currently in use and those in development. Of special note is the final section, titled "Additional Help and Information." It will be useful for anyone connected with those afflicted with mental illness. Names and addresses of organizations, a glossary of terms, services for veterans, and sources for additional reading are located in this section. A comprehensive, alphabetically arranged index can be found at the back of the book. This reference source is well organized and well written for its target audience of nonprofessionals investigating all aspects of mental disorders. It is suitable for public library collections and academic libraries with undergraduate programs in psychology. —**Marianne B. Eimer**

471. **Psychology.** Bethel, Conn., Grolier Educational, 2002. 6v. illus. index. $379.00/set. ISBN 0-7172-5662-6.

Psychology is a six-volume set produced by Grolier Educational that explores the various components found within the field of psychology. Geared for a high school level and above researcher, the articles included contain concise information, with a multitude of photographs, charts, and illustrations that supplement the text. The publisher has incorporated a color-coded box system that highlights important information for the reader, such as key points for a chapter summary, key theories, works or dates related to the topic covered, experimental work that fostered theory development, or in-depth studies by field researchers in that particular area of psychology.

Broken into six main categories, starting with the history of psychology, each volume has its own focus, such as developmental or social psychology. Chapters such as "Mental Disorders" (found in volume 6, "Abnormal Psychology") investigate subtopics of the main subject. All have a cross-reference box titled "Connections," which provide links to related topics in other chapters. Conveniently located in each volume is both an identical glossary, which provides the psychological definition of terms used in the chapters, and an alphabetically arranged keyword set index. Another opportunity to provide further research is a section titled "Resources Section," which contains three types of resources (print sources, Websites for that subject category, and quotation information for that volume). Ease of use, quality of each volume, good binding, bright colors, and easily read fonts all contribute in recommending this as a worthwhile basic reference set in psychology for all libraries, and as a necessary acquisition for those libraries serving high school students and above.—**Marianne B. Eimer**

472. **Psychology Basics.** Frank N. Magill, ed. Pasadena, Calif., Salem Press, 1998. 2v. index. $118.75. ISBN 0-89356-963-1.

This 2-volume set of *Psychology Basics* breaks all the rules for an introductory text. It has no color photographs, self-tests, graphs, exercises, or questions for discussion. With all these exceptions to the norm, one might wonder if these books are something that all college libraries need. The answer is a definite yes. *Psychology Basics* contains the information undergraduates need for their term papers or to delve deeper into a favorite subject. The editor came up with the right format for each article and kept a tight rein on the 90 contributors. Each 6-page article contains sections that review, apply, and show the larger context of 101 important psychological topics and 9 theorists. A short annotated bibliography follows each article, and every confusing term is defined at the outset and in the glossary. There are, however, some problems. The contributors, who are excellent teachers giving their favorite lectures, cite classic studies and leading theorists, but, with annoying regularity, do not cite any of the original works. Contributors also have a variety of interpretations as to applications or the larger context. Some nail the distinctions; others think they are being asked for an advanced overview. Writing styles vary, but most articles are clearly written and interesting. Some names like Robert Zajonc and terms like *dementia praecox* cry out for a pronunciation guide. This 2-volume set is highly recommended. [R: BL, 1 June 98, p. 1816]—**Pete Prunkl**

473. **Stevens' Handbook of Experimental Psychology.** Hal Pashler, ed. New York, John Wiley, 2002. 4v. illus. index. $900.00/set. ISBN 0-471-44333-6.

As the preface of this work states, the field of experimental psychology has progress substantially in the 10 years since this work was last published (1988). This new edition has grown from two volumes to four. The editors have broadened the scope of the work to include a volume created exclusively for methodology, intended for those doing new research in the field. The set also focuses on the "marked increase in efforts to link psychological phenomena to neurophysiological foundations."

Arranged into four volumes, each volume covers a specific area of experimental psychology. Volume 1 discusses sensation and perception. It has 17 essays written by leaders in the field, which discuss such topics as attention, motor control, and speech perception. Volume 2 is titled "Memory and Cognitive Processes" and covers such topics as the different kinds of memory, psycholinguistics, and reasoning. Volumes 3 and 4 cover the areas of methodology and learning, motivation, and emotion. Each essay provides references and each volume has both author and subject indexes.

This work is very scholarly in scope and is intended for those with advanced degrees in psychology. It will be appropriate for university libraries offering advanced degrees in this area of study.—**Shannon Graff Hysell**

Author/Title Index

Reference is to entry number.

Subject Index

Reference is to entry number.